A Practitioner's Guide
to Clinical Occupational Therapy

# A Practitioner's Guide to Clinical Occupational Therapy

*Second Edition*

*Edited by*
Donna Weiss,
Marlene J. Morgan,
*and*
Moya Kinnealey

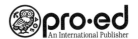

An International Publisher

8700 Shoal Creek Boulevard
Austin, Texas 78757-6897
800/897-3202
Fax 800/397-7633
www.proedinc.com

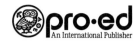

© 2012, 2004 by PRO-ED, Inc.
8700 Shoal Creek Boulevard
Austin, Texas 78757-6897
800/897-3202    Fax 800/397-7633
www.proedinc.com

**Library of Congress Cataloging-in-Publication Data**

A practitioner's guide to clinical occupational therapy / edited by
Donna Weiss, Marlene J. Morgan, and Moya Kinnealey.— 2nd ed.
      p. cm.
   Rev. ed. of: A practitioner's guide to clinical occupational therapy /
Moya Kinnealey, Donna Weiss, Marlene J. Morgan. c2004.
   Includes bibliographical references.
      ISBN 978-1-4164-0499-6
      I. Weiss, Donna (Donna F.) II. Morgan, Marlene J. III. Kinnealey, Moya.
IV. Kinnealey, Moya. Practitioner's guide to clinical occupational therapy.
   [DNLM: 1.  Occupational Therapy.  WB 555]
   LC  Classification not assigned
   615.8'515—dc23
                                                    2011044997

Art Director: Jason Crosier
Designer: Jan Mullis
This book is designed in Sabon and Vectora LH.

Printed in the United States of America
1  2  3  4  5  6  7  8  9  10      20  19  18  17  16  15  14  13  12  11

*The editors and contributors gratefully acknowledge the community of academic and clinical scholars who achieve, on a daily basis, the client-centered integration of theory and practice.*

# Contents

# Contributing Authors

**Nancy Beck, MA, OTR/L**
Director, Rehabilitation Services
Belmont Center for Comprehensive
    Treatment
Philadelphia, Pennsylvania

**Roberta T. Ciocco, OTR/L**
Bucks County Schools Intermediate
    Unit #22
Doylestown, Pennsylvania

**Meryl S. Cooperman, MS, OTR/L**
Bucks County Schools Intermediate
    Unit #22
Doylestown, Pennsylvania

**Kendall Daly, OTR/L**
Director, Rehabilitation Services
Elder Service Plan of the North Shore
Lynn, Massachusetts

**James Foster, MS, OTR/L**
Facility Rehabilitation Coordinator
ProStep Rehabilitation
Suburban Woods Health and
    Rehabilitation
Norristown, Pennsylvania

**Steven M. Gagajewski, DOT, OTR/L**
Senior Staff Therapist
Nazareth Hospital
Philadelphia, Pennsylvania

**Michael J. Gerg, MS, OTR/L, CHT,
    CEES, CWCE**
Instructor, Occupational Therapy
    Program
Department of Rehabilitation Sciences
College of Health Professions and
    Social Work
Temple University
Philadelphia, Pennsylvania

**Gail E. Huecker, OTR/L**
Director/Owner, OT 4 Kids
Crystal River, Florida

**Nancy Allen Kauffman, EdM, OTR/L**
Director, Occupational Therapy
    Programs
Newtown Square, Pennsylvania

**Christine L. Hischmann, MS, OTR/L,
    FAOTA**
Director, Occupational Therapy
Clarks Summit State Hospital
Clarks Summit, Pennsylvania

**Deborah Humpl, OTR/L**
Outpatient Occupational Therapy Team
    Leader/Seating Clinic Coordinator
Children's Hospital of Philadelphia
Philadelphia, Pennsylvania

**Arley Johnson, MS, OTR/L**
Site Manager
Pennsylvania Hospital
Good Shepherd Penn Partners
Philadelphia, Pennsylvania

**Moya Kinnealey, PhD, OTR/L,
    FAOTA**
Director, Occupational Therapy Program
Department of Rehabilitation Sciences
College of Health Professions and
    Social Work
Temple University
Philadelphia, Pennsylvania

**William Lambert, MS, OTR/L**
Faculty Specialist, Occupational and
    Physical Therapy
Panuska College of Professional Studies
The University of Scranton
Scranton, Pennsylvania

**Rosalyn Lipsitt, PhD, OTR/L**
Staff Therapist
Wesley Enhanced Living
Philadelphia, Pennsylvania

**Josette Merkel, MBA, OTR/L**
Chief, Occupational Therapy Section
Physical Medicine and Rehabilitation
    Department
Temple University Hospital
Philadelphia, Pennsylvania

**Marlene J. Morgan, EdD, OTR/L**
Director, Occupational Therapy
    Program
Panuska College of Professional Studies
The University of Scranton
Scranton, Pennsylvania

**Jonathan Niszczak, MS, OTR/L**
Senior Occupational Therapist,
    Occupational Therapy Section
Physical Medicine and Rehabilitation
    Department
Temple University Hospital
Philadelphia, Pennsylvania

**C. Thomas North, PhD, OTR/L**
Associate Professor, Occupational
    Therapy Program
Department of Rehabilitation Sciences
College of Health Professions and
    Social Work
Temple University
Philadelphia, Pennsylvania

**Beth Pfeiffer, PhD, OTR/L, BCP**
Associate Professor, Occupational
    Therapy Program
Department of Rehabilitation Sciences
College of Health Professions and
    Social Work
Temple University
Philadelphia, Pennsylvania

**Ellen Rosenberg Pitonyak, MS,
    OTR/L**
Fieldwork Coordinator, Occupational
    Therapy Assistant Program
Harcum College
Bryn Mawr, Pennsylvania

**Scott Rushanan, MS, OTR/L**
Lead Therapist, Inpatient Rehabilitation
    Services
Pennsylvania Hospital
Philadelphia, Pennsylvania

**James Siberski, MS, CMC**
Assistant Professor, Social Work
Coordinator of Gerontology Education
Misericordia University
Dallas, Pennsylvania

**Fern Silverman, EdD, OTR/L**
Assistant Professor, Occupational
    Therapy Program
Department of Rehabilitation Sciences
College of Health Professions and
    Social Work
Temple University
Philadelphia, Pennsylvania

**Mary Squillace, DOT, OTR/L**
Clinical Assistant Professor,
    Occupational Therapy Program
Stony Brook University
New York, New York

**Dana L. Weiss, MS, LPC**
Licensed Professional Counselor
Sewell, New Jersey

**Donna Weiss, PhD, OTR/L, FAOTA**
Associate Professor Emeritus,
    Occupational Therapy Program
Department of Rehabilitation Sciences
College of Health Professions and
    Social Work
Temple University
Philadelphia, Pennsylvania

**Stephen G. Whittaker, PhD, OTR/L,
    CLVT**
Moss Rehabilitation Hospital
Moore Eye Foundation
Philadelphia, Pennsylvania

# Introduction | *Donna Weiss*

Occupational therapists are concerned with the anatomical and physiological substrate of human behavior, the in-depth analysis of human occupation throughout the lifespan, and the effects of disabling conditions on functional behavior. Whether they are engaged in institution- or community-based practice, occupational therapists must analyze, synthesize, and relate complex arrays of observational and evaluative data and design intervention strategies that facilitate their clients' meaningful participation in the tasks of life. Experienced clinicians have learned that attention to the client's personal context facilitates clinical problem solving and the development of relevant and effective intervention strategies.

This book is based on an ecological approach to the practice of occupational therapy, in which the therapist's knowledge of theory and clinical conditions is interwoven with the client's personal experience and aspirations. The evaluation, interventions, and related outcomes of treatment are viewed as interacting determinants of one another. Successful application of theory to practice requires that occupational therapists use abstract skills, such as critical thinking, clinical reasoning, and clinical problem solving.

The manner in which practitioners engage in the clinical reasoning process has been described and operationalized in the literature (Mattingly & Fleming, 1994; Schell, 2009). The simultaneous employment of procedural, conditional, narrative, and ethical aspects of the clinical reasoning process requires the therapist to interweave theoretical knowledge of disabling conditions with the individual client's aspirations and personal experience, in order to create a relevant and viable treatment program (Mattingly & Fleming, 1994; Schell, 1998).

Critical thinking, clinical reasoning, and clinical problem solving are complex processes that are central to the practice of occupational therapy but not readily visible to the learner. The hallmark of the progression from novice to expert is an increase in the efficiency of the clinical reasoning process—the speed, flexibility, and accuracy with which contextual data, clinical problem definition, evaluation, and the design of the treatment plan are integrated and implemented. The keys to expert performance are experience, organization of knowledge, efficiency in gathering and organizing data, and reflectivity (Johnson, 1988; Mattingly & Fleming, 1994). The primary task as one progresses toward expertise is not only to amass knowledge but also to develop increasingly more efficient strategies for organizing and manipulating that knowledge for problem solving (Bruer, 1993; Lave & Wenger, 1991).

The traditional method of transgenerational transmission of professional information has been based on an apprenticeship model, in which the expert clinician "makes thinking visible" (Collins, Brown, & Holum, 1991, p. 6). The components of apprenticeship—modeling, scaffolding, fading, and coaching—represent a progression from demonstrated problem solving, to guided problem solving, and then to independent problem solving.

First, the expert *models* the target process, often showing the novice what to do. Then, the expert provides a *scaffold*, or support, as the novice carries out a task. The level of support can vary from carrying out a task with the novice to giving occasional hints as to what to do next. *Fading* refers to the gradual removal of support as the novice assumes more and more responsibility. *Coaching* is an ongoing effort by the expert to oversee the novice's learning by choosing and structuring tasks, providing hints, diagnosing problems, offering encouragement, and giving feedback (Collins et al., 1991).

Metacognitive strategies, such as conceptual frameworks, help to reify expert thought processes and provide a tangible model of expert thinking for the novice (Bruer, 1993; West, Farmer, & Wolff, 1991). Reification of thought processes facilitates teacher and student interaction and can help the student become more cognizant of efficient methods for ordering and using information for clinical reasoning and independent problem solving (Lave & Wenger, 1991; Resnick, 1987; West et al., 1991).

The trend away from institutional toward community-based services and administrative downsizing in all arenas, including health care, leaves novice occupational therapists and experienced therapists who have transitioned to new practice areas with diminished access to expert on-site supervisors. As a result, there are fewer opportunities for the interactions described above, which are inherent in a progressive, interactive apprenticeship.

## ❧ Purpose and Format

Although the written word cannot replace the interactive relationship between a novice and an expert practitioner, it is hoped that this book will provide the reader with the opportunity to see how some expert occupational therapists think. Each chapter is divided into five sections:

1. Synopsis of Clinical Condition
   - Prevalence and etiology

- Common characteristics and symptoms
- Target areas for intervention

2. Contextual Considerations
- Clinical
- Family
- Practice setting
- Sociopolitical
- Lifestyle/lifespan

3. Clinical Decision-Making Process
- Defining focus for intervention
- Establishing goals for intervention
- Designing theory-based intervention
- Evaluating progress
- Determining change in or termination of treatment

4. Case Study
- Description
- Long- and short-term goals
- Therapist goals and strategies
- Activity
- Treatment objectives

5. Resources
- Internet resources
- Print resources

The structure of the book is consistent with the multimodal nature of the clinical reasoning process (Mattingly & Fleming, 1994). The synopsis of the clinical condition reflects the procedural aspects of clinical reasoning, and the contextual considerations make up the narrative or conditional aspects. The contributing authors identify the theories and/or frames of reference that inform their decision-making processes. They also indicate what frames of reference or theoretical models may be employed, either alone or in combination, depending on the clinical, family, practice setting, and lifestyle/lifespan context. In the Clinical Decision-Making Process section, the experts make their thinking visible (Collins et al., 1991) and model how they relate theory to practice. Finally, just as the master craftsperson introduces an apprentice to the rubrics of a craft by providing an example of a completed product, the experts provide a reification of their thought processes by providing a case study that includes an assessment and interpretation of contextual data, an action plan, and expected outcomes.

The book encourages readers to structure their thinking and become more efficient—more expert—in data gathering and analysis and in designing intervention that is grounded in theory and relevant to the context of the client.

# Structured Reflectivity:
# The Relationship of Research to Practice

As noted earlier, reflectivity is an important component of expert practice. Evidence-based practice, outcomes measurement, and research are the functional manifestations of reflectivity and are necessary for the vitality of the occupational therapy profession (Holm, 2000; Laver-Fawcett, 2007). Reflectivity requires both the critical analysis of existing literature to inform practice decisions and the structured examination of the outcomes of treatment methodologies to assess their efficacy. Both practices simultaneously edify the individual clinician and the profession as a whole by evaluating and expanding the compendium of literature that informs and supports practice.

The *Occupational Therapy Practice Framework* (American Occupational Therapy Association [AOTA], 2008) identified occupation as both a means and an end, as well as the hallmark of occupational therapy. The *Framework* further defines the domains of concern for occupational therapy (areas of occupation, client factors, performance skills, performance patterns, context and environment, and activity demands) and helps define the unique outcomes of occupational therapy treatment to individual and institutional consumers.

Specification of the expected outcomes of occupational therapy intervention (occupational performance, adaptation, health and wellness, participation, prevention, quality of life, self-advocacy, and occupational justice) helps clarify the choice of measurement tools that will provide an accurate means of collecting and reporting data regarding the efficiency and efficacy of occupational therapy intervention.

Health policy–making bodies have articulated guidelines for acceptable methods of data collection and reporting that provide documentation with a patient-centered orientation. In other words, the focus is on reporting a more holistic picture of health that is rooted in the context of the patient's/client's ability to function in daily life (AOTA, 2007; World Health Organization, 2010). Provision of clear outcome measures allows policy makers to make decisions regarding the inclusion and reimbursement of services.

In daily practice, therapists are required to make decisions regarding the type and duration of therapy and to make predictions regarding outcomes. The constituencies who pay for services will require more than intuition and experience as rationales for services. The primary challenge for occupational therapy practitioners is to create assessment processes that provide a comprehensive picture of the person–environment interaction and how that impacts the person's occupational performance.

Concepts such as occupational performance, role balance, and quality of life are difficult to quantify. Qualitative measures, which often incorporate observations and interviews, provide a method for systematically examining occupational performance. Both qualitative and quantitative assessment tools must be critically evaluated for reliability, validity, trustworthiness, and clinical utility.

In all arenas, the call for accountability and proof of efficacy of service reinforces the fact that institutional viability will depend on the reliability, validity, and clinical utility of assessment processes. The literature is replete with resources that provide comprehensive critiques regarding the reliability, validity, and clinical utility of a vast array of assessment tools (Law, Baum, & Dunn, 2005; McDowell, 2006). It is important to remember that there is no one perfect indicator of anything—what is important is "settling upon a consistent and intelligent method of assessing your output results, and then tracking your trajectory with rigor . . . what matters is that you systematically assemble evidence—qualitative or quantitative—to track your progress" (Collins, 2005, p. 8).

Clinicians who systematically cultivate their clinical curiosity by asking questions regarding the variables that affect and are affected by treatment are more likely to develop an evidence-based practice (Holm, 2000). The availability of electronic databases (e.g., MEDLINE, CINAHL, Cochrane Database of Systematic Reviews, ACP Journal Club, Evidence-Based Medicine Reviews, ERIC, PsychLit, OT Search) facilitates the search for evidence regarding the relationships among variables, such as populations, frequency, and duration of intervention and treatment outcomes. This curiosity, in tandem with clinical expertise, contributes to the development and maintenance of expert practice.

The evidence-based practitioner, through the systematic use of reliable and valid assessment tools, gathers and analyzes data that validate or question available evidence and contribute to the body of knowledge, documents client progress, and identifies the unique focus of occupational therapy: "supporting health and participation in life through engagement in occupation" (AOTA, 2008, p. 626).

The perspectives shared in this book are based on the clinical expertise of the contributors and on the current supporting literature. Since practice is contextual and evolutionary, it is expected that there will be myriad viable treatment methodologies applicable in each of the presented clinical situations.

The challenge to the practitioner is to evaluate these methods through literature review, systematically examine the outcomes of evidence-based practice, and contribute their findings to the knowledge base of the profession. With that in mind, it would be prudent for the reader to consider this book the beginning of a professional dialogue about treatment, rather than the last word.

## References

American Occupational Therapy Association. (2007). *AOTA fact sheet on Transmittal 63: New Medicare documentation requirements for evaluations*. Retrieved from http://www.aota.org/Practitioners/Advocacy/Federal/Highlights/39837.aspx

American Occupational Therapy Association. (2008). Occupational therapy practice framework: Domain & process. *The American Journal of Occupational Therapy, 62*(6), 625–683.

Bruer, J. (1993, Summer). The mind's journey from novice to expert: If we know the route, we can help students negotiate their way. *American Educator, 17*(2), 6–15, 38–46.

Collins, A., Brown, J., & Holum, A. (1991, Winter). Cognitive apprenticeship: Making thinking visible. *American Educator, 15*(3), 6–11, 38–46.

Collins, J. (2005). *Good to great and the social sectors: Why business thinking is not the answer* [Monograph]. New York, NY: Harper Collins.

Holm, M. (2000). Our mandate for the new millennium: Evidence-based practice. *The American Journal of Occupational Therapy, 54*(6), 575–584.

Johnson, S. (1988). Cognitive analysis of expert and novice troubleshooting performance. *Performance Improvement Quarterly, 1*(3), 38–54.

Lave, J., & Wenger, E. (1991). *Situated learning: Legitimate peripheral participation.* New York, NY: Cambridge University Press.

Laver-Fawcett, A. J. (2007). *Principles of assessment and outcome measurement for occupational therapists and physiotherapists: Theory, skills and application.* Chichester, England: John Wiley & Sons, Ltd.

Law, M., Baum, C., & Dunn, W. (2005). *Measuring occupational performance: Supporting best practice in occupational therapy.* Thorofare, NJ: Slack, Inc.

Mattingly, C., & Fleming, M. (1994). *Clinical reasoning: Forms of inquiry in a therapeutic practice.* Philadelphia, PA: FA Davis.

McDowell, I. (2006). *Measuring health: A guide to rating scales and questionnaires.* New York, NY: Oxford University Press.

Resnick, L. (1987). *Education and learning to think.* Washington, DC: National Academy Press.

Schell, B. (2009). Professional reasoning in practice. In E. Crepeau, E. Cohn, & B. Schell (Eds.), *Willard & Spackman's occupational therapy* (11th ed., pp. 314–327). Philadelphia, PA: Lippincott, Williams & Wilkins.

West, C., Farmer, J., & Wolff, P. (1991). *Instructional design: Implications from cognitive science.* Boston, MA: Allyn and Bacon.

World Health Organization. (2010). *International classification of functioning, disability and health (ICF).* Retrieved from http://www.who.int/classifications/icf/en/

# Prematurity | *Mary Squillace*

## 🌿 Synopsis of Clinical Condition

### Prevalence and Etiology

The length of a normal pregnancy is considered to be 40 weeks from the date of conception, and infants born before 37 weeks gestation are considered premature. An estimated 13 million babies worldwide are born premature, and 1 million of these do not live. In 2008, 12.3% of babies born in the United States were premature. Prematurity is the leading cause of newborn death, and many who survive have lifelong health challenges (March of Dimes, 2011). Although the underlying etiology is usually unknown, premature labor can be brought on by several different conditions. These include placental abruption, in which the placenta detaches from the uterus; placenta previa, in which the placenta grows too low in the uterus; premature rupture of membranes, in which the amniotic sac is torn; incompetent cervix, in which the cervix opens too soon; and maternal toxemia or infection. Premature labor is more common with a multiple pregnancy (i.e., twins, triplets, etc.) and for mothers with a history of past premature births or miscarriages. Social and behavioral issues may also contribute to the onset of preterm labor. One identifiable cause of prematurity is maternal drug abuse, particularly cocaine abuse (Edgren, 1998).

Premature infants are typically classified in two ways: by gestational age and by birth weight. Gestational age is the number of weeks an infant is born after conception. Classification by gestational age is as follows:

- 🌿 Full term = 37–42 weeks
- 🌿 Preterm = 28–<37 weeks

The editors gratefully acknowledge the contributions of Janene P. Benson.

- Extremely preterm = <28 weeks
- Postterm = >42 weeks

Classification by birth weight is as *average* or *low*. Low birth weight is broken down into three additional subcategories:

- Average = >2,500 grams
- Low birth weight (LBW) = 1,500–2,500 grams
- Very low birth weight (VLBW) = 1,000–1,499 grams
- Extremely low birth weight (ELBW) = <1,000 grams
- Micro-preemies = <800 grams

Additionally, newborn infants can be classified by the relationship of birth weight to postconceptual age. This is determined by plotting the birth weight by gestational age on a standardized graph. Newborn age/weight classifications are as follows:

- GA = gestational age; total number of weeks the infant was in utero before birth
- AGA = appropriate for gestational age (between the 10th and 90th percentiles)
- SGA = small for gestational age (below the 10th percentile. *Note.* SGA is a better predictor of poor outcome than low birth weight for infants who are classified as AGA)
- LGA = large for gestational age (above the 90th percentile)
- PCA = postconceptual age; this is the infant's age in relation to conception (gestational age + number of weeks of age) and is calculated until the infant reaches 40 weeks
- Chronological age = infant's actual age
- Corrected age = how old the infant would be if full term; calculated until age 2 years for assessment and intervention purposes

## Common Characteristics and Symptoms

Characteristics of the premature infant at birth will vary based on gestational age. Physical characteristics may include the presence of lanugo, which is lost in utero at approximately 38 weeks gestation. The skin may appear red, mottled, and/or translucent, with the vessels close to the surface. Little fat or muscle is present below the skin, and the infant may lack mature breast buds and ear cartilage, which appear at approximately 34 weeks gestation. Extremely premature infants may have eyelids that are still fused shut. The plantar creases of the feet that develop in utero at approximately 32 weeks gestation may be absent (Dubowitz & Dubowitz, 1981).

Neurological characteristics include hypotonia and lack of active flexor tone. The flexor muscles begin to develop in utero at approximately 32 weeks gestation, when the infant begins to grow and the confined space of the uterus requires the infant to flex in the fetal position. Premature infants are typically very hyperextensible and may lack full flexor range of motion (ROM). Flexor tone develops in a caudocephalic progression before 40 weeks and in a cephalocauda progression after 40 weeks. Many primitive reflexes do not begin to appear until after 28 weeks gestation and therefore may not be present in the premature infant. Sucking reflex usually is not strong enough until 32 weeks gestational age. As the reflexes emerge, they are usually weaker than those found in a healthy, full-term infant. Active movement of the premature infant is usually dominated by extensor patterns and appears disorganized, jerky, and/or tremulous. Premature infants' movements are wider, less modulated, and more frequent than those of full-term infants.

Neurobehavioral, or state, characteristics refer to an infant's level of awareness and interactive behavior. State behavior will influence the infant's response to the environment and can help determine when interaction with the infant is appropriate. Brazelton (1984) classified six neurobehavioral states of newborns that are typically used for infants of 32 weeks gestation and older, as well as for full-term infants.

### Sleep states

- Deep sleep: The infant's eyes are closed, the infant demonstrates regular breathing, and there are no spontaneous movements, except for startles or jerky movements at quiet intervals. External stimulation may produce startles with some delay but no eye movement (Vegara & Bigsby, 2004).

- Light sleep (also called *active sleep*): The infant will sleep with his or her eyes closed, with sometimes rapid eye movement and body movements. The infant displays low activity, with random movements and startles; sucking movements occur. Movements are smoother and more monitored (Lester & Tronick, 2005; Vegara & Bigsby, 2004). Minor twitches and stretching movements may be presented as movement of the limbs, and the infant may respond to voices and other noises (Lubbe, 2009).

- Drowsy: The infant's eyelids are fluttering, and there will be a variable activity level with an occasional mild startle. The infant's eyes may be heavy lidded or closed. The infant may have delayed reaction to sensory stimuli; movements are usually smooth and may appear dazed and minimally reactive with eyes open (Lester & Tronick, 2005; Vegara & Bigsby, 2004). The infant's breathing is faster and shallower than in quiet sleep, and the infant may exhibit increased movement, with mild startles (Lubbe, 2009).

### Wake states

- Quiet alert (also called *quiet awake*): The infant has a bright look with a focused attention on stimulation and minimal motor activity. He or she may show appropriate facial expressions in response to stimulation and may focus on visual auditory stimulation (Lester & Tronick, 2005; Vegara & Bigsby, 2004). A premature infant may spend time in a quiet alert state normally after 32 weeks gestation, but before this time, he or she may be awake for a maximum of 2 minutes a day.

- Active awake (also called *active alert*): This is the stage when the infant's eyes are usually open and he or she will demonstrate generalized movements that are accompanied by grimacing or brief vocalizations (Lubbe, 2009).

🖖 Crying: This can be intense, loud, rhythmic, and sustained crying that is difficult to stop with stimulation. The infant may show a high level of motor activity (Lester & Tronick, 2005; Vegara & Bigsby, 2004).

Young, premature infants spend much of their time in the light sleep and drowsy states. The *NICU Network Neurobehavioral Scale* (Lester & Tronick, 2005) discusses modifications that may be necessary to accommodate infants from 23 to 33 weeks gestation because of their fragile state.

In addition to sleep–wake states, premature infants exhibit behavioral cues or signals that indicate responses to stimulation or stress. These cues reflect the infant's readiness to interact, tolerance of handling, and tolerance of the environment. Self-regulatory signals (i.e., approach signals) suggest that the premature infant is able to interact and tolerate stimulation. Stress signals (i.e., avoid signals) suggest that the premature infant is unable to cope with interaction or tolerate stimulation. Common behavioral cues identified in premature infants are listed below.

### Stress (avoid) signals

🖖 oxygen desaturation

🖖 color changes

🖖 change in heart rate

🖖 change in respiration

🖖 vomiting or spitting up

🖖 seizures

🖖 arching

🖖 limb extension

🖖 twitching

🖖 finger or toe splaying

🖖 saluting

🖖 sitting on air

🖖 grimacing

🖖 frowning

🖖 gaze aversion

🖖 yawning

🖖 sneezing

🖖 hiccups

🖖 generalized hypotonia

🖖 glassy eyes

🖖 irritability

🖖 diffuse sleep or wake states with whimpering sounds, facial twitching, or discharge

🖖 smiling

🖖 eye floating

- active averting
- staring
- strained fussing or crying
- worry or panic

A premature infant can be helped to reach self-regulation if the caregiver offers skin-to-skin contact, positive touch techniques, positioning, and protection (Lubbe, 2009). These techniques may be used when an infant is presenting with stressor cues during interactions. When stressors appear, the infant should be given a rest from the interaction, and intervention or interaction with the infant can resume at a later time. Vegara and Bigsby (2004) stated that self-regulation includes the infant's ability to protect his or her sleep or acclimate to the repeated stimulation; tolerate painful or stressful stimulation or basic care; demonstrate minimal physiological responses to social interactions with caregivers; and make good efforts to self-regulate during states of arousal.

Well-regulated infants will present with the following (Als, 1982; Vegara & Bigsby, 2004):

- adaptation and maintenance of a relaxed and flexed posture
- regulation of their own heart and respiration rates in order to continue interacting with stimulation within their environment
- maintenance of a state of quiet alertness
- respond to stressful situations with stress cues and may employ self-regulation strategies in order to calm themselves, such as foot bracing, bringing hand to the face, or thumb sucking
- stable digestion
- good, stable color

Infants who are able to organize or regulate themselves are able to return to a more balanced posture and physiological baseline faster than infants who are unable to self-regulate. If there is a lack of ability to self-regulate, caregiver intervention may be required to regain a physiological state or motor stability. If an infant is unable to self-regulate after caregiver intervention or a break from the assessment, the evaluation process may have to be stopped until another time. But, if he or she is calmed and regulated, then the stimulation was well tolerated and the assessment may be continued. The following are signs of appropriate self-regulation:

### Self-regulatory (approach) signals

- stable heart rate
- stable respiratory rate
- stable color
- relaxed limbs
- "ooh" face
- leg bracing

- hand or foot clasp
- grasping
- sucking on fingers
- hands to mouth
- minimal motor activity
- alertness
- relaxed facial expression (Als, Lester, Tronick, & Brazelton, 1982)

Prematurity now surpasses birth defects as the leading cause of death in neonates, accounting for 23% of deaths in the first month of life (Smith, 2003). Because of advances in medical technology and care for the neonate, babies born as early as 23 weeks gestation and at birth weights as low as 500 grams are now surviving. Babies born prematurely face a greater risk of serious health problems, generally proportionate to gestational age. This is due in part to low birth weight, less developed organs, and decreased ability to fight infection. Extremely premature infants have the highest risk for complications and long-term disabilities, including cerebral palsy, intellectual disability, lung and gastrointestinal disorders, and vision and hearing loss. The following are common complications frequently seen in premature infants.

- *Respiratory distress syndrome* (RDS) is the most common problem seen in premature infants. Most infants born before 34 weeks gestation will suffer from RDS. The likelihood and severity of the disease are proportionate to gestational age—the more premature the infant, the more likely RDS will occur, and the more severe it will be. RDS is caused by immaturity of the infant's lungs, which lack the protein *surfactant*. Surfactant creates a protective film that prevents the alveoli in the lungs from collapsing. Lack of surfactant results in ineffective breathing, which is referred to as RDS. Infants with RDS are treated with artificial surfactant at birth. Depending on the severity of the RDS, many premature infants require additional respiratory support in the form of mechanical ventilation, nasal continuous positive airway pressure, or nasal canula.

- *Bronchiopulmonary dysplasia* (BPD) is a chronic lung disorder that primarily affects premature infants who require prolonged mechanical ventilation for the treatment of RDS. These infants develop lung damage as a result of fluid in the lungs and the development of scar tissue. The presence of scar tissue causes small areas of the lungs to collapse and other areas to overexpand, leading to spasms and constrictions, which create breathing difficulties. Depending on the severity of the BPD, treatment ranges from supplemental oxygen to a tracheotomy with continued ventilator support. These infants' lungs usually heal over the first 2 years of life; however, some severely affected infants will develop a chronic lung disease similar to asthma.

- *Intraventricular hemorrhage* (IVH), commonly referred to as a *bleed*, is a serious and fairly common complication of prematurity. IVH is characterized by ruptured blood vessels, resulting in bleeding in the brain near or into the ventricles. Although this bleeding can occur before birth or later, it usually occurs within the first 4 days of life, when the more premature infant is at higher risk. IVH is diagnosed via ultrasound and graded for severity on a scale of I to IV, characterized as follows:

  - Grade I—small amount of bleeding limited to the area around the ruptured blood vessels near the ventricle

- Grade II—bleeding extends into the ventricle, but no ventricle enlargement occurs
- Grade III—bleeding extends into the ventricle, resulting in the enlargement of the ventricle
- Grade IV—a large amount of bleeding extends into the ventricle, resulting in the enlargement of the ventricle and bleeding into the surrounding brain tissue

The most common IVHs are mild (Grades I and II). Most of these resolve on their own and do not cause identifiable brain damage. These infants have no or few long-term deficits related to their IVH. More severe IVHs (Grades III and IV) can cause the ventricles to expand rapidly, creating pressure on the surrounding brain tissue, which can lead to brain damage. In some cases, the ventricle continues to enlarge, causing a condition known as *posthemorrhagic hydrocephalus*, which may require surgical placement of a shunt system to redirect excess fluid collecting in the ventricle. Infants with severe IVH are at high risk for long-term deficits, including cerebral palsy, motor and coordination deficits, seizures, hearing loss, vision deficits, and learning disabilities.

✺ *Periventricular leukomalacia* (PVL) is a condition in premature infants in which there is softening of the brain tissue as a result of cell death of the white matter around the ventricles. PVL is caused by decreased blood flow to the brain and decreased oxygen in the blood. PVL can occur alone or in conjunction with severe IVH. In severe cases of PVL, porencephalic cyst formation, ventricle scarring, and cerebral atrophy can occur. Because PVL usually affects the motor tracts of the brain, these infants are at high risk for long-term motor deficits and cerebral palsy. They may also have hearing loss, vision deficits, learning disabilities, and seizures.

✺ *Retinopathy of prematurity* (ROP) occurs primarily in infants born before 32 weeks gestation, with more premature infants at higher risk. ROP is an abnormal development of the blood vessels in the eyes, which can lead to bleeding and scar formation that can damage the retina. Most cases heal on their own with little or no vision loss. More severe cases require intervention and can result in vision loss or blindness. ROP has been associated with high oxygen concentrations delivered during mechanical ventilation.

✺ *Necrotizing enterocolitis* (NEC) is a potentially dangerous condition that can develop in premature infants in which a portion of the infant's intestines becomes necrotic and is destroyed. NEC occurs when blood supply to the intestines is decreased or interrupted, allowing bacteria that are normally present to invade the area, causing further damage. Depending on the severity of the disease, bowel damage can range from minimal to extensive. Treatment also depends on severity. Some cases can be treated by allowing the infant to eat nothing by mouth, possibly for several weeks, to give the bowel complete rest and time to heal. More severe cases may require surgery to remove the necrotic bowel and create a temporary ostomy to allow the bowel to heal. In the most severe cases, the infant may develop short gut syndrome. Short gut occurs when there is not enough healthy bowel remaining to adequately absorb nutrition. As a result, the infant will require intravenous nutrition for a prolonged period and may eventually require special formula. Feeding problems, both physiological and behavioral in nature, can occur in infants with NEC. Infants who require multiple surgeries as a result of NEC may also experience weakening of the abdominal muscles, which can affect later acquisition of motor skills.

Due to premature infants' immature immune systems, infections are common and include pneumonia, sepsis, and meningitis. Infections occur in three ways:

intrauterine/congenital, perinatal, and acquired. Intrauterine infections occur during pregnancy. They are not common but can be serious. If the infection occurs early in gestation, it can result in nervous system or tissue abnormalities and even brain damage. These infections include toxoplasmosis, rubella, cytomegalovirus, herpes simplex, and HIV. Perinatal infections occur during delivery through the birth canal. These include group B streptococcus, *E. coli*, chlamydia, and hepatitis B. Acquired infections occur after birth through contact. These include *S. epidermidis* (staph epi), *S. aureus* (staph aureus), pseudomonas, and respiratory syndrome. Infections are typically treated with antibiotics or antiviral drugs. The problems resulting from infection depend primarily on the severity and type of infection. One problem commonly related to infection is hearing loss.

## Target Areas for Intervention

Precautions associated with premature infants depend greatly on gestational age, postconceptual age, medical stability, complications, and the infant's state and interactive behaviors. It is important to have an understanding of the equipment used frequently in the NICU. Knowledge of physiological parameters for premature infants is essential. Understanding the meaning of premature infants' neurobehavioral states and cues is also essential. Universal precautions and strict handwashing practices should always be observed to prevent infection in these fragile infants.

Although premature infants may require occupational therapy intervention at various stages of their lives, this chapter will focus on intervention during the initial acute hospitalization in the NICU. The primary goal for intervention with the premature infant is to enhance and optimize development. The occupational therapist in the NICU can assume many roles while working with the premature infant, including those of developmental specialist, educator, and advocate. There are five typical areas of focus for intervention with the premature infant in the NICU:

- positioning
- caregiver–infant interaction/caregiver education
- sensory intervention/environmental adaptations
- developmental/motor intervention
- feeding

Positioning intervention with the premature infant is an important and often early focus of the occupational therapist in the NICU. Goals for positioning are to minimize motor disorganization, promote physiological flexion, discourage arching and rigidity, prevent cranial molding, and counteract emerging stereotypical postures. Other goals for positioning are to encourage midline orientation and provide boundaries and containment to promote self-regulation. Such interventions support development by providing the infant with positive input without prolonged direct handling or undue stress. With the appropriate and accurate observation and documentation of the subsystems and their interaction—the autonomic system, the motor system, the state organizational system, the attention and interaction system, and the self-regulatory system—an appropriate individualized intervention plan can be developed. The stabilization and integration of the various systems are interdependent and contribute to the infant's overall ability to self-regulate (Als et al., 1982).

Promoting caregiver–infant interaction and caregiver education is another important and early focus of the occupational therapist in the NICU. The birth of an infant with special needs can be a trying experience for any parent. A range of reactions and emotions, including fear, denial, anger, guilt, loss, frustration, and powerlessness, are common. In addition, the NICU can be a very overwhelming environment for parents. Parents can often feel like "secondary caregivers" in this acute setting. These feelings, coupled with the medical condition of the infant, can create barriers to parent–infant bonding. Early identification and remediation of parent–infant interaction difficulties are important to maximizing the infant's developmental outcome.

Olson and Baltman (1994) stated that the role of the parent within the NICU may first seem to be that of a technician, with parents reading and watching monitors, interpreting ventilator pressures, and becoming proficient at maintaining the surrounding tubing and hosing. This is very different from the role they would expect to play as parents of a child without medical issues. These parents must adjust to the loss of the idea of the perfect child and learn to resolve their inner conflicts of blame, biological ineptitude, and ambivalence about their new infant in the NICU. By educating the parents on their infant's states and behavioral cues as well as general development, and by assisting parents in interactions with their infant, occupational therapists can have a positive impact on parent–infant bonding and developmental outcomes.

The most important goal for intervention with parents and family members is to promote interactions and caregiving skills with their infant. The interventionist can act as a role model and help in reducing parents' fears of handling their child. The interventionist should reinforce the bonding between the parent and infant, focus on the infant's strengths, and discuss the best way of consoling the infant. Positive reinforcement should be encouraged from the parents when the infant smiles or gazes at the parent.

Premature infants do not have mature neural systems and therefore have difficulty synthesizing all of the sensory input they receive (Peterson-DeGroff, 1996). A focus of the occupational therapist in the NICU is frequently on sensory intervention and environmental adaptation. The NICU environment can be very overstimulating to a premature infant's immature sensory system and can elicit stress behaviors. Therefore, early sensory intervention focuses more on adapting the infant's environment to reduce stimulation than on providing stimulation. When the infant becomes more physiologically stable and the neural system matures, the focus of sensory intervention includes providing carefully graded stimulation to enhance the infant's auditory, visual, tactile/proprioceptive, and vestibular skill development (Vergara, 1993). Sensory stimulation should be offered based on the infant's level of stress and the infant's reaction to stimulation.

A therapist must observe the infant's response to the stimulation to ensure that it is not overwhelming. Handling can be synchronized with various sensory inputs, such as with visual and auditory stimulation. These stimulations encourage parent–infant interactions (Als, 1982). Anderson and Auster-Liebhaber (1984) suggested the following techniques and tips:

- ᴪ Treatment sessions may include handling and treatment sequencing.
- ᴪ Use visual stimulation (e.g., toys, mirrors, faces) to elicit exploration and tracking skills.
- ᴪ Use tactile stimulation activities (e.g., hand-to-hand, foot-to-hand, knee-to-foot, or foot-to-foot stimulation).
- ᴪ Tactile input can include placing the infant on sheepskin to allow for input during movements.
- ᴪ Use proprioceptive input (e.g., treatment sequencing with weight-bearing activities, swaddling, giving input during holding).
- ᴪ Swaddling occurs toward the end of a treatment session. The infant is wrapped tightly in a blanket after a specific bundling sequence, with the amount of flexion depending on the infant's tolerance to the swaddle and medical condition.
- ᴪ Vestibular stimulation (the use of a rocking chair while positioned on the caregiver's lap) is useful with infants who are distressed with transitions in movement.
- ᴪ Movement must be done only after swaddling.
- ᴪ Movement is used when the infant is distressed, disorganized, and hypertonic and is done in a slow, rhythmic anterior–posterior plane to decrease tone and soothe.
- ᴪ Use gradually introduced quicker movements in handling to increase tone and level of alertness.
- ᴪ Periodic interruptions of vestibular input are necessary to observe behavior and state of arousal.
- ᴪ Side lying and prone positions may be used for the more medically stable infant.
- ᴪ An inverted position can be used after the 29th week of gestation.
- ᴪ Slow and rhythmic input should be used with infants suffering neonatal seizures.
- ᴪ Rotary rocking must be avoided with the NICU neonate.

Premature infants are at risk for developing abnormal motor patterns and developmental delay. Another important area of focus for the occupational therapist in the NICU is on preventing the development of abnormal posture and movement patterns, while facilitating normal development through handling and therapeutic exercise appropriate to the infant's developmental level. The primary goals for intervention are to facilitate flexion; decrease extension of the neck, trunk, and extremities; decrease shoulder elevation and retraction; and promote weight bearing and weight shifting. Positioning is known to have an effect on an infant's body systems; proper positioning will promote an infant's engagement in normal sensorimotor experiences, such as bringing the hand to the mouth. Incorrect positioning can cause behavioral disorganization and physiological distress and can compromise soft tissue integrity, shoulder and pelvic girdle activity, and postural alignment (Vegara & Bigsby, 2004). Infants in the NICU usually suffer from abnormal tonal issues and lack of normal reflexes, causing them to avoid social interactions by falling asleep or averting their eyes (Olson & Baltman, 1994). Because of the low percentage of positive tactile input that occurs in the incubator of an infant who is less active and has low postural tone, the infant will engage in less self-exploration and self-engagement of tactile stimulation as well. Medications that result in lethargy contribute to less active movement of the infant. The main outcome of positioning within the NICU is to provide postural and self-regulatory supports that will help normalize the infant's sensorimotor experiences regardless of the medical equipment or restrictions (Vegara & Bigsby, 2004). It is important to encourage normal newborn postures (i.e., flexor postures) with the NICU neonate because these infants are usually unable to maintain a flexed posture, which is key for self-regulation and proper muscular development. By placing an infant in a flexed position with a blanket roll, padding, or the hands, an interventionist or parent is promoting both motor stability and organization (Fay, 1998). Goldberg-Hamblin, Singer, Singer, and Denney (2007) stated that positioning in flexion with the limbs drawn toward the middle of the body during sleep using blanket rolls, padding, commercial positioning devices, or loose swaddling can help achieve a flexed position. Hypotonia occurs with NICU preterm infants because they spend an extended period of time in a supine position, where gravity will force a relatively extended position and may lead to possible extensor tone if the infant is not placed in a flexed position periodically. Positions must be varied throughout the course of a day, should not interfere with medical care, and must be convenient for other medical staff to perform when the therapist is not available.

The evaluation and treatment of feeding problems in premature infants is another essential focus of the occupational therapist in the NICU. Infants rely on sucking as their primary source of feeding. This is a very complex task, especially for the premature infant. In addition to needing adequate oral-motor control to suck, the infant must also be able to coordinate sucking, swallowing, and breathing; have mature rooting, sucking, and swallowing reflexes; have normal oral tone and flexor tone; have strong sucking pads to be able to tolerate the stimulation involved with feeding; and have adequate endurance to sustain feeding. Contributing factors for feeding problems would be increased extensor tone and decreased flexor tone, immature reflexes, poor lip seal, poor alertness, and oral hypersensitivity. Most premature infants do not exhibit all of the characteristics of optimal oral-motor readiness for feeding until approximately 36 weeks gestation (Long, 1997). The primary goals for intervention are to promote the appropriate tactile responses, state control, motor control, oral-motor control, physiological control, coordination of suck–swallow–breathe, and endurance necessary for safe and efficient feeding. Caregiver education is also an important aspect of feeding intervention in the NICU.

## ❦ Contextual Considerations

### Clinical

The purpose of the clinical occupational therapy assessment of the premature infant in the NICU is to delineate the infant's strengths, weaknesses, and needs in order to plan a program. The clinical evaluation must include information on neurobehavioral organization, neuromuscular status, and developmental status (including sensory processing). When indicated, the evaluation should also include information on feeding.

The neurobehavioral evaluation includes information on the infant's state behavior, self-regulatory abilities (including approach signals), tolerance for stimuli and handling (including stress signals), temperament, and interactive abilities. Collection of this information is done primarily through observation and may require several sessions to gain an accurate picture. There are several assessment tools available, including the *Neonatal Behavioral Assessment Scale* (Brazelton, 1984), the *Neonatal Neurobehavioral Examination* (Dubowitz & Dubowitz, 1981), the *Neurobehavioral Assessment of Preterm Infant* (Dubowitz & Dubowitz, 1981), the *Assessment of Preterm Infant Behavior* (Als et al., 1982), and the *Naturalistic Observation of Newborn Behavior* (Als, 1986), which provide information regarding the neurobehavioral status of the premature infant.

The neuromuscular evaluation includes information regarding the infant's muscle tone, ROM, posture, reflex development, and motor activity. This information is collected through handling and observation. Assessment tools available include the *Neonatal Neurological Examination* (Dubowitz & Dubowitz, 1981) and *INFANIB* (Ellison, 1994), which will provide neuromuscular information about movement, tone, and reflexes.

The developmental evaluation includes information regarding the infant's visual, auditory, tactile, vestibular, proprioceptive, and motor development, and the developmental level achieved within each area. This information is also collected through handling and observation. Assessment tools available include the *Bayley Scales of Infant Development–III* (Bayley, 2005), *Peabody Developmental Motor Scales–Second Edition* (Folio & Fewell, 2000), and *Alberta Infant Motor Scale* (Piper & Darrah, 1994), which will provide information on the general development of the infant.

The feeding evaluation includes information regarding oral-motor reflexes, muscle tone and strength, postural stability, oral-motor coordination, coordination of suck–swallow–breathe, response to tactile input, physiological control, and endurance. Most therapists evaluate feeding with self-developed criterion-referenced evaluations that include the aforementioned basic feeding components (Vergara, 1993). It is important to note that many assessment tools require specialized training and/or certification.

---

## Family

It is important to remember that the parents of premature infants have had the responsibility of parenting thrust upon them earlier than expected. In addition to being denied the expected preparation time, parents are faced with an infant who is physically and behaviorally different from the full-term infant they anticipated. The occupational therapist can play a key role in helping the parents adapt to the NICU environment and understand their infant's unique behaviors in order to interact effectively, promote bonding, and optimize development.

Since the mid to late 1980s there has been a philosophical shift from child-centered to family-centered provision of services. Although it can be difficult to shift focus from the critically ill infant to the family as a whole, family-centered care principles should be employed by a therapist dealing with families of premature infants. The key elements of family-centered care include the following:

- recognizing that the family is a constant in the infant's life
- facilitating parent–professional collaboration at all levels of health care
- honoring the racial, ethnic, cultural, religious, and socioeconomic diversity of families
- recognizing family strengths and individuality and respecting different methods of coping
- sharing complete and unbiased information with parents on a continuing basis and in a supportive manner
- encouraging family-to-family support and networking

A major goal of family-centered care is to support parents in the caregiver role (Long, 1997). The manner in which medical and nursing care is given often sets up barriers to providing family-centered care in the NICU. Valuing parent–professional collaboration and incorporating it into NICU care can assist professionals in meeting the needs of both the infant and the parents by removing some of these barriers (Kreibel, Munsick-Bruno, & Lowe, 1991). Although changing the dynamics of providing care in the NICU may be difficult, establishing collaborative relationships with parents should be a primary focus of the occupational therapist (Holloway, 1994).

In preparing for discharge from the NICU, the occupational therapist can educate the family about ways to promote their infant's development at home. Referral to a NICU follow-up clinic, early intervention, and/or outpatient occupational therapy services is often also warranted.

## Practice Setting

Although this chapter focuses on the NICU as the primary practice setting, occupational therapists may also encounter premature infants in a variety of other settings at various stages in the infant's life. Home-based early intervention services to promote developmental milestones and, later, school-based services to promote academically related skills are often required. Some infants may benefit from inpatient and/or outpatient rehabilitation. Occupational therapists working in home care often provide intervention to former premature infants. When disabilities related to prematurity are severe, some infants may eventually require care in a long-term-care facility.

## Sociopolitical

Two primary laws apply to premature infants and their families. The Family and Medical Leave Act of 1993 (FMLA, 1993) mandates that most employers provide up to 12 weeks of unpaid leave for the birth of a child or the care of a seriously ill family member with continuation of the employee's health benefits (Zaichkin, 1996). Under the Individuals With Disabilities Education Act (IDEA, 1997), programs were developed for infants and toddlers with disabilities (from birth to 3 years) and their families. All 50 states and Puerto Rico have statewide early intervention programs to address the needs of infants and toddlers who are developmentally delayed or at risk for delay and their families.

In addition, premature infants and their families may qualify for benefits under other government programs. These include Social Security, Medicaid, and Women, Infants, and Children (WIC) programs. These programs provide financial, medical, and nutritional assistance to qualifying persons.

## Lifestyle/Lifespan

It is important to assist parents in understanding the possible short-term and long-term issues related to their premature infant. Issues may be medical, developmental, financial, and familial.

The premature infant's gestational age and hospital course will greatly influence medical issues after discharge. Needs can include tube feeding, medications, monitors, tracheostomy care, and ostomy care. Some families may require cardiopulmonary resuscitation (CPR) training. Some infants may require follow-up with any number of medical specialists, including neurology, ophthalmology, cardiology, and surgery. Infants who are discharged with complex medical needs may qualify for nursing services in the home to assist the parents.

Gestational age and medical complications also influence developmental issues. Premature infants are at higher risk for developmental delay than are healthy, full-term infants. Severe IVH and PVL can greatly affect the motor tracts of the brain and are red flags for possible future motor and speech delays. Former preemies account for approximately one third of children with cerebral palsy. Approximately 60% are considered "normal," 24% have mild disabilities (e.g., learning disabilities, attention-deficit disorder, vision deficits, mild cerebral palsy), and 16% have severe disabilities (e.g., spastic quad cerebral palsy, intellectual disabilities; Long, 1997). Although it is impossible to accurately predict outcomes, it is important to make the parents aware of the developmental issues for which their premature infant may be at risk.

The family's economic resources and the infant's medical needs will influence financial issues. Sicker infants may require a longer NICU stay, and infants with chronic illnesses may require frequent hospitalizations after NICU discharge. Some families' employment or financial situations may not allow time off from work during these times. The medical needs of the infant may require 24-hour care, which may make it necessary for one parent to leave his or her job. Some equipment and nursing care may not be covered under medical insurance. Day care for an infant or child with medical needs or a disability can be expensive and difficult to find, if available at all. All of these issues have the potential to cause financial strain on a family.

The birth of a premature child can be devastating to families. The stress of having a sick infant can strain familial relationships and can cause feelings of both physical and emotional separation. Parents, as well as other family members, may be employing all their resources to cope with the situation personally and may not have any energy left to support one another (Zaichkin, 1996). Siblings may feel neglected if the infant's care requires an excessive amount of a parent's time. An infant's social environment includes the infant's interaction with family and caregivers. The infant's physiological stability and state of arousal must be observed and documented during and after the caregiver's interaction. It must be noted if the infant is depleted in energy after given care or being handled by the caregivers. Certain family members or caregivers may elicit an optimal response with a state of arousal and may bring out the infant's best performance or cause a withdrawal affect. Timing of social interactions must be considered and may influence the infant's state of arousal or physiological stability. A therapist may have to schedule off-work hours in order to observe family visitations, or a schedule for visitation may have to be created in order to synchronize with the infant's best time for interaction. These factors may offer the best assessment approaches for the infant.

## 📖 Clinical Decision-Making Process
### Defining Focus for Intervention

The focus for the occupational therapy intervention will depend on a variety of factors, including timing of the referral, gestational and postconceptual ages, and medical stability. If an infant is very premature, very sick, and in the first few weeks of life, occupational therapy will focus on environmental adaptations to reduce stress, positioning to promote physiological flexion and provide containment, developmentally supportive care, and parent education. A complete evaluation is often too stressful for the infant at this early stage. Observation and screening are often the best methods to determine the needs for the aforementioned focus areas. Though educating the parents should always be a focus of intervention, it is particularly important at this time. Most parents of preemies will be overwhelmed by the NICU and will need thorough orientation to the unit, equipment, staff, and their baby's unique issues.

As the infant grows and becomes more medically stable, a more complete evaluation will be possible. Areas of focus for evaluation will be neurobehavioral status (stress signals, state behavior, self-regulatory skills, etc.), neuromuscular status (ROM, tone, quality of active movements, reflexes, etc.), and developmental status (visual skills, auditory skills, etc.). Focus for intervention includes promoting state control and self-regulatory skills, improving tolerance for handling, promoting normal muscle tone and movement patterns, and promoting developmentally appropriate skills. Another important focus is on parent–infant interaction. Getting a parent to use *kangaroo care* (providing skin-to-skin contact by placing the infant on the parent's chest) is a good way to promote bonding, and studies have shown it to be physiologically beneficial for the infant as well (Luddington-Hoe, Thompson, Swinth, Hadeed, & Anderson, 1994).

When medically and developmentally appropriate, feeding is often a main focus for intervention with premature infants. Typically, these infants need to work on sucking, coordination of suck–swallow–breathe, and endurance. Environment, positioning, nipple selection, oral-motor stimulation, and oral-motor skills are focuses within feeding intervention. Since it is impossible for the occupational therapist to be present during all feedings, it is essential to educate parents and nursing staff about the guidelines for safe and efficient feeding of the infant.

When the infant is ready to leave the hospital, discharge planning is the final focus of the occupational therapist working in the NICU. It may be necessary to provide the family with a home program for ROM, feeding, and/or developmental stimulation. A referral to early intervention or outpatient services may be required.

Last, it may be necessary to adapt the infant's car seat for safe transport home. More often than not, even the smallest of infant car seats are too large for preemies. It may be necessary to provide a commercially available car seat insert or to use blanket rolls around the infant's head, along the sides, and between the legs to prevent the infant from sliding down or to the side in the seat, which could potentially restrict breathing.

## Establishing Goals for Intervention

Goals for intervention will also be dictated by timing of referral, gestational and postconceptual ages, and medical stability. For example, nipple feeding would not be a goal for a 2-week-old, 24-week-gestation preemie but could be for a 9-week-old, 28-week-gestation preemie. It is important to consider the infant's neurobehavioral strengths and weaknesses when establishing goals. State control, self-regulatory skills, and tolerance for handling will usually be initial goals, as these skills are the foundation for addressing other goals. It would be impossible to work on a goal of visual tracking, for example, if the infant screams uncontrollably when handled.

## Designing Theory-Based Intervention

There are many different frames of reference applicable to this population. These may include syntactic theory of development/developmental care, biomechanical, developmental, neurodevelopmental treatment, and sensory integration.

Intervention with premature infants should be based on the theory of developmental care. The premise of developmental care is the synactive theory of development, pioneered by psychologist Heidelise Als and associates after extensive research with premature infants (Als, 1986). This theory is much too complex to address in detail within the confines of this chapter. In short, the synactive theory of development outlines how infants interact with the environment through various hierarchically organized behavioral subsystems: physiological (autonomic), motor, state, interactive/attentional, and self-regulation. Stability in the lower subsystems is necessary for higher level functioning (Vergara, 1993). From this theory emerged the approach known as *individualized developmental care*. The theory indicates that assessing the infant's ability to cope with the environment and stimulation will provide the caregiver with information to modify each infant's environment and form treatment strategies to maximize positive outcomes. Developmental care should encompass all disciplines, including occupational therapy. The occupational therapist is often the person who assesses and designs each infant's individualized developmental care program and adapts/modifies the environment accordingly. This plan then becomes the foundation for all intervention, including therapeutic, nursing, and medical intervention.

The biomechanical frame of reference is used with premature infants who frequently have neuromuscular or musculoskeletal issues, since they typically lack physiological flexion and exhibit low muscle tone and abnormal movement patterns. For example, knowledge and understanding of biomechanical neurodevelopmental and developmental principles are necessary for intervention with a preemie whose lack of flexion and predominant extensor movement patterns and resulting structural changes make it difficult for the infant to get his or her hands to his or her face or mouth for self-calming.

The developmental frame of reference is used in this population as in any other pediatric population. It is necessary to have a good understanding of normal development in order to identify emerging atypical development and promote achievement of developmental milestones. For example, does a 14-week-old, 28-week-gestation preemie who is able to hold his head up for extended periods truly have good head control? Or is increased extensor tone allowing him to hold his head up? Knowledge of developmental principles suggests that a 2-week-old infant (the infant's corrected age) does not have enough head control to maintain an erect head and neck; therefore, extensor tone is likely the underlying cause. Premature infants are at high risk for developmental delay, and early identification and intervention are key to improving developmental outcomes.

Neurodevelopmental treatment principles are often used to treat the older preemie population. Positioning principles and handling techniques of this approach can be beneficial in treating infants who demonstrate neurological and motor problems. Keep in mind that neurodevelopmental treatment is frequently used with children with cerebral palsy, and many premature infants who are later diagnosed with this condition show early neuromuscular problems.

Use of the sensory integration approach with premature infants can be beneficial, but sensory input must be carefully graded and monitored. Although these techniques are not appropriate for use with the young preemie, they can be applied to the older preemie, whose neural system is more mature and able to tolerate the stimulation. For example, sensory integration principles and techniques may be useful when working on feeding with an infant who demonstrates tactile defensiveness of the face and mouth after prolonged intubation.

## Evaluating Progress

Progress is evaluated by achievement of established goals. Because preemies can change and develop so rapidly, evaluation and reevaluation of progress is an ongoing process. Improved physiological status, decreased ventilator requirements, weight gain, decreased medication requirements, and increased awake/alert time can be less obvious signs of progress.

## Determining Change in or Termination of Treatment

Change in or termination of treatment is warranted when the infant fails to progress or has met all of the goals established.

### Case Study

*Description*

BW is a 2-week-old infant born at 26 weeks gestation, weighing 775 grams, to a 32-year-old mother with good prenatal care. BW's parents have a 4-year-old daughter at home, which makes frequent visitation difficult. BW was intubated at delivery because of poor respiratory effort and continues to require mechanical ventilation for RDS. A head ultrasound revealed a right Grade II IVH. BW had an intravenous line in his right arm. Episodes of apnea, bradycardia, and oxygen desaturation have been documented.

Occupational therapy evaluation found BW to have poor state control and poor tolerance for environmental stimulation. BW demonstrated significant stress signs with caregiving and poor self-calming skills. Supine resting position was with legs in slight flexion, arms extended at the sides, and neck rotated to the right and extended. Active movements were disorganized, jerky, and predominated by extension. BW was able to open his eyes for brief periods when the lights were dimmed.

*Long- and Short-Term Goals*

The long-term goal of intervention for BW is to enable him to improve his state control, increase his tolerance for environment, and develop self-calming skills. These goals will be reached in part through successfully achieving the following short-term goals:

1. Transition smoothly from sleep state to quiet alert state.
2. Tolerate diaper change with minimum signs of stress.
3. Self-calm with moderate therapist assistance.
4. Maintain an optimally flexed position with assistive devices.

### Therapist Goals and Strategies

The therapist's goals include the following:

1. Promote physiological flexion and midline orientation.
2. Promote state control and self-calming.
3. Minimize positional deformities, abnormal tone, and abnormal movement patterns.
4. Provide an environment that reduces infant stress and promotes self-regulatory behaviors.
5. Educate family and caregivers on infant's abilities and weaknesses and how to optimally interact with the infant.
6. Promote infant–parent bonding.

The therapist's strategies include the following:

1. Use positioning aids to facilitate flexion and midline orientation, to provide containment and boundaries, and to reduce cranial molding.
2. Take pictures and leave bedside instructions to promote carryover of optimal positioning with caregivers.
3. Employ four-handed care techniques whenever possible during caregiving and routine procedures.
4. Adapt the infant's environment to reduce stressful stimuli (e.g., provide an isolette cover to shield the infant from light and visual stimuli, dim lights, reduce noise).
5. Explore calming techniques that work best with the infant.
6. Provide parents with opportunities to observe their infant's various states and signals to promote understanding of behaviors.
7. Provide parents with opportunities for positive interactions with their infant.

### Activity: Kangaroo Care

BW's mother will hold him skin to skin on her chest in a private, quiet, and dimly lit area of the nursery (since BW is still intubated, a screen will be provided around his warmer bed and the tube taped to Mom to prevent accidental extubation). Mom will be guided in holding BW in a flexed position with opportunities for hands-to-face and hands-to-mouth contact, skills important for self-calming in infants. Initially, this therapeutic holding would be for a short period with close supervision, giving Mom the opportunity to identify BW's stress and approach signals, assist him in self-calming, and gain confidence in her ability to interact with her infant. As the infant becomes more able to tolerate sensation and self-regulate and Mom becomes more confident and comfortable, the activity can be graded to increase time, handling, and stimulation.

*Treatment Objectives*

   1. BW will tolerate handling and his environment for 10 minutes.

   2. Mom will correctly identify BW's stress and approach signals and respond appropriately.

# Resources

## Internet Resources

American Association of Premature Infants: www.aapi-online.org

Association for Retinopathy of Prematurity and Related Diseases: www.ropard.org

Institute for Patient- and Family-Centered Care: www.familycenteredcare.org

March of Dimes: www.marchofdimes.com

Come Unity Parenting Support: www.comeunity.com/premature/preemiepgs.html

Premature Infant: www.premature-infant.com

## Print Resources

Gross, R., Spiker, D., & Haynes, C. (1997). *Helping low birthweight, premature babies: The infant health and development program.* Stanford, CA: Stanford University Press.

Klein, A. (1998). *Caring for your premature baby.* New York, NY: Harper Resources.

Ludington-Hoe, S. (1993). *Kangaroo care: The best you can do to help your preterm infant.* New York, NY: Bantam Books.

Wyly, V. (1995). *Premature infants and their families: Developmental interventions.* San Diego, CA: Bantam Books.

Zaichkin, J. (1996). *Newborn intensive care—What every parent needs to know.* Santa Rosa, CA: NICU Ink Books.

# References

Als, H. (1982). Toward a synactive theory of development: Promise for the assessment and support of infant individuality. *Infant Mental Health Journal, 3*(4), 229–243.

Als, H. (1986). A synactive model of neonatal behavioral organization: Framework for the assessment of neurobehavioral development in the premature infant and for support of infants and parents in the neonatal intensive care environment. In J. K. Sweeney (Ed.), *High risk neonate: Developmental therapy perspectives* (pp. 1–55). New York, NY: Hawthorn Press.

Als, H., Lester, B. M., Tronick, E. Z., & Brazelton, T. B. (1982). Toward a research instrument for the assessment of preterm infants' behavior (APIB). In H. Fitzgerald, B. M. Lester, & M. S. Yogman (Eds.), *Theory and research in behavioral pediatrics* (Vol. 1, pp. 35–132). New York, NY: Plenum.

Anderson, J., & Auster-Liebhaber, J. (1984). Developmental therapy in the neonatal intensive care unit. *Physical and Occupational Therapy in Pediatrics, 4*(1), 89–106.

Bayley, N. (2005). *Bayley scales of infant and toddler development* (3rd ed.). San Antonio, TX: The Psychological Corporation.

Brazelton, T. B. (1984). *Neonatal behavioral assessment scale*. Philadelphia, PA: Lippincott, Williams & Wilkins.

Dubowitz, L., & Dubowitz, V. (1981). *The neurological assessment of the pre-term and full-term newborn infant*. Philadelphia, PA: Lippincott, Williams & Wilkins.

Edgren, A. (1998). Prematurity. In *Gale Encyclopedia of Medicine*. Detroit, MI: Gale Group.

Ellison, P. H. (1994). *The INFANIB*. San Antonio, TX: Therapy Skill Builders.

Family and Medical Leave Act of 1993, 29 U.S.C. § 2654 *et seq.* (1993) (P.L.103-3; FMLA)

Fay, M. J. (1988). The positive effects of positioning. *Neonatal Network*, 23–28.

Folio, M. R., & Fewell, R. R. (2000). *Peabody developmental motor scales* (2nd ed.). Austin, TX: PRO-ED, Inc.

Goldberg-Hamblin, S., Singer, J., Singer, G. H. S., & Denney, M. K. (2007). Early intervention in neonatal nurseries: The promising practice of developmental care. *Journal of Infants and Young Children, 20*(2), 163–171.

Holloway, E. (1994). Parent and occupational therapist collaboration in the neonatal intensive care unit. *American Journal of Occupational Therapy, 48,* 535–538.

Individuals With Disabilities Education Act of 1990, 20 U.S.C. § 1400 *et seq.* (1990) (amended 1997).

Kreibel, R., Munsick-Bruno, G., & Lowe, R. (1991). NICU infants born at developmental risk and the individualized family service plan/process. *Children's Health Care, 20*(1), 26–33.

Lester, B. M., & Tronick, E. (2005). *The NICU network neurobehavioral scale*. Baltimore, MD: Paul H. Brookes.

Long, T. (1997, September). *Therapeutic intervention in the neonatal intensive care unit*. Workshop presented by Pacific Coast Seminars, San Francisco, CA.

Lubbe, W. (2009). *Little steps NICU program*. Retrieved from http://www.littlesteps.co.za/

Luddington-Hoe, S. M., Thompson, C., Swinth, J., Hadeed, A. J., & Anderson, G. C. (1994). Kangaroo care: Research results and practice implications and guidelines. *Neonatal Network, 13,* 19–27.

March of Dimes. (2011). *PeriStats*. Retrieved from www.marchofdimes.com/peristats

Olson, J. A., & Baltman, K. (1994). Infant mental health in occupational therapy practice in the neonatal intensive care unit. *The American Journal of Occupational Therapy, 48*(6), 499–505.

Peterson-DeGroff, M. (1996). *Developmental care: Overstimulation and your premature baby*. Retrieved from http://www.prematurity.org/overstimulation.html

Piper M. C., & Darrah, J. (1994). *Motor assessment of the developing infant*. Philadelphia, PA: Saunders.

Vergara, E. (1993). *Foundations for practice in the neonatal intensive care unit and early intervention: A self-guided practice manual.* Rockville, MD: American Occupational Therapy Association.

Vergara, E. R., & Bigsby, R. (2004). *Developmental and therapeutic interventions in the NICU.* Baltimore, MD: Paul H. Brookes.

Zaichkin, J. (1996). *Newborn intensive care—What every parent needs to know.* Santa Rosa, CA: NICU Ink Books.

# Regulatory Disorders

*Moya Kinnealey*

## 🌿 Synopsis of Clinical Condition

### Prevalence and Etiology

Self-regulation is an important foundation for human adaptation in all aspects of life. Self-regulation is the ability to react to change, recover from the reaction, and maintain regulatory capacity (Shonkoff & Phillips, 2000). Regulatory disorders are presumed to be constitutionally or biologically based. Although some cases may have a genetic link, many cases have no clear precipitating factor. Negative temperamental predispositions are often exacerbated by caregiver patterns and early maturational factors, such as prematurity, drug exposure in utero, difficult births, and low birth weight.

### Common Characteristics and Symptoms

Regulatory disorder is diagnosed in children in infancy and early childhood (National Center for Clinical Infant Programs [NCCIP], 1994). It is characterized by difficulties in regulating physiological, sensory, attentional, motor, or affective processes and maintaining a calm, alert, and emotionally positive state. Presenting problems include sleep disturbances, behavioral lethargy or hyperactivity, feeding difficulties, fearfulness of changes in routine or environment, and impaired ability to play alone or with others. The diagnosis involves distinct behavioral patterns and sensory, sensorimotor, or organizational processing difficulties. Some of the sensorimotor processing difficulties include difficulty with sensory modulation, such as over- or undersensitivity to auditory or visual stimuli, temperature, or odors; hypersensitivity to tactile stimulation, movement, and food textures and tastes; and underreactivity to pain. Motor difficulties include diminished ability to coordinate oral musculature and tolerate movement challenges because of poor muscle tone and decreased postural stability, motor disorganization, and stimulus craving. Consequentially, deficits appear in the quality and control of motor activity, the performance of gross and fine motor skills, verbal articulation, and the use of visual–spatial cues. There are qualitative difficulties in attending, relating, and interacting with people other than the primary caregiver (NCCIP, 1994).

Regulatory disorders impact arousal, attention, affect, and action in early childhood (Williamson & Anzalone, 2001). In later childhood, they may be identified as dysfunction in sensory integration or dysfunction in sensory modulation, which can be further categorized as sensory sensitivity; sensory avoidance; sensory seeking (Dunn, 2002, 2007); and language, somatosensory, or vestibular-based dyspraxia. There are four types of regulatory disorders based on predominant characteristics. These are Type I: Hypersensitive; Type II: Underreactive; Type III: Motorically Disorganized; and Type IV: Other.

## Type I: Hypersensitive

The two distinct behavioral patterns that are typical of Type I: Hypersensitive are (a) fearful and cautious or (b) negative and defiant. The fearful and cautious child is sensitive to sensory stimuli, and sensory input may have a cumulative effect. The child is easily upset and unable to soothe him- or herself, and cannot quickly recover from frustration. Although auditory verbal processing abilities are intact, the child overreacts to touch, movement, light, and noise. The negative and defiant child is often fearful and cautious and overreactive to touch and sound. The child also tends to be stubborn and controlling but not necessarily aggressive. The child has great difficulty with change or making transitions, may be compulsive and perfectionist, and may be slow to engage. Auditory processing and fine motor control may be problematic, but visual–spatial orientation and postural control are usually good (NCCIP, 1994).

## Type II: Underreactive

Children in the Type II: Underreactive category are typically withdrawn, difficult to engage, and self-absorbed. Characteristic behaviors of the withdrawn child include disinterest in exploring relationships or the environment and the appearance of apathy or exhaustion. The child is often underreactive to sound and movement but either over- or underreactive to touch. Visual–spatial processing, motor planning, and explorative abilities may be compromised (NCCIP, 1994). The self-absorbed child may be creative and imaginative and tend to focus on personal sensations, thoughts, and emotions rather than attend to or communicate with other people. The child may demonstrate a fantasy life with enormous imagination and creativity and use it to avoid challenges or competition. Auditory–verbal processing and other sensory and motor capacities may be diminished.

## Type III: Motorically Disorganized

A child who is Type III: Motorically Disorganized demonstrates inaccurate, jerky, or impulsive motor behavior that may include a craving of sensory input. The child may appear disorganized, fearless, aggressive, or impulsive. Motor and sensory patterns are characterized by sensory underreactivity to touch and sound and decreased ability to modulate movement. As a result, auditory or visual–spatial processing is disorganized and motor performance is often unfocused and diffused (NCCIP, 1994).

### Type IV: Other
This category is for children who have motor and sensory processing difficulty but whose behavioral patterns are not adequately described by one of the other three types.

## Target Areas for Intervention

The focus for occupational therapy intervention is (a) normalization of the infant's response to sensory stimulation, (b) improvement in motor organization and development, and (c) establishment of positive sensory, emotional, and social interactions between infant and caregiver. Some conditions, such as eczema and food allergies, may cause symptoms similar to regulatory disorders. It is also important to rule out maternal mental illness, as this may impact behavior and regulation. Medical causes of irritability and eating problems, such as reflux and cleft pallet, need to be considered separately.

Note that if an infant is medically fragile and has regulatory disorders, time and care must be taken in handling so the infant can maintain self-regulation. Regulatory disorders can interfere with mother–infant bonding and parental attachment in the infant. In many cases, the child's irritability, behavioral difficulties, and eating and sleeping disorders may impact the functioning of the entire family.

## Contextual Considerations
### Clinical

The child with regulatory disorders may be referred to community- or home-based early intervention programs because of developmental delay and sensory-based behavioral problems. Failure to thrive because of feeding difficulties that have a sensory base may necessitate referral to a medical facility, and behavioral and emotional difficulties may prompt referral to a mental health facility. The diagnosis of regulatory disorders is relatively new, and its root sensory and physiological bases are not readily apparent. The occupational therapist must pay special attention to the presenting symptomatology and referral complaints.

A hypersensitive child may be identified as requiring intervention because of extreme irritability, including poor eating and sleeping routines and delayed motor and/or play and social development. The child may be easily startled, be upset by movement, arch and pull away when held or handled, and react strongly to sounds and noise in the environment. Eating and sleeping are frequently of concern when the infant, disliking the feeling of being held or the oral stimulation of the nipple, may suck briefly but not enough to be satiated. The resultant sensation of hunger may impede the child's ability to fall asleep and stay asleep for predictable periods of time.

A child who is gravitationally insecure and wary of movement may experience gastrointestinal upset when moved and may not move from one position to the next to explore his or her environment. The aversion to movement may result in family members' being concerned and cautious about physical interactions and inadvertently limiting opportunities for movement. The paucity of movement experience fosters tonal abnormalities that hinder motor development. Of equal concern is the underreactive child who may be described as very good and sleeps a great deal but is difficult to engage. This child may not be developing as expected because more than the usual amount of sensorimotor stimulation is required to achieve an alert state. On the other hand, the motorically disorganized child may not appear delayed until he or she is walking and expected to explore his or her environment and manipulate toys or eating utensils in a developmentally appropriate manner.

Evaluation is done primarily through parent and/or caretaker interview, observation, and handling of the child. Assessing responses to touch, movement, and other environmental stimuli is essential. Several published tests, including the *Infant/Toddler Sensory Profile* (Dunn, 2002), the *Test of Sensory Functions in Infants* (DeGangi & Greenspan, 1989), and the *Hawaii Early Learning Profile* and *HELP Strands* (HELP; Furuno, O'Reilly, Hosaka, Zeisloft, & Altman, 1984), can assist in the examination and identification of the sensory bases of behavioral response patterns that emerge.

## Family

The goodness of fit between the caretaker and the child is one of the most important factors affecting positive developmental outcomes. It is important to help family members understand and interpret the child's responses to the sensory environment and learn techniques to help foster self-regulation in the child and provide a sensory diet in the daily environment to enable his or her self-regulation.

## Practice Setting

Since children from birth to age 3 years are expected to have early intervention services provided to them in their natural environments, they are most frequently seen by the occupational therapist at home with their parent or caretaker. They may also be seen in day care centers, medical settings, and mental health centers.

## Sociopolitical

The Individuals With Disabilities Education Act (IDEA, 1997) mandates that children from birth to age 3 years be seen in their natural settings, most typically at home with parents or caretakers, or in day care centers. Early intervention services are coordinated and provided at state and local levels through Interagency Coordinating Councils and the designated lead agency for the state. Depending on the state, this may be the Department of Education or the Department of Human Services. There are federal guidelines with which all states must comply, which emphasize interagency coordination of early identification. Additionally, intervention should be family centered, community based in natural environments, and culturally sensitive. Intervention strategies should be embedded within family routines. Some states may have additional state requirements and regulations and may have adopted specific models for intervention, such as a transdisciplinary model.

According to federal regulations, occupational therapy is considered a primary service for children from birth to age 3 years. It may be the only service provided or one of several services. Other mandated services include service coordination, special instruction, speech and language therapy, physical therapy, nursing, nutrition, and family training (IDEA, 1997). Eligibility for services is determined by (a) the multidisciplinary team that includes the family and (b) the diagnosis and/or percentage of delay in one of the developmental domains, according to results on a standardized measure. Early learning guidelines have been developed in many states and generally address four developmental domains: physical/motor, social/emotional, language/communication, and cognitive/knowledge (Scott-Little, Kagan, Frelow, & Reid, 2009). The Individualized Family Service Plan (IFSP), the legal document for intervention, is guided by the family's goals and priorities. In addition, the federal government mandates that programs under IDEA report progress for children in three outcome areas: (a) social and emotional skills; (b) acquisition of knowledge, including language and communication; and (c) appropriate behavior for meeting their needs (Scott-Little et al., 2009).

## Lifestyle/Lifespan

After the age of 3 years, children are no longer diagnosed as having regulatory disorders. Effective intervention by the parents and professionals may mitigate the disorder, and the child may be developing normally by age 3 years. If the disorder persists into early childhood and adolescence, a variety of diagnoses may be rendered by medical, psychological, or educational personnel, depending on the symptoms and age of the child. These diagnoses include autistic spectrum disorder, attention-deficit/hyperactivity disorder, behavior problems or social skill deficits, psychological diagnosis, and learning disabilities. These diagnoses may have underlying sensory integration or sensory processing problems, and many children respond well to an occupational therapy program based on a sensory integration approach. The literature supports the notion that regulatory disorders and disrupted patterns of attachment in early childhood can contribute to mental health issues, requiring psychotherapy in adulthood (DeGangi, 2000).

Dysfunction in sensory integration and sensory modulation disorders are not presently medical or psychological diagnoses, although awareness regarding the cause, identification, and treatment of these disorders is growing among health and education professionals.

## 🌿 Clinical Decision-Making Process

### Defining Focus for Intervention

The chief complaint of the parent or referral source should be the focus of intervention, but insight into the child's constitutional needs, the interactive patterns between the child and the human and non-human environment, and sensory processing issues is crucial. The most effective intervention strategies are designed by the occupational therapist to be home based and to reflect the values, beliefs, and resources of the family. Interventions are expected to be embedded within the family's routines, such as mealtime, bath time, and community outings. Intervention strategies for other settings, such as hospital or day care settings, will be designed to reflect the institutional mission, programs, and resources but should always include follow-up activities that are relevant to the abilities and needs of the primary caregivers in those settings.

### Establishing Goals for Intervention

The following should be kept in mind when establishing goals for intervention:

- 🌿 Assess the goodness of fit between the child and caregiver by examining the sensory, emotional, and social interaction between the caregiver and the child.
- 🌿 Help the family read and interpret the child's behavior in terms of sensory systems affected, modulation patterns, and self-regulatory ability.
- 🌿 Establish whether the child is hypersensitive or underresponsive to environmental stimuli.

### Designing Theory-Based Intervention

A family-centered intervention based on a sensory integration frame of reference is the most appropriate for addressing regulatory disorders. Sensory integration treatment involves addressing sensory hypersensitivities through a variety of modulating sensory inputs, such as touch pressure and proprioception; enhancing the sensory responsiveness of underreactive children through carefully chosen stimulation; facilitating a calm, alert state through expanding conditions for self-regulation; and enhancing purposeful activity through graded play activities. The child's interest, motivation, and abilities develop in a playful atmosphere that promotes self-direction and mastery. For example, activities such as swaddling and rocking that provide deep pressure touch and graded movement are effective ways to calm a child who is hypersensitive to touch, sound, and movement. Light touch, unpredictable movement, and loud noise should be avoided. Intervention outcomes are enhanced by extending therapy goals and techniques into daily activities and family routines.

## Evaluating Progress

Progress can be tracked by identifying improvements in the child's overall mood and adaptability. With progress, the child is happier; less irritable; more amenable to interaction with family; better able to sustain a calm, alert state; and more engaged in environmental exploration and play behaviors. Behavior and activity charts and family logs can be effective for measuring change.

## Determining Change in or Termination of Treatment

Changing the goals of treatment is warranted when the child appears bored or unmotivated or is not making steady progress toward his or her goals. After self-regulation and a calm, alert state conducive for learning are routinely observed, the child's goals should address developmentally appropriate motor, play, and social skills. Termination of services may be recommended when (a) the multidisciplinary team, using a standardized measure, determines that the child no longer meets the eligibility criteria to warrant services or (b) the child turns 3 years old and is transitioned to another service provider system. Termination of service is appropriate when the child's developmental and behavioral goals have been achieved and environmental supports are such that they continuously foster the child's development. For example, some families intuitively and accurately interpret the child's signals and behaviors and provide ongoing appropriate stimulation through play, self-care, and eating and sleeping routines. Family outings become possible as regulation is achieved, thereby providing additional opportunities for integration of new skills at playgrounds, in playgroups, and with other children.

### Case Study

*Description*

BF was referred at 1 month of age to the early intervention system because of delayed development. She was discharged to home weighing 3.8 pounds, in the third percentile of weight for her age. She was hearing impaired and was irritable most of the time. Any movement or touch exacerbated her irritability. BF would fuss unless she was held against her mother's chest, neck, or stomach. BF ate small amounts of formula at a time and took medication for reflux. Bathing was extremely difficult because BF was very stressed by getting undressed to get in and out of the bath. However, once she was in the bath, it was one of the few times that she seemed to relax.

*Long- and Short-Term Goals*

The long-term goal of intervention for BF is to enable her to increase food intake and gain weight. The short-term goals of intervention for BF are to help her achieve a calm, alert state and foster stress-free parent–infant interaction.

## Therapist Goals and Strategies

The therapist's goals include the following:

1. Reduce BF's negative response to touch and movement.
2. Promote self-regulation.
3. Reduce family stress resulting from care of BF.

The therapist's strategies include the following:

1. Teach parent to read and respond appropriately and effectively to BF's behavioral signals.
2. Encourage deep pressure touch, skin-to-skin contact, and gentle up-and-down movements to reduce negative response to the sensory environment.
3. Limit stimulation to one modality at a time to reduce sensory overload.

## Activity

Encourage holding by the mother, swaddling to reduce hypersensitivity to touch, and gentle up-and-down movements that BF can tolerate. Place BF under a warm baby blanket before dressing and undressing. To reduce agitation, perform an infant massage with warm baby oil under a warm baby blanket.

## Treatment Objectives

1. BF will become increasingly tolerant of touch and movement.
2. BF will be able to tolerate position changes.

# Resources

Earlychildhood.com: www.earlychildhood.com

Family Education (parenting information): www.familyeducation.com

National Association for the Education of Young Children (professional resources): www.naeyc.org

Zero to Three: www.zerotothree.org

# References

DeGangi, G. (2000). *Pediatric disorders of regulation in affect and behavior.* New York, NY: Academic Press.

DeGangi, G. A., & Greenspan, S. I. (1989). *Test of sensory functions in infants.* Los Angeles, CA: Western Psychological Services.

Dunn, W. (2002). *Infant/toddler sensory profile manual.* San Antonio, TX: The Psychological Corporation.

Dunn, W. (2007). The impact of sensory processing abilities on the daily lives of young children and their families: A conceptual model. *Infants and Young Children, 9*(4), 23–25.

Furuno, S., O'Reilly, K., Hosaka, C. M., Zeisloft, B., & Altman, T. (1984). *Hawaii early learning profile.* Palo Alto, CA: VORT.

Individuals With Disabilities Education Act of 1990, 20 U.S.C. § 1400 *et seq.* (1990) (amended 1997).

National Center for Clinical Infant Programs. (1994). *Diagnostic classification 0–3: Diagnostic classification of mental health and developmental disorders of infancy and early childhood.* Arlington, VA: Zero to Three.

Scott-Little, C., Kagan, L., Frelow, V. S., & Reid, J. (2009). Infant and toddler learning guidelines. *Infants and Young Children, 22*(2), 87–99.

Shonkoff, J. P., & Phillips, D. A. (Eds.). (2000). *From neurons to neighborhoods: The science of early childhood development.* Washington, DC: National Academy Press.

Williamson, G. G., & Anzalone, M. E. (2001). *Sensory integration and self-regulation in infants and toddlers: Helping very young children interact with their environment.* Arlington, VA: Zero to Three.

# Autism Spectrum Disorders

*Beth Pfeiffer*

## 🕮 Synopsis of Clinical Condition

According to the fourth edition of the *Diagnostic and Statistical Manual of Mental Disorders–Fourth Edition* (*DSM-IV*; American Psychiatric Association [APA], 1994), pervasive developmental disorders include autism, pervasive developmental disorder—not otherwise specified (PDD-NOS), Asperger's disorder, Rett's disorder, and childhood disintegrative disorder. These disorders have similar diagnostic criteria, but certain characteristics vary and symptoms range from mild to severe. The varying degrees of symptoms have led to the use of the term *autism spectrum disorder* (ASD), which typically describes the three most common conditions—autism, PDD-NOS, and Asperger's disorder—all of which are addressed in this chapter. These three have commonalities in their diagnostic criteria and share many clinical features and interventions.

### Prevalence and Etiology

The Centers for Disease Control and Prevention (2007), after completing a multisite study in the United States, identified ASD prevalence estimates at approximately 1 in 150 children and determined that it is 3 to 4 times more prevalent in boys than in girls. It is now a common developmental childhood condition.

*Comorbidity* is the co-occurrence of conditions that may or may not be causally related (Ghaziuddin, 2002). Individuals with ASD commonly develop comorbid conditions throughout the course of a lifetime. The most common of these are attention-deficit/hyperactivity disorder, obsessive–compulsive disorder, anxiety and mood disorders, tic disorders, seizure disorders, and sleep disorders (Tsai, 2000).

There is no known single cause for ASD, although there are well-documented associations with abnormalities in brain structure or function. Many studies identify neuropathologies in both the temporal lobe and the limbic system (Bauman & Kemper, 1985, 1994). These two systems work together to mediate social–emotional functioning, a primary area of concern for individuals with pervasive developmental disorders. Specifically, abnormalities were found in the size and density of tissue in the temporal lobe and limbic system. The limbic system includes the structures of the amygdala and hippocampus (Lundy-Ekman, 1998), both of which are located in the temporal region. Abnormalities in the amygdala are of particular interest and importance in individuals with ASD. It is strongly believed that the amygdala "plays a critical role in emotional arousal, assigning behavioral significance to environmental stimuli, and attaching emotional relevance to stimuli" (Schultz, Romanski, & Tsatsanis, 2000, p. 187). Social–emotional problems and abnormal responses to environmental stimuli are all characteristics of ASD.

The cortical and subcortical frontal lobe region is also associated with ASD. Two studies have identified decreased frontal lobe perfusion in individuals with autism (George, Costa, Houris, Rang, & Ell, 1992; Zilbovicius et al., 1995). One section of the frontal lobe, the orbital–medial prefrontal cortex (PFC), has a key role in social–emotional functions. This section is interconnected with limbic areas, such as the amygdala. It is speculated that a faulty connection between the amygdala and the orbital–medial PFC could contribute to the inappropriate emotional and social behavior associated with ASD (Schultz et al., 2000).

Research has also explored myelin in the brains of individuals with ASD (Koul, 2005). Results identified that myelin is not fully mature in individuals with ASD. This may have a significant impact on the developing brain and contribute to the abnormalities identified in the brains of individuals with ASD.

It has been theorized that ASD etiologies are genetic and environmental. Recent research has identified that genetic factors increase the risk of ASD (Glessner et al., 2009; Ma, 2009; Wang et al., 2009). These studies revealed that there are many genes that contribute to an increased risk and that the interaction of genes and environmental factors is often the cause of ASD. Research has indicated that ASD aggregates in families. There is an extremely high rate of concordance of ASD in identical versus fraternal twins and a higher rate of siblings with the condition (Miller-Kuhaneck & Glennon, 2001). Chromosomal studies have identified further support for genetic links. Chromosomal alterations are present in a fairly large number of individuals with ASD, although the alterations are not consistent. More recent research (Glessner et al., 2009; Ma, 2009; Wang et al., 2009) has identified variants of genes involved in cell adhesion in individuals with ASD. The National Institutes of Health (2009) stated that "in the developing brain, cell adhesion proteins enable neurons to migrate to the correct places and to connect with other neurons" (para. 11). This connects genetic factors to abnormal brain structures and development identified in ASD.

There have been various speculations about the environmental etiology of ASD, and further research is warranted. Some believe that prenatal exposure to toxins—in particular, pesticides and polychlorinated biphenyls—is the cause of abnormal brain development in children with ASD. Researchers have explored the possibility that an abnormal immune system response to vaccinations leads to the regression in skills that children with autism and PDD-NOS often present with around ages 2 to 3 years (Miller-Kuhaneck & Glennon, 2001), and viruses have been researched as a possible etiology. Initial animal models of virus-induced autism have been supported (Pletnikov & Carbone, 2005), although further research is needed.

Autoimmune disorders are more common in the family members of children who have ASD (Comi, Zimmerman, Frye, Law, & Peedan, 1999), and there are documented autoimmune abnormalities in certain individuals with ASD (Miller-Kuhaneck & Glennon, 2001). Gastrointestinal issues were suspected in many individuals with ASD, although research has not identified an increased prevalence when compared to neurotypical populations (Fombonne & Chakrabarti, 2001; Taylor et al., 2002). Much of the research in these areas is inconclusive, and therefore the etiologies of ASD continue to be speculative in nature. Based on the current research, it is thought that ASD is a complex disorder with multiple interactive etiologies, including both genetic and environmental factors.

## Common Characteristics and Symptoms

For a child to be diagnosed with autism, he or she must present with delays in social interactions, social communications, or symbolic or pretend play prior to 3 years of age. The child must meet a total of six or more items from three main areas in the *DSM-IV*, with at least two from Category 1 and one each from Categories 2 and 3 (APA, 1994). The three main areas include a qualitative impairment in social interactions; a qualitative impairment in communication; and restricted, repetitive, or stereotyped patterns of behavior, interests, and activities.

Qualitative impairments in social interactions include impairments in the use of nonverbal behaviors, limitations in peer relationships, a lack of social or emotional reciprocity, and a lack of spontaneous initiative to share enjoyment, interests, or achievements with others. Qualitative impairment in communication includes a delay or lack of development of spoken language, impairment in the ability to initiate or sustain conversations with others (for those that do speak), stereotyped and repetitive use of language, and limitations in pretend or social imitative play for their age. Restricted, repetitive, or stereotyped patterns of behavior include a restricted interest of abnormal intensity and focus (preoccupation), inflexibility in certain rituals or routines, motor patterns that are stereotypical or repetitive, and a preoccupation with parts of objects.

For a child to meet the criteria for PDD-NOS, certain criteria for autism must be met, but not the full criteria (APA, 1994). These children have features of autism that are not due to other disorders. Asperger's disorder also has many features of high-functioning autism disorder, but such children differ in cognitive and language functions. An individual with Asperger's disorder has average to above-average cognitive abilities and often develops expressive language within normal developmental ranges (Attwood, 1998). Social interactions and functioning are significantly impaired in all three disorders. There is ongoing controversy in diagnosing ASD because of the overlap and the high rate of comorbidity with other childhood conditions. Professionals have recently expanded the terminology to include the term *autism phenotype*, which identifies a group of individuals who have characteristics that are nontypical in the areas of personality, language, and social skills but who do not meet the criteria for ASD. Research has identified that family members of individuals with ASD are more likely to have characteristics of these broader autism phenotypes (Piven, Palmer, Jacobi, Childress, & Arndt, 1997).

A child with an ASD may or may not have verbal language delays, but nonverbal language delays are almost always present (Attwood, 1998). Individuals with autism or PDD-NOS frequently experience delays in expressive language development, although this characteristic is absent in Asperger's disorder. Social development does occur but is often qualitatively different. Deficits in communication contribute to delays in social development. Eye contact and responsiveness to another person may be decreased, as well as an understanding of the pragmatic aspects of communication (i.e., the practical ability to use language in social situations). Children with ASD have a decreased interest in interacting with others and prefer isolated activities. They often have a limited range of representational play activities, along with restricted interests (Miller-Kuhaneck & Glennon, 2001). For example, they may be resistant to change and insist on certain routines and rituals. They may also engage in stereotypical or self-stimulatory behaviors.

Although it has been estimated that 75% of individuals with autism demonstrate some level of intellectual disability (Huebner & Dunn, 2001), it is likely that this estimate is extremely high. Intelligence often differentiates autism and Asperger's disorder, as there are no cognitive deficits associated with Asperger's disorder. As individuals with autism have difficulty completing standardized IQ measures because of characteristics not related to intelligence, the results of many of these tools may be questionable and therefore misrepresent the true intellect of the person.

Although not yet part of the diagnostic criteria for ASD according to the *DSM-IV*, sensory processing and integration issues are common (Mayes & Calhoun, 1999; Ornitz, 1974). Kientz and Dunn (1997) compared the sensory processing of children with autism to that of children without autism and identified significant differences in their patterns of processing sensory information. The children with autism demonstrated significant tactile sensitivity compared with the control group. Other researchers have also supported these findings. In one study, as many as 70% of children diagnosed with pervasive developmental disorders demonstrated disturbances in sensory modulation (Ornitz, 1974). Another study showed that 100% of children diagnosed with pervasive developmental disorders demonstrated somatosensory (tactile, vestibular, and proprioceptive) disturbances and 50% demonstrated hyper- or hyposensitivity to sensory input (Mayes & Calhoun, 1999).

Motor problems vary in individuals with ASD. Clumsiness and incoordination are identified as common characteristics in individuals with Asperger's disorder (Volkmar et al., 1994), and issues in motor planning can be found across the autism spectrum. It is important to note that characteristics and degree of symptoms can vary significantly among individuals.

## Target Areas for Intervention

The role of an occupational therapist working with an individual with ASD varies depending on contextual factors such as age, intervention setting, and the primary reason for referral. Pervasive developmental disorders suggest multiple areas of focus. Over the course of a person's lifetime, an occupational therapist may focus interventions on almost all areas of occupation, including activities of daily living, instrumental activities of daily living, education, work, play, leisure, and social participation. For the person with ASD, treatment interventions may focus on sensory processing and integration, sensorimotor function, and social–emotional development.

One of the interventions most widely used by occupational therapists in the treatment of ASD is sensory integration (Watling, Deitz, Kanny, & McLaughlin, 1999). Used in combination with other interventions, including behavioral and developmental approaches, a primary focus is frequently on the modulation of sensory input, as many individuals with ASD tend to under- or overrespond to sensory input or demonstrate a mixed reactivity. This, in turn, affects behavior, communication, and functional skills. Other areas of specific occupational therapy interventions include improving the motor planning necessary for play and daily living activities, as well as interventions focused on promoting social skills.

## ◖ Contextual Considerations

### Clinical

Autism spectrum disorders are pervasive developmental disorders that frequently affect many areas of functioning. To clarify/identify the diagnosis, the *Pervasive Developmental Disorders Screening Test–Second Edition* (PDDST-II; Siegel, 2004) can be useful. An evaluation must address the primary concerns of the referral source and the family and could include many domains of occupational therapy practice. A top-down evaluation process promotes occupationally based interventions. Using this approach, evaluation must initially collect information on the occupational profile of the individual through interviews and observations (Fisher, 1998). Along with identifying relevant and meaningful occupations, this involves collecting information about the individual's or family's concerns, problems, and priorities. Observing the individual engaging in targeted occupations is important for identifying the discrepancies between the demands of the task and the skills of the individual. After identifying the primary problems and priorities, the next stage involves using assessment tools that focus more specifically on areas of occupation, performance skills, and client factors. Pervasive developmental disorders affect many areas of function, and there are a variety of assessment tools that are appropriate for individuals with ASD. Because many individuals are not able to complete standardized assessments, caregiver interviews or questionnaires and clinical observation are sometimes the most appropriate assessment measures for people with ASD. A number of individuals with ASD can complete more formalized assessment procedures, and therefore both kinds are discussed.

Adaptive behavior measures provide a method for evaluating many areas of occupational function. Frequently, the general areas of social, self-help, motor, and communication skills are assessed. The *Vineland Adaptive Behavior Scales–Second Edition* (Sparrow, Cicchetti, & Balla, 2005) specifically measures the areas of communication, daily living skills, socialization, motor skills, and maladaptive behaviors. It is appropriate for use with individuals from birth to 18 years 11 months and for low-functioning adults. There are norms based on all of these age groups. The scales are completed through an interview with the parent or caregiver.

The *Adaptive Behavior Assessment System–Second Edition* (ABAS-II; Harrison & Oakland, 2003) uses a rating form to assess the areas of communication, community use, functional academics, school living, health and safety, leisure, self-care, self-direction, social skills, and work. There are parent, teacher, and adult versions of the ABAS-II. Caregivers or the adults themselves can complete the adult rating scale. It is a norm-referenced test for individuals from school age through adulthood. Adaptive behaviors are highly correlated with cognitive deficits, although these scales also provide important information regarding the function of individuals with ASD who do not have cognitive deficits.

General developmental scales, such as the *Hawaii Early Learning Profile* (Furuno, O'Reilly, Hosaka, Zeisloft, & Allman, 1984) and the *Early Learning Accomplishment Profile* (Glover, Preminger, & Sanford, 1988), are helpful in assessing overall development in young children from birth to 5 years of age. These types of general developmental scales are often used to determine eligibility for early intervention services and can be completed through observation and parent/caregiver interview.

There are documented differences in play in children with ASD. Restricted representation play is a common characteristic of ASD. As play is the main occupation of preschool children, the *Revised Knox Preschool Play Scale* (Knox, 1997) provides an observational measure assessing space and material management, pretense/symbolic aspects of play, and participation in play. This is a tool that has a history of use with preschool children diagnosed with ASD.

If a child is referred for a school-based assessment, the *School Function Assessment* (SFA; Coster, Deeney, Haltiwanger, & Haley, 1998) can guide intervention planning for children with ASD who are in elementary school. The SFA has three main parts assessing participation in school-related settings, the task supports needed for participation, and activity performance. Activity performance has 21 separate scales measuring a variety of functions necessary for optimal school performance. These include functional communication, written work, clothing management, school travel, and behavioral regulation, to name only a few. This is a questionnaire that can be completed in sections, by one individual who is familiar with the child or by a team of professionals.

Social–emotional measures are particularly relevant to the ASD population because of the nature of the condition. The *Functional Emotional Assessment Scale* (Greenspan, DeGangi, & Wieder, 1996) is an observation assessment looking at the infant's or young child's social–emotional functioning with parents or caregivers. It also provides information on the related motor, sensory, language, and cognitive capabilities.

The *Social Responsiveness Scale* (Constantino & Gruber, 2005) is a rating scale completed by a parent or caregiver for children between the ages of 4 and 18 years. It measures social impairments, including the components of social awareness, social information processing, capacity for social communication, social anxiety/avoidance, and autism preoccupations and traits. It was specifically developed for use in assessment of children with ASD.

Dysfunction in sensory processing and integration is prevalent in individuals with ASD. Some of the most helpful tools for providing insight into sensory processing in relationship to everyday functioning and behavior are the *Infant/Toddler Sensory Profile* (Dunn, 2002), the *Sensory Profile* (Dunn, 1999), the *Sensory Profile School Companion* (Dunn, 2006), and the *Adolescent/Adult Sensory Profile* (Brown & Dunn, 2002). These four profiles cover the ages from birth to adulthood and a variety of settings, including home, school, and community. For each profile, with the exception of the *Adolescent/Adult Sensory Profile,* the caregiver, parent, or teacher completes standardized questionnaires. For the *Adolescent/Adult Sensory Profile,* the individual completes the questionnaire, unless he or she is unable to do so, in which case a caregiver can do so.

The *Sensory Processing Measure* is a rating scale that assesses sensory processing issues, praxis, and social participation in children from the ages of 5 to 12 years (Parham & Ecker, 2007). There is a Home Form, completed by the parents, and a Main Classroom and School Environments Form, completed by school personnel.

The *Test of Sensory Function in Infants* (TSFI; DeGangi & Greenspan, 1981), the *DeGangi–Berk Test of Sensory Integration* (TSI; Berk & DeGangi, 1983), and the *Sensory Integration and Praxis Test* (SIPT; Ayres, 1989) are all standardized tests assessing sensory integration. These require the child to participate in more formal testing procedures. The TSFI is a criterion-referenced rating scale intended to be a screening tool for sensory integration dysfunction in infants between 4 and 18 months of age. The TSI is a norm-referenced test designed to assess sensory integration dysfunction in preschoolers. The SIPT is a battery of

17 tests specifically assessing sensory integration and praxis for children between the ages of 4 years and 8 years 11 months. Administration and interpretation of the SIPT requires specialized training and certification.

The *Peabody Developmental Motor Scales–Second Edition* (PDMS-2; Folio & Fewell, 2000) and the *Bruininks–Oseretsky Test of Motor Proficiency–Second Edition* (Bruininks & Bruininks, 2005) are helpful tools for assessing overall motor function. The *Quick Neurological Screening Test–Second Edition* (Mutti, Martin, Sterling, & Spalding, 1998) assesses certain motor and perceptual functions related to neurological integration.

The *Developmental Test of Visual Perception–Second Edition* (Hammill, Pearson, & Voress, 1993) and the *Beery–Buktenica Developmental Test of Visual–Motor Integration–Sixth Edition* (Beery, Buktenica, & Beery, 2010) may also help identify underlying performance deficits in the areas of visual–motor and perceptual skills. Finally, clinical observations are an essential part of the evaluation process.

## Family

Intervention strategies for the child need to be supplemented with ongoing family education. Parents, siblings, and caregivers require information regarding the nature of the child's conditions, the ramifications of the condition on functional behavior, the scope and purpose of occupational therapy, and other components of the intervention program. They also require guidance regarding additional supportive services and resources that are available in the local community (Galvin, 2001). This could include referrals for other services, including speech and language therapy, physical therapy, psychologists, developmental pediatricians, nutritionists, and neurologists. ASD support groups frequently meet in community settings and serve as both a support system and a place for families to acquire knowledge.

Collaboration with a multidisciplinary team that includes families is essential for the most effective interventions. Recent law and policies promote the involvement of the parents in the intervention process. For example, laws guiding early intervention services mandate family-focused interventions. Due in part to these laws, parents are becoming more educated in the service delivery systems and often serve as advocates for their children. Being provided resources and education allows parents to be more successful advocates. With education, families can also implement important interventions in the context of the home and community settings. For example, a child with a sensory processing dysfunction often benefits from a sensory diet implemented into daily routines. Education is essential in helping the family successfully integrate and modify these interventions.

As mentioned previously, many children with ASD are unable to attend or participate fully in formalized assessment procedures; therefore, families serve as important informants for their children. Inclusion of the family in all evaluation procedures encourages an understanding of the family's priorities, culture, and dynamics, along with the development of viable and relevant intervention plans.

## Practice Setting

Individuals with ASD can receive occupational therapy services in a variety of settings, including early intervention services in the home or community, schools, outpatient rehabilitation or private practice facilities, and community living centers or adult day programs. They may receive services in more than one setting at a time.

Early intervention services are for children primarily between the ages of birth through 5 years. Children who qualify for occupational therapy from birth through age 3 years typically receive these services in their homes or in community settings, such as day care centers. The occupational therapist's role is to provide family-focused intervention, which often involves family education. Occupational therapy is considered a primary service for children from birth to 3 years and is most commonly provided directly and individually. In many states, intervention funding switches to the school system when a child turns 3 years old. Typically, a child will enter into a preschool program. The family continues to be an important component of the service delivery process, which focuses on the development of school readiness skills and the facilitation of school participation. Direct services can be provided individually or within a group setting. Consultation may also be provided to the classroom teacher or other professional working with the child. Typically, the treatment of ASD is guided by a developmental model focused on sensorimotor development, play skills, social–emotional development, and self-help skills.

School-based occupational therapy is one of the largest practice areas in the profession. Many children and adolescents with ASD will receive occupational therapy services in the school system in order to support successful performance and participation. Services can be provided in varying forms, including consultation, monitoring, and direct intervention, both in groups and individually. The occupational therapist, in consultation with other professionals, such as teachers, physical therapists, and speech therapists, may provide suggestions on how to improve a child's writing, attention span, and/or social skills.

Children and adults with ASD can receive private therapy through outpatient pediatric rehabilitation facilities or private practice therapy clinics. Certain clinics may specialize in an area of practice, such as providing sensory integration therapy specifically for individuals with ASD. Adults with ASD sometimes receive services within community living centers or adult day programs. These services often focus on helping the individual develop the ability to modulate and regulate sensory input, in order to improve attention and decrease secondary behaviors, and engage successfully in self-maintenance and vocational training.

## Sociopolitical

Legislation significantly influences intervention funding for children with ASD. The Individuals With Disabilities Education Improvement Act (IDEIA; 2004) is probably the most influential legislation regarding the provision of services for children and adolescents with ASD. Part C of IDEIA defines services for children between the ages of birth and 2 years 11 months. Part B defines services for children and adolescents in special education from 3 to 21 years of age (U.S. Department of Education, 2009). Part B of IDEIA stipulates that a child must fall under one of the categories of disability identified in IDEIA. Autism is included as a category of disability.

The legislation further identifies services as either *primary* or *related*. A service that is considered primary may be provided in the absence of other services. Occupational therapy is a primary service under Part C of IDEIA, but it is a related service under Part B. In the latter case, the child must be receiving special education with an Individualized Education Program (IEP) in order to be eligible for occupational therapy. Funding is provided from both federal and state governments in order to implement programs under IDEA and IDEIA. IDEA was reauthorized and renamed the Individuals With Disabilities Educational Improvement Act, and the changes enable schools to help students make progress in the general education curriculum. One of the most significant additions to the act was "Response to Intervention," which influences both assessment and how interventions are provided in school settings. Response to Intervention (RTI) allows schools to identify students at risk for failing and provide learning support through monitoring progress, providing science-based interventions, and adjusting the intensity and nature of intervention depending on the student's needs and response to the intervention. Occupational therapists are legally required to implement evidence-based practice and document the progress of the students we treat.

Other legislation influencing the provision of services for individuals with ASD includes the Rehabilitation Act of 1973 (revised 1986) and the Americans With Disabilities Act of 1990. The Rehabilitation Act requires reasonable accommodations to be made in schools so that the needs of individuals with disabilities can be met as adequately as those of individuals without disabilities (de-Bettencourt, 2003). Children with ASD who do not qualify for services under the Individuals With Disabilities Education Act (IDEA) can sometimes qualify for occupational therapy services under Section 504 of the Rehabilitation Act. Under this law, a child does not need to receive special education services to qualify for occupational therapy.

Funding for outpatient rehabilitation or services conducted in private practice settings often comes from family resources or medical insurance. Certain medical insurance providers identify ASD as a developmental disorder and thus will not cover occupational therapy interventions for it. Although this is not the case for all medical insurance, education continues to be necessary when working with insurance providers concerning the roles and scope of occupational therapy. Some states have recently approved legislation requiring that insurance companies cover occupational therapy services for children with ASD.

## Lifestyle/Lifespan

ASD is considered a lifelong condition, but intensive services provided in childhood and adolescence appear to have resulted in a large population of individuals with ASD integrating into their communities and living productive and functional lives (Howlin, 2000). Occupational therapists are often involved in the development of programs that assist the transition of a child with ASD from early intervention to school and, finally, to the world of work. Transitions can be particularly challenging for both the child and the family, and consistent professional support and ongoing education is paramount. As the child progresses from early intervention settings to adulthood, the focus of service and intervention changes from the home or community environment to a school and community environment. It also often changes from direct and individual treatment to primarily indirect or group treatment.

The role of the occupational therapist is to prepare and educate the family and the child and to promote the skills necessary for optimal performance when making the transition into each setting. For instance, parental separation issues may emerge as the child moves from early intervention to preschool, while the move to elementary school requires a transition from a part-time to a full-time program. Another major school transition is into the junior high or high school environment, where the student may be expected to function more independently and often with less structure. Preparations for transitions from the school setting to adult life in the community start as early as elementary school, in terms of preparation for future adult roles. For example, a focus on independent daily living activities provides an individual with ASD a foundation for participation in future adult roles. Encouraging families to have children participate in household chores and take on other responsibilities is important for future transitions (Miller-Kuhaneck & Glennon, 2001).

IDEIA requires that the IEP address formal postschool transition planning, which must begin when the child turns 16 years old and must be readdressed annually and include goals addressing transition based on transition assessments. These often include goals focused specifically on life after high school and services required in the transitional process. The student, along with professionals and the family, is involved in setting goals and identifying priorities. Community involvement, social skills, behavioral concerns, and vocational skills are often the primary focus of occupational therapy in the high school years. Occupational therapy interventions may continue into adulthood, addressing similar issues in order to further promote independence.

Along with transition planning, it is important to understand family dynamics and supports across the lifespan of the individual. For instance, the sibling of a child with ASD may face certain challenges. Families may have difficulty managing the balance of care between the child with ASD and his or her siblings. In certain communities, support groups are available for siblings of children with disabilities or, more specifically, with ASD. Obtaining necessary services and resources for a child with ASD can inflict financial stress on the family.

Along with occupational therapy, individuals with ASD may benefit from speech and language therapy, physical therapy, special education, psychological services, behavioral interventions, and dietary interventions. Interventions often involve complementary approaches. A list of alternative and complementary approaches (Lerner, 2001) is identified in Table 4.1. Some of these approaches are considered controversial because limited research has been conducted, while others are supported by solid effectiveness research.

## 🦋 Clinical Decision-Making Process

### Defining Focus for Intervention

The focus for home-based treatment may include promoting optimal interactions with family members, modulating responses to sensory stimulation, and fostering developmentally appropriate skills. For example, treatment interventions may focus on correcting feeding and eating issues related to oral hypersensitivity or decreasing self-stimulatory behaviors interfering with play and interactions. In the school environment, treatment interventions might focus on the development of social skills for peer interaction and sensorimotor skills for computer usage, handwriting, and physical education.

In adolescence and adulthood, treatment interventions often focus on promoting independence in activities of daily living, vocational skills, and the social skills necessary to live in the community. In general, treatment interventions can vary greatly and must be determined by individual needs, family priorities, and cultural beliefs. As pervasive developmental disorders occur on a spectrum, children can vary greatly in their individual needs.

### Establishing Goals for Intervention

Goals are established based on the results of the evaluation and the reason for referral. It is also important to consider the priorities of the individual and the family. Including the individual and the family in the goal-writing process can promote successful outcomes. The service delivery model has a significant impact on the goal-writing process. Goals for a child receiving services through early intervention are developed by the family or caregivers during the Individualized Family Service Plan meeting. The parents or caregivers identify the goals toward which they would like to see the child work, and these are documented in the exact language presented. The role of the occupational therapist in this process

**Table 4.1** Common and Alternative Treatment Interventions for Individuals
With Autism Spectrum Disorders

| Intervention | Types or methods |
|---|---|
| Structural therapy | Osteopathy<br>Cranial-sacral therapy<br>Chiropractic |
| Treatments to boost immune system | Dietary modifications<br>  Feingold diet<br>  Gluten- and casein-free diet<br>  Yeast-decreasing diet<br>Nutritional supplements<br>  Vitamins and minerals<br>  Amino acids<br>  Essential fatty acids<br>  Probiotics and antifungals<br>Immunotherapy<br>  Intravenous immune globulin therapy<br>  (often used when children have high titers<br>  believed to be related to vaccines)<br>Secretin |
| Treatments addressing sensory processing | Sensory integration<br>Vision therapy<br>Auditory integration training |
| Facilitated communication | A facilitator provides physical support to the hand, arm, or wrist while the child or adolescent points to a picture or letter or types |
| Medication | Psychostimulants<br>Antidepressants<br>Hypertensives<br>Anticonvulsants<br>Antipsychotics |
| Applied behavioral analysis/discrete trial training | Repetitive teaching trials based on providing a stimulus and reinforcing the response; structured curriculum of skill-based tasks |
| Floortime/Development, Individual and Relationship-Based (DIR) intervention | Focused on affective and relationship-based interventions to address social, communication, cognitive, play, sensory, and motor planning issues |
| Miller method | Teaches communication and cognition while focusing on physical organization |
| Treatment and Education of Autistic and Related Communication Handicapped Children (TEACCH) | Structured teaching approach focused on provision of environmental modifications, concrete visual presentation of information, and use of routine |

is to educate the family in goal development and to identify strategies and objectives that support the goals identified by the family. In contrast, goals established in the school setting are developed by the occupational therapist with input from the family and educational professionals. These goals need to be measurable and relate to school performance.

ASD can affect many areas of functioning, including social skills, communication, motor skills, cognition, sensory processing, and activities of daily living. These may all be areas of concern identified during the evaluation process, but the goal-writing process needs to focus on the most significant areas of concern, and goals may have to be prioritized. Sociopolitical factors such as funding sources also impact the goal-writing process. For example, insurance companies may require that goals be written in a specific format and that they address only those areas relevant to medical intervention, such as activities of daily living or motor skills. However, all goals should be functional and promote participation in the occupation and roles of the individual.

## Designing Theory-Based Intervention

In general, multiple theoretical frameworks are used to guide intervention planning. The developmental theory is particularly applicable to this population. It is based on the premise that individuals develop certain life skills in both a parallel and sequential fashion that promotes adaptive functioning (Walker & Ludwig, 2004). For example, children simultaneously develop motor and cognitive skills but learn to sit before they learn to walk. ASD can delay the development of skills in many areas, including psychosocial, cognitive, language, motor, sensory processing, and daily living. Using developmental theory to inform treatment, an occupational therapist might structure situations that require parallel play and progress to more active interaction with peers.

Sensory integration theory is also widely used to design interventions for individuals with ASD. It is well documented that individuals with ASD are more likely to experience dysfunctions in sensory integration and modulation (Kientz & Dunn, 1997; Mayes & Calhoun, 1999; Ornitz, 1974). This theory is based on the assumption that meaningful registration of sensory input must occur for an individual to make an adaptive response. Another assumption is that the brain has plasticity and, therefore, intervention can change the way the brain responds to sensory input. Dysfunction in sensory integration and modulation is manifested in hypersensitivity to touch and/or sound, avoidance behaviors, sensory-seeking activities such as self-stimulation or self-injurious behaviors, attention disorders, and an inability to make effective adaptive responses. Modulation of sensory responses through structured sensory motor experiences is often the focus of intervention.

The acquisitional frame of reference is used to teach functional skills. It assumes that the learning of functional skills is based on reinforcement (Royeen & Duncan, 1999). Another assumption is that learning a skill results in the belief that one has competence and can influence the environment. This approach is often used in skill-based learning programs and in programs designed to modify behavior. Applied behavioral analysis and discrete trial training are popular approaches with this population.

The psychosocial frame of reference has its theoretical base in developmental theories related to temperament, attachment, social skills, play, and coping abilities (Olson, 1999). It focuses on peer and family interactions. By addressing and understanding those areas (e.g., temperamental qualities, attachment relationships, interactional patterns, play skills), intervention focuses on promoting optimal interactions between peers and family members. One example is the developmental, individual difference, and relationship-based (DIR) model. This is particularly relevant to the ASD population, as communication and social abilities are frequently areas of concern.

## Evaluating Progress

Observations and interviews are very important aspects of identifying progress in individuals with ASD. In some instances, progress cannot be measured by more formal assessment procedures but can only be observed or identified by caregivers. For example, after treating an individual with ASD for sensory modulation dysfunction, there may be changes in flexibility and less need for control. Such changes involve the overall quality of life and are not typically addressed in formal assessment procedures.

Documenting progress and, essentially, the effectiveness of interventions is not only ethical but also a legal requirement by some of the largest funding sources for occupational therapy. The IDEIA of 2004 requires practitioners to document the effectiveness of interventions and adjust interventions accordingly. As standardized assessments are often difficult to administer validly to many children with ASD, measurable goals are essential. Goal attainment scaling (GAS) is a method that can be very helpful in the reassessment process and in identifying progress for children with ASD. In GAS, individualized goals are established for the child in collaboration with either the parents or a professional who knows the child well. Each goal is then graded as *below expectations*, *expected level of achievement*, or *above expectations* and provided a number from −2 to +2. Total scores can be converted into a standard score to determine progress. GAS is able to depict functional and meaningful outcomes that are often challenging to assess using standardized measures (Mailloux et al., 2007).

Evaluation of progress is ongoing and based on established goals and the treatment plan. In most practice settings, anecdotal records are kept along with more formal documentation methods. For example, 3-, 6-, and 9-month progress notes are often required, as are formal annual reviews, for the early intervention population. The service delivery model (along with funding sources) determines the specific guidelines for documenting progress.

## Determining Change in or Termination of Treatment

Change in treatment is warranted if the primary concerns for the individual have deviated, if there is minimal progress toward goals, or if goals have been achieved.

For example, a transition to a community living arrangement may signal the achievement of goals for self-care independence but may also signal the need for new goals, such as the use of public transportation.

Termination of treatment occurs when the individual has met his or her goals or if there has been a plateau of progress over time. It is also important to identify when there is a plateau in progress and reevaluate whether changes in intervention strategies or a continuation of occupational therapy services are warranted. At this point, a referral to other professionals for alternate interventions may be appropriate. Once again, both the service delivery model and the funding sources help to determine termination or changes. For example, a family may need to discontinue services after 30 treatment sessions if that is all that is covered by the insurance company.

## Case Study

### Description

JT is a 4-year-old boy who has been diagnosed with PDD-NOS. He lives with his mother, an older sister, and a younger brother. For half a day 5 days a week, JT attends a special education program, where he receives 1 hour of speech therapy a week in the classroom setting. He received occupational therapy in his home at the age of 2 years through an early intervention program but no longer qualified when he turned 3 years old and transitioned into a preschool setting. JT's teacher is concerned with JT's unusual responses to sensory activities and his delayed play and motor skills, and she recently referred him for an occupational therapy evaluation. She reported that he also has a difficult time attending to sit-down group activities. JT was evaluated through clinical and classroom observations and interviews with his mother and classroom teacher. He also completed the PDMS-2.

JT does not like to be touched by other people and will often pull away when someone attempts to touch him. He prefers to play by himself away from the other children during free-play time and engages in limited reciprocal play. JT frequently cries during messy play and insists on washing his hands immediately. During snack time, he will only eat crunchy or chewy foods and avoids all foods that have soft textures or varying consistencies. JT's mother reported that he has a very limited food repertoire at home and that he is extremely fussy during grooming tasks, such as brushing his teeth and hair. He refuses to have his hair cut by anyone other than his mother. JT is easily distracted by sensory stimuli in the environment and often is unable to attend for more than a few minutes during group activities because of sensory distractions. Sensory defensiveness appears to be influencing JT's ability to participate fully in his classroom setting.

Along with this, motor planning difficulties appear to further impact JT's play skills. He engages in very little symbolic play with other children and tends to use the same play schemes with most of his toys. JT will imitate a simple symbolic play scheme when one is introduced by an adult, but he does not come up with these schemes on his own. He prefers to stack or line up objects. Motor planning deficits also impact JT's overall motor skills. On the PDMS-2, JT performed fine motor skills in the 25th percentile and gross motor skills in the 30th percentile for his age range.

## Long- and Short-Term Goals

The long-term goal of intervention for JT is to help him participate in classroom activities with other children for the designated activity time. The short-term goals of intervention for JT are as follows:

1. Attend to group activities in the classroom setting 80% of the time.
2. Initiate and participate in reciprocal play activities with other children in the classroom during 70% of the free-play time.
3. Expand play skills in order to sequence five or more ideas during symbolic play.
4. Eat and enjoy a variety of foods with varying textures during snack time 80% of the time.

## Therapist Goals and Strategies

The therapist's goals include the following:

1. Decrease JT's sensory defensiveness.
2. Increase JT's body awareness for motor planning.
3. Educate the family and professionals on techniques to expand play skills.

The therapist's strategies include the following:

1. Engage in activities that provide calming and inhibitory sensory input, including deep pressure, proprioception, and slow linear vestibular sensory input to decrease hypersensitivity.
2. Provide home instruction and classroom in-service on floortime techniques to foster reciprocal and symbolic play skills.
3. Engage in activities that provide proprioceptive and vestibular feedback to increase the body awareness necessary for motor planning.
4. Provide consultation on classroom modifications in order to decrease extraneous sensory stimuli.
5. Provide opportunities for play time initially with one other child in a safe and structured format and then in less structured play settings.
6. Model appropriate play schemes.
7. Implement an oral sensory-stimulation program.

## Activity

JT will choose activities to complete in an obstacle course during free-play time. The choices will include equipment that provides deep pressure tactile, proprioceptive, or inhibitory vestibular sensory input. He will then help set up the course, to expand motor planning schemes and participate in the obstacle course on his own. Eventually, he will be asked to choose a doll or toy to maneuver through the course with him, to expand pretend and symbolic play schemes with objects such as a doll, a stuffed animal, or a toy car/truck. He will also choose one other child to participate in the obstacle course with him and then expand this to a group of children. Suggestions will be made to parents and teachers on games that can be carried out at home and school, as well as toys that foster symbolic and reciprocal play.

This activity was chosen because it addresses multiple areas of needs and allows for the integration of other children into the activity when appropriate. JT's involvement in the development and choice of equipment to be included fosters ideational and motor planning aspects of praxis. The equipment and toys that are available for the obstacle course all provide some form of enhanced tactile, proprioceptive, and/or vestibular sensory input to decrease sensory hypersensitivity and increase body awareness, which is necessary for improved motor planning. Symbolic toys are incorporated into the activity to provide opportunities to model pretend play and for JT to practice the modeled play. The modeling can be done by either the therapist or another child involved in the activity. Throughout the session, the therapist can grade and adapt the activity to promote a challenge that will enhance praxis while allowing the child to be successful. Including other children in the play activity will provide opportunities for JT to expand his social skills with support as needed. As with any skill, if it is not practiced and generalized, participation across settings is limited. Therefore, it is essential to provide suggestions to the teachers and parents on what interventions would benefit JT across settings for enhanced occupational performance and participation in the home, school, and community settings.

### Treatment Objectives

1. JT will complete four new motor schemes with minimal assistance as needed.
2. JT will participate in symbolic play, requiring the sequence of at least two new play schemes.
3. JT will interact with at least one other child to successfully guide that child through the obstacle course he developed.

# Resources

## Internet Resources

The National Autism Association: www.nationalautismassociation.org

Autism Society: www.autism-society.org

## Print Resources

Huebner, R. A. (2001). *Autism: A sensorimotor approach to management.* Gaithersburg, MD: Aspen.

Miller-Kuhaneck, H., & Watling, R. (Eds.). (2010). *Autism: A comprehensive occupational therapy approach* (3rd ed.). Bethesda, MD: American Occupational Therapy Association.

Murray-Slutsky, C., & Paris, B. A. (2000). *Exploring the spectrum of autism and pervasive developmental disorders: Intervention strategies.* San Antonio, TX: Therapy Skill Builders.

Myles, B. S., Cook, K. T., Miller, N. E., Rinner, L., & Robbins L. A. (2001). *Asperger syndrome and sensory issues: Practical solutions for making sense of the world.* Shawnee Mission, KS: Autism Asperger Publishing Co.

Sicile-Kira, C. (2004). *Autism spectrum disorders: The complete guide to understanding autism, Asperger's syndrome, pervasive developmental disorder, and other ASDs.* New York, NY: Perigee.

# References

American Psychiatric Association. (1994). *Diagnostic and statistical manual of mental disorders* (4th ed.). Washington, DC: Author.

Americans With Disabilities Act of 1990, 42 U.S.C § 12101 *et seq.* (1990).

Attwood, T. (1998). *Asperger syndrome: A guide for parents and professionals.* London, England: Jessica Kingsley Publishers.

Ayres, A. J. (1989). *Sensory integration and praxis test.* Los Angeles, CA: Western Psychological Services.

Bauman, M. L., & Kemper, T. L. (1985). Neuroanatomic observations of the brain in early infantile autism. *Neurology, 35,* 866–874.

Bauman, M. L., & Kemper, T. L. (1994). Neuroanatomic observations of the brain in autism. In M. L. Bauman & T. L. Kemper (Eds.), *The neurobiology of autism* (pp. 119–145). Baltimore, MD: Johns Hopkins University Press.

Beery, K. E., Buktenica, N. A., & Beery, N. A. (2010). *Beery–Buktenica developmental test of visual–motor integration* (6th ed.). San Antonio, TX: Pearson Assessments.

Berk, R., & DeGangi, G. (1983). *DeGangi–Berk test of sensory integration.* Los Angeles, CA: Western Psychological Services.

Brown, C., & Dunn, W. (2002). *Adolescent/adult sensory profile.* San Antonio, TX: The Psychological Corporation.

Bruininks, R. H., & Bruininks, B. D. (2005). *Bruininks–Oseretsky test of motor proficiency* (2nd ed.). San Antonio, TX: Pearson Assessments.

Centers for Disease Control and Prevention. (2007). Prevalence of autism spectrum disorders—Autism and developmental disabilities monitoring network, 14 sites, United States, 2002. *Morbidity and Mortality Weekly Report, 56,* 12–27.

Comi, A., Zimmerman, A., Frye, V., Law, P., & Peedan, J. (1999). Familiar clustering of autoimmune disorders and evaluation of medical risk factors. *Journal of Child Neurology, 14,* 388–394.

Constantino, J. N., & Gruber, C. P. (2005). *Social responsiveness scale manual.* Los Angeles, CA: Western Psychological Services.

Coster, W., Deeney, T., Haltiwanger, J., & Haley, S. (1998). *School function assessment.* San Antonio, TX: The Psychological Corporation.

deBettencourt, L.U. (2003). Understanding the difference between IDEA and Section 504. *Teaching Exceptional Children, 34*(3), 16–2.

DeGangi, G., & Greenspan, S. (1981). *Test of sensory functions in infants.* Los Angeles, CA: Western Psychological Services.

Dunn, W. (1999). *Sensory profile.* San Antonio, TX: The Psychological Corporation.

Dunn, W. (2002). *Infant/toddler sensory profile.* San Antonio, TX: The Psychological Corporation.

Dunn, W. (2006). *Sensory profile school companion*. San Antonio, TX: The Psychological Corporation.

Fisher, A. G. (1998). Uniting practice and theory in an occupational framework. *American Journal of Occupational Therapy, 52*, 509–520.

Folio, R., & Fewell, R. (2000). *Peabody developmental motor scales* (2nd ed.). Austin, TX: PRO-ED, Inc.

Fombonne, E., & Chakrabarti, S. (2001). No evidence for a new variant of measles-mumps-rubella-induced autism. *Pediatrics, 108*, E58.

Furuno, S., O'Reilly, K., Hosaka, C. M., Zeisloft, B., & Allman, T. (1984). *The Hawaii early learning profile*. Palo Alto, CA: VORT.

Galvin, D. (2001). The family of a child with autism. In H. Miller-Kuhaneck (Ed.), *Autism: A comprehensive occupational therapy approach* (4th ed., pp. 43–53). Bethesda, MD: AOTA.

George, M. S., Costa, D. C., Houris, K., Rang, H. A., & Ell, P. J. (1992). Cerebral blood flow abnormalities in adults with infantile autism. *Journal of Nervous and Mental Disease, 180*, 413–417.

Ghaziuddin, M. (2002). Asperger syndrome: Associated psychiatric and medical conditions. *Focus on Autism and Other Developmental Disabilities, 17*, 138–144.

Glessner, J. T., Wang, K., Cai, G., Korvaqtska, O., & Kim, C. E. (2009). Autism genome-wide copy number variation reveals ubiquitin and neuronal genes. *Nature, 459, 569–573.*

Glover, M. E., Preminger, J. L., & Sanford, A. R. (1988). *The early learning accomplishment profile (ELAP)*. Winston-Salem, NC: Kaplan Press.

Greenspan, S., DeGangi, G., & Wieder, S. (1996). *Functional emotional assessment scale*. Bethesda, MD: The Interdisciplinary Council on Developmental and Learning Disorders.

Hammill, D., Pearson, N. A., & Voress, J. K. (1993). *Developmental test of visual perception* (2nd ed.). Austin, TX: PRO-ED, Inc.

Harrison, P. L., & Oakland, T. (2003). *Adaptive behavioral assessment system* (2nd ed.). San Antonio, TX: The Psychological Corporation.

Howlin, P. (2000). Outcome in individuals with autism or Asperger syndrome. *Autism, 4*(1), 63–83.

Huebner, R. A., & Dunn, W. (2001). Introduction and basic concepts. In B. A. Huebner (Ed.), *Autism: A sensorimotor approach to management* (pp. 3–35). Gaithersburg, MD: Aspen.

Individuals With Disabilities Education Act of 1990, 20 U.S.C. § 1400 *et seq.* (1990) (amended 1997).

Individuals With Disabilities Education Improvement Act of 2004, 20 U.S.C § 1400 *et seq.* (2004).

Kientz, M. A., & Dunn, W. (1997). Comparison of the performance of children with and without autism on the sensory profile. *American Journal of Occupational Therapy, 51*, 530–537.

Knox, S. (1997). Development and current use of the Knox preschool play scale. In L. Parham & L. S. Fazio (Eds.), *Play in occupational therapy for children* (pp. 35–51). St. Louis, MO: Mosby.

---

Koul, O. (2005). Myelin and autism. In M. L. Bauman & T. L. Kemper (Eds.), *The neurobiology of autism* (2nd ed., pp. 150–163). Baltimore, MD: Johns Hopkins University Press.

Lerner, P. S. (2001). Alternative and complementary approaches in the treatment of autism. In H. Miller-Kuhaneck (Ed.), *Autism: A comprehensive occupational therapy approach* (pp. 237–268). Bethesda, MD: AOTA.

Lundy-Ekman, L. (1998). *Neuroscience fundamentals for rehabilitation*. Philadelphia, PA: Saunders.

Ma, D. (2009). A genome-wide association study of autism reveals a common novel risk locus at 5p14.1. *Annals of Human Genetics, 73,* 263–273.

Mailloux, Z., May-Benson, T. A., Summers, C. A., Miller, L. J., Brett-Green, B., Burke, J. P., . . . Schoen, S. A. (2007). Goal attainment scaling as a measure of meaningful outcomes for children with sensory integration disorders. *American Journal of Occupational Therapy, 61*(2), 254–259.

Mayes, S. D., & Calhoun, S. (1999). Symptoms of autism in young children and correspondence with DSM. *Infants and Young Children, 12*(2), 90–97.

Miller-Kuhaneck, H., & Glennon, T. J. (2001). An introduction to autism and pervasive developmental disorders. In H. Miller-Kuhaneck (Ed.), *Autism: A comprehensive occupational therapy approach* (pp. 1–23). Bethesda, MD: AOTA.

Mutti, M. C., Martin, N. A., Sterling, H. M., & Spalding, N. V. (1998). *Quick neurological screening test manual* (2nd ed.). Novato, CA: Academic Therapy Publications.

National Institutes of Health. (2009, April 28). *Risk of autism tied to genes that influence brain cell connections.* Retrieved from www.nih.gov/news/health/apr2009/ninds-28.htm

Olson, L. J. (1999). Psychosocial frame of reference. In P. Kramer & J. Hinohosa (Eds.), *Frames of reference for pediatric occupational therapy* (2nd ed., pp. 323–376). Philadelphia, PA: Lippincott, Williams & Wilkins.

Ornitz, E. M. (1974). The modulation of sensory input and motor output in autistic children. *Journal of Autism and Childhood Schizophrenia, 4*(3), 197–215.

Parham, L. D., & Ecker, C. (2007). *Sensory processing measure manual.* Los Angeles, CA: Western Psychological Services.

Piven, J., Palmer, P., Jacobi, D., Childress, D., & Arndt, S. (1997). Broader autism phenotype: Evidence from a family history study of multiple-incidence autism families. *American Journal of Psychiatry, 154,* 185–190.

Pletnikov, M. V., & Carbone, K. M. (2005). An animal model of virus-induced autism: Borna disease virus infection of the neonatal rat. In M. L. Bauman & T. L. Kemper (Eds.), *The neurobiology of autism* (2nd ed., pp. 190–206). Baltimore, MD: Johns Hopkins University Press.

Rehabilitation Act of 1973, 29 U.S.C. § 701 *et seq.* (1973) (amended 1986).

Royeen, C. B., & Duncan, M. (1999). Acquisitional frame of reference. In P. Kramer & J. Hinohosa (Eds.), *Frames of reference for pediatric occupational therapy* (2nd ed., pp. 377–400). Philadelphia, PA: Lippincott, Williams & Wilkins.

Schultz, R. T., Romanski, L. M., & Tsatsanis, K. D. (2000). Neurofunctional models of autistic disorder and Asperger syndrome: Clues from neuroimaging. In A. Kiln,

F. R. Volkmar, & S. S. Sparrow (Eds.), *Asperger syndrome* (pp. 159–171). New York, NY: Guilford Press.

Siegel, B. (2004). *Pervasive developmental disorders screening test* (2nd ed.). Sydney, Australia: Pearson Clinical Assessment.

Sparrow, S. S., Cicchetti, D. V., & Balla, D.A. (2005). *Vineland adaptive behavior scales* (2nd ed.). Circle Pines, MN: American Guidance Service.

Taylor, B., Miller, E., Lingam, R., Simmons, A., Stowe, J., & Waight, P. (2002). Measles, mumps and rubella vaccination and bowel problems or developmental regression in children with autism: Population study. *British Journal of Medicine, 324,* 393–396.

Tsai, L. (2000). Children with autism spectrum disorders: Medicine today and in the new millennium. *Focus on Autism and Other Developmental Disabilities, 15,* 138–145.

U.S. Department of Education. (2009). *Building the legacy: IDEA 2004.* Retrieved from http://idea.ed.gov/explore/home

Volkmar, F. R., Klin, A., Siegel, B., Szatmari, P., Lord, C., Campbell, M., & Kline, W. (1994). *DSM–IV* autism/P.D.D. field trial. *American Journal of Psychiatry, 151,* 1361–1367.

Walker, K., & Ludwig, F. (2004). *Perspectives on theory for the practice of occupational therapy* (3rd ed.). Austin, TX: PRO-ED, Inc.

Wang, K., Zhang, H., Ma, D., Bucan, M., Glessner, J. T., Abrahams, B. S., . . . Hakonarson, H. (2009). Common genetic variants on 5p14.1 associate with autism spectrum disorder. *Nature, 459,* 528–533.

Watling, R., Deitz, J., Kanny, E. M., & McLaughlin, J. F. (1999). Current practice of occupational therapy for children with autism. *American Journal of Occupational Therapy, 53,* 498–505.

Zilbovicius, M., Garreau, B., Samson, Y., Remy, P., Barthelemy, C., Syrota, A., & Lelord, G. (1995). Delayed maturation of the frontal cortex in childhood autism. *American Journal of Psychiatry, 152,* 248–252.

# Attention-Deficit/ Hyperactivity Disorder

*Gail E. Huecker*

## 🌿 Synopsis of Clinical Condition

### Prevalence and Etiology

Attention-deficit/hyperactivity disorder (ADHD) is manifested by limitations in impulse control and attention span (Hempel, 2003). ADHD is commonly described as *childhood hyperactivity*. The fourth edition of the *Diagnostic and Statistical Manual of Mental Disorders–Fourth Edition* (*DSM-IV*) reports an ADHD prevalence of 3% to 5% in school-age children (American Psychiatric Association [APA], 1994).

The *DSM-IV* also reports that ADHD occurs much more frequently in male children than in female children, with male-to-female ratios ranging from 4:1 to 9:1. However, some researchers believe that girls with ADHD are not accurately identified by these statistics because the problems of hyperactive girls are not as visible or as troublesome to adults as are the problems of hyperactive boys (Berry, Shaywitz, & Shaywitz, 1985). The exact etiology of ADHD is unknown, although ADHD has been linked to body chemistry, the structure and function of nerve cells, maternal alcohol and drug use, and genetic and environmental factors.

### Common Characteristics and Symptoms

The *DSM-IV* describes the following signs of inattention: becoming easily distracted by irrelevant sights and sounds, failing to pay attention to details and making careless mistakes, rarely following instructions carefully and completely, and losing or forgetting things. Signs of hyperactivity and impulsivity are described as follows: feeling restless; often fidgeting with hands or feet; squirming, running, climbing, or leaving a seat in situations where sitting or quiet behavior is expected; blurting out answers before hearing the whole question; and having difficulty waiting in line.

In confirming the diagnosis of ADHD, the *DSM-IV* states that "the essential feature of ADHD is a persistent pattern of inattention and/or hyperactivity-impulsivity that is more frequent and severe than is typically observed in individuals at a comparable level of development" (APA, 1994, p. 78). The *DSM-IV* further classifies subtypes of ADHD into the following three categories: (a) ADHD, combined type; (b) ADHD, predominantly inattentive type; and (c) ADHD, predominantly hyperactive–impulsive type. The *DSM-IV* clearly specifies that to be accurately diagnosed with one of the above three subtypes, some symptoms have to be present before the age of 7 years, there must be impairment from the symptoms in two or more settings (e.g., school and home), and there must be clinically significant impairment in social, academic, or occupational functioning.

There is a high prevalence of sensory processing or sensory integration dysfunction in children with ADHD (Huecker & Kinnealey, 1998; Mangeot et al., 2001; Shochat, Tzischinksy, & Engel-Yerger, 2009; Yochman, Parush, & Ornoy, 2004). Miller et al. (2006) reported that of a group of children referred with ADHD or sensory processing disorder, 60% reported symptoms of both. Furthermore, Reynolds and Lane (2009) reported that children with comorbid ADHD and sensory processing disorder overresponsively demonstrated higher levels of anxiety than did those without comorbidity.

## Target Areas for Intervention

When there is significant impairment in social, academic, or occupational functioning, some children with ADHD may be referred for occupational therapy intervention. The therapist must decipher the underlying sensorimotor and sensory integrative problems that may be contributing to the child's inability to attend. The primary areas to be addressed are reaction to sensory stimuli and antigravity movement, motor planning, and social–emotional responses. All of these areas impact social, academic, and/or occupational functioning.

The inattention, hyperactivity, and impulsivity most commonly associated with ADHD are related to abnormal sensory integrative and sensorimotor processing and the consequent disorder in the ability to transmit, interpret, and respond appropriately to sensory stimulation from the environment (Ayres, 1979; Greenspan, 1992). Characteristic symptoms include sensory hypo- or hypersensitivity, sensory defensiveness, unusual patterns of arousal, dyspraxia, and emotional and social difficulties (Burpee, 1994; Cermak, 1988a, 1988b; Oetter, 1986a, 1986b; Wilbarger & Wilbarger, 1991).

Ayres (1979) described a variety of behaviors that can result from increased sensory sensitivity. These behaviors include excess emotional reactions and hyperactivity, along with other behavioral manifestations, including excessive fighting, the inability to sit quietly at a school desk, and increased motor activity. The inability to enjoy contact comfort with a significant other has also been described by Royeen (1985).

*Sensory registration* refers to an individual's ability to accurately perceive incoming sensory information. Sensory registration deficits occur when an individual exhibits significant delays in responding to sensory information or when there is an apparent failure to notice sensory stimulation at all (Lane, 2002; Oetter, 1986a, 1986b).

Clinically, children with sensory registration deficits may appear to have a heightened pain tolerance or may brush off bruises or scratches as if nothing ever happened. They may also be described as the children who have poor safety awareness, and they often seek out movement activities that can interfere with their personal safety (e.g., jumping from high places).

Another focus for occupational therapy intervention is the child's postural attention, or the ability to receive consistent information about the body and its relationship to the environment in terms of space, place, and time (Oetter, 1986a, 1986b). Because postural control should be an automatic process, it can be difficult for the child with postural deficits to attend, since they may have to focus on their inability to maintain an erect posture as opposed to attending to the task at hand.

Dyspraxia can occur when a child has underlying difficulty processing somatosensory (tactile and proprioceptive) information and when there is inadequate postural control to allow smooth, coordinated movement when executing a task (Cermak, 1988a, 1988b). When somatosensory processing deficits are apparent within a child with dyspraxia, his or her difficulty with perceiving touch and pressure can lead to difficulty registering sensory input. This, in turn, can contribute to the child's attention issues, since he or she may be unaware that there is even anything to attend to.

Individuals with ADHD may also experience fluctuations in levels of alertness and arousal, which are related to sensory processing disturbance. These fluctuations can be reflected by disorganized sleep patterns or by fluctuations in the individual's ability to attend during interactions with unfamiliar people, tasks, and environments that the individual perceives as overstimulating (Oetter, 1986a, 1986b).

Vestibular-related disorders, specifically, shortened duration of postrotary nystagmus (PRN), are another sensory integrative deficit that has been linked to resultant attentional deficits. Children with a shortened duration of PRN also demonstrate poor balance, difficulty maintaining antigravity postures, and low muscle tone (Cermak, 1988a, 1988b). Kimball (1986) proposed that a large percentage of children with ADHD have an underresponsive vestibular system, which contributes to their attention deficits. Huecker and Kinnealey (1998) confirmed Kimball's research in a descriptive study, by reporting a vestibular processing disorder in more than 50% of the children with ADHD studied, making them hyporesponsive or underreactive to vestibular stimulation. It has also been suggested that children with ADHD who demonstrate sensory integration deficits report a high incidence of social–emotional challenges, including poor frustration tolerance; difficulty making friends; rigid personalities; and feelings of anxiousness, anxiety, or depression (Huecker & Kinnealey, 1998).

Many children with attention disorders also exhibit auditory processing deficits, commonly diagnosed as a central auditory processing disorder (CAPD; Greenspan, 1992). Many children with auditory processing deficits are frequently accused of not following directions or not listening, and they may fail to get their work completed on time. It is important to understand the relationship between CAPD and attention deficits, since CAPD may actually be one of the underlying causes of the child's inability to focus or attend.

It is estimated that 50% or more of children with ADHD have a learning disability (Stahl, 1995). Between 15% and 20% of children and adolescents with learning disabilities have ADHD (Silver, 1990). Because ADHD can interfere with a child's ability to concentrate and pay attention, this diagnosis—in conjunction with the diagnosis of learning disability—can make it exceptionally difficult for a child to function in school.

Another condition sometimes found in conjunction with ADHD is a rare disorder called *Tourette syndrome*. Children diagnosed with Tourette syndrome typically have tics and other uncontrolled movements, such as eye blinks, facial twitches, grimacing, shrugging, or sniffing. Typically, this syndrome is controlled with medications. One of the most disabling aspects of Tourette syndrome is that in 90% of cases, it exists in conjunction with some other disorder, with the most frequent co-occurring condition being ADHD (University of Calgary, 2009). Furthermore, Nass and Bressman (2002) estimated that tics and Tourette syndrome occur in as many as 50% of children diagnosed with ADHD and that ADHD is even more common in Tourette syndrome, with comorbidity reported as high as 90%.

It has been estimated that almost half of all children with ADHD are boys, and these children are sometimes diagnosed with oppositional defiant disorder (ODD). Children with this disorder reportedly exhibit behaviors that include lashing out at others; acting stubborn, belligerent, or defiant; and having significant temper tantrums. If a child with ADHD and ODD does not receive proper medical treatment, he or she may progress to more serious behaviors and may then be diagnosed with a conduct disorder. Children with this disorder typically take unsafe risks and break laws. They may steal, set fires, destroy property, or harm. Eventually, these children may become involved with the juvenile justice system on account of their uncontrolled behavior.

Many children with ADHD may also be diagnosed with anxiety disorder or depression. An estimated one fourth of children with ADHD feel anxious and/or depressed.

# Contextual Considerations

## Clinical

The clinical evaluation of a child who has ADHD should assess sensory processing, motor control, praxis/cognition, developmental status, communication, activities of daily living (ADL), and social–emotional functioning. By assessing these areas, the occupational therapist should be able to determine if the child demonstrates soft neurological processing deficits and if there is impairment in function at home and/or at school. For children ages 4 years to 8 years 11 months, the *Sensory Integration and Praxis Test* (SIPT; Ayers, 1989) is extremely helpful in determining if sensory integration and praxis/motor planning problems are present.

The SIPT has been described as a sophisticated and psychometrically sound assessment tool designed to provide diagnostic and descriptive information related to sensory integrative and practic functions (Mailloux, 1990). The SIPT consists of 17 subtests that assess abilities related to praxis and various aspects of sensory processing, including vestibular, proprioceptive, kinesthetic, tactile, and visual processing (Ayres, 1991). In addition to the 17 subtests of the SIPT, both a sensory history and clinical observations are necessary supplements for a complete assessment of sensory integrative dysfunction.

Other sensory processing deficits that children with ADHD may exhibit are assessed through clinical observations and a sensory history. Most standard clinical observations include general assessment of activity level; response to touch; visual control; coordination; praxis or motor planning; and postural responses, including reflexes and balance reactions. The most commonly used sensory history is the *Sensory Profile* (Dunn, 1999). It is most appropriate to use the *Sensory Profile* for children between the ages of 5 and 10 years. The *Sensory Profile* is completed by a parent or caregiver and includes information regarding sensory processing, modulation, and behavioral and emotional responses. The *Sensory Profile* is standardized and can be use to provide baseline data and assess progress.

The *Quick Neurological Screening Test–II* (QNST-II; Mutti, Martin, Sterling, & Spalding, 1998) is a quick and accurate instrument for detecting the soft neurological signs often associated with learning disabilities. It is designed for use with children as young as 5 years but can also be used for older children, adolescents, and adults. Because it can be completed in 20 to 30 minutes, the QNST-II is easy to use in a variety of settings, including outpatient, private practice, school, or home.

Other assessments for the school-age child may be needed to further evaluate visual motor skills, visual perception, and fine and gross motor coordination. Common examples include the *Beery–Buktenica Developmental Test of Visual–Motor Integration–Sixth Edition* (Beery, Buktenica, & Beery, 2010), the *Developmental Test of Visual Perception* (Hammill, Pearson, & Voress, 1993), the *Bruininks–Oseretsky Test of Motor Proficiency–Second Edition* (Bruininks & Bruininks, 2005), and the *Test of Visual Perceptual Skills–Third Edition* (Martin, 2006). The *Pediatric Examination of Educational Readiness–Revised* (Levine & Schneider, 1983) and the *Pediatric Examination of Educational Readiness at Middle Childhood–Revised* (Levine, 1985) are also beneficial in assessing soft neurological processing deficits and academic performance.

For the younger child with ADHD, a developmental assessment can be helpful to determine developmental levels in the areas of motor skills, cognition, language, self-help skills, and social–emotional functioning. Examples of general developmental assessments include the *Peabody Developmental Motor Scales– Second Edition* (Folio & Fewell, 2000), the *Hawaii Early Learning Profile* (Furuno et al., 1991), and the *Pediatric Evaluation of Disability Inventory* (Haley, Coster, Ludlow, Haltiwanger, & Andrellos, 1992). Most of these developmental assessments are completed through use of both clinical observation and parent interview.

In assessing ADL skills in the child with ADHD, the occupational therapist should focus on the areas most affected by the regulation of sensory input, including sleep cycles, bowel and bladder control, and feeding/eating. Sensory processing deficits or a sensory processing disorder can significantly affect a child's ability to self-regulate within these areas. Children with ADHD and sensory processing deficits often have difficulty winding down to get to sleep or awaken frequently throughout the night. Nightmares are also commonly reported. Disturbed sleep patterns can only add to their difficulty focusing and attending throughout the day.

Some children are delayed in bowel/bladder control, and for these children bed-wetting can be a common occurrence. If bed-wetting continues to persist into later childhood, this can contribute to social–emotional concerns, including anxiety and poor self-esteem. For example, the older child with bed-wetting issues may formulate excuses to refuse sleepovers with peers to avoid the possibility of an embarrassing situation. It is the occupational therapist's role to become aware of treatment approaches that address sensory regulation and modulation deficits, as these factors may contribute to the root cause of sleeping, toileting, or feeding delays.

Children with ADHD and a sensory processing disorder who have feeding/ eating deficits or delays are often picky eaters, which is possibly caused by oral hypersensitivity. These children can gag easily on foods and may therefore limit their diet to only a few textures. It is also common for parents to report that their child "overstuffs" or "pockets" food in his or her mouth when eating. If a child exhibits hypo- or underresponsiveness to sensory input, then poor oral sensory awareness can be a factor contributing to difficulty processing when his or her mouth is full. This can create a choking hazard, and oral motor intervention should be a definite focus of the treatment plan. Poor oral sensory awareness can also contribute to other developmental concerns, including poor articulation; oral motor delays, such as drooling, difficulty sucking, and/or blowing; and oral praxis deficits. Although these issues are often treated in occupational therapy, it may become the therapist's role to refer the child to speech therapy for further assessment and treatment if it has not already been indicated.

Other areas that should be assessed in reference to ADL skills include grooming, bathing, and dressing. Sensory defensiveness can significantly contribute to grooming issues, including difficulty tolerating haircutting, nail trimming, toothbrushing, or face washing. Bathing issues may include anxiety caused by having water in the face, hair washing, or lying backward in the bathtub, which can occur secondary to postural or vestibular deficits. As a result of varying sensory processing deficits or sensory defensiveness, the child may become quite rigid with his or her grooming or bathing routine, possibly in an attempt to avoid uncomfortable or threatening situations.

Sensory processing, specifically sensory overresponsiveness, can also affect dressing skills. Some children can be averse to certain clothing textures or tags in their clothes or to the seams in their socks. In addition, dyspraxia, fine motor deficits, and poor body awareness can all interfere with a child's ability to dress independently. Children may not notice if their clothing is on inside out or backward, or they may be unable to manipulate fasteners on clothing because of fine motor delays. All of these issues are typically frustrating for the parent and child, and it becomes the therapist's role to help the child form the foundational skills necessary for these skills to develop more naturally.

## Family

When interviewing the family of a child with ADHD who exhibits sensory processing deficits, an occupational therapist should be empathetic and sensitive. Parents are frequently frustrated and believe their child is only being difficult, stubborn, or lazy, and they may be unaware that the behaviors their child exhibits may have a neurological base. The occupational therapist's role should include educating parents and families that using negative terms such as *lazy* or *stubborn* when referencing their child can only contribute to the child's already poor self-confidence and self-esteem, as well as to negative behaviors.

It can be difficult to discipline a child with ADHD, and some parents may ask for suggestions in this area. When providing suggestions, it is important for the occupational therapist to be sensitive to cultural issues regarding discipline. Parents may feel guilty that their child is having social or developmental delays and may not set enough limits for behavior. This can be difficult for children with ADHD, who thrive on structure and routine to help with organizational skills.

Another consequence of a parent feeling guilty about his or her child is that the parent may be fostering dependency without being aware of it. For example, if the child with ADHD is frustrated about having difficulty dressing, a parent may do it for him or her, causing the child to develop learned helplessness. Therefore, it is important to model independent behaviors and empower the child for success. The therapist can teach families methods of empowering, such as blaming the object instead of the child, especially when the child is frustrated over an inability to perform a task independently. Empowering success in the child and the parent will hopefully help increase self-confidence and decrease self-blame and feelings of guilt.

Unavoidable excessive guilt often leads to depression. If depression does occur, it is important for the occupational therapist to be able to recognize this in parents and refer them to the appropriate professionals. If the parent is depressed to the point of being unable to function as a caregiver, it can interfere with the child's ability to develop the foundations for organizational skills and independent functioning.

## Practice Setting

Occupational therapists may work with children with ADHD in a variety of settings, including private practice, home, school, and early intervention centers or day care centers. In a private practice, there should be a variety of specialized equipment available to meet the needs of the child. Direct/individualized treatment may be the most beneficial in the early stages of care, whereas treatment in small groups may be beneficial in the later stages, to help address social–emotional concerns.

Specialized equipment may not be readily available for an occupational therapist working in the home. The therapist should help parents establish home activities that utilize the equipment already available. Examples may include enhanced deep pressure activities, such as wheelbarrow walking, jumping on mattresses, swinging outdoors, rearranging furniture, or carrying in groceries. These types of gross motor activities that provide movement and deep pressure input to the child's nervous system can be calming or inhibitory in nature and therefore may be used to help improve focus and attention. It is especially important to formulate a sensory diet of activities for the child in the home setting, including these types of gross motor tasks, in addition to fine motor, oral motor, and respiratory challenges. Examples may include engaging in deep blowing and or sucking activities, chewing gum or other resistive textures, as well as squeezing or pulling resistive hand fidgets. The goal in providing the child with a sensory diet in the home can be to promote more organized behavior or more focused behavior during homework tasks.

The school-based occupational therapist must provide services that are educationally relevant in terms of the child's academic functioning. The Individuals With Disabilities Education Act (IDEA, 1997) mandates that all children have the right to a free, appropriate public education in the least restrictive environment. If the child with ADHD is having academic difficulty, he or she may be referred to an occupational therapist as a supportive service. The occupational therapist's role may be to address the child's fine motor delays, handwriting problems, problems focusing and attending during seated work, poor organizational and sequencing skills, and sensory processing deficits as they relate to social interaction (i.e., interaction with other children on the playground).

In 2006, the United Nations Convention on the Rights of Persons With Disabilities called on all states to ensure an "inclusive education system" at all levels, as does the Individuals With Disabilities Education Improvement Act. This means that it is now mandatory to include the child with special needs in classrooms with nondisabled students. Because students with disabilities such as ADHD are no longer separated from students without disabilities, the occupational therapist may find it beneficial to plan appropriate therapeutic activities for the whole class, as opposed to singling out the individual child with ADHD. For example, the occupational therapist could use *Handwriting Without Tears* (Olsen, 2001) to teach handwriting to the entire class, rather than removing the child with ADHD out of the classroom to work singly on improving handwriting skills.

For preschool-age children, the occupational therapist may work not only within the school setting but also within an early intervention center or day care center for individuals who are age 3 to 5 years. In these settings, it is important for the therapist to be a team member and use a transdisciplinary approach while working with other professionals. As with the school-age child, instead of pulling the preschool-age child out of his or her classroom for therapy, the therapist can use the inclusion model to integrate functional needs into the daily routine. In using the inclusion model within these settings, the occupational therapist should be cognizant of the role of the other members of the professional team, which can include psychologists, speech–language pathologists, teachers, social workers, and physicians. All these professionals can be helpful in addressing the needs of the child with ADHD.

## Sociopolitical

As mentioned earlier, IDEA mandates a free, appropriate public education for children with disabilities (IDEA, 1997). Since children with ADHD may have learning disabilities, school-based occupational therapists may be involved in the development of legally required Individualized Education Programs (IEPs). Some children with ADHD may not qualify for services under IDEA but may qualify for classroom adaptations under the Rehabilitation Act, Section 504 (Rehabilitation Act, 1973), which defines *disability* more broadly than does IDEA. The occupational therapist providing direct services to the child with ADHD may be expected to write specific IEP goals for maintaining attention for a specific period of time (e.g., 10–15 minutes without requiring physical cues for redirection). In contrast, the child with ADHD who does not qualify for direct occupational therapy but still requires classroom strategies to improve, for example, attention or focus, could have a 504 Plan in place. The occupational therapist's role in this case may be to suggest sensory diet activities for the whole classroom that can help increase attention, such as chewing gum, using hand fidgets, or using a visual barrier to block out environmental distractions.

It is imperative that the occupational therapist working in private practice consult with and provide education for pediatricians and other physicians who may refer the child with ADHD for therapy. It is important for the therapist to discuss with the referring physicians the possible neurological processing deficits that may be interfering with the child's function. Since ADHD is viewed as a behavioral diagnosis, some insurance companies may not deem to be occupational therapy treatment as medically necessary. By educating the physician, they may be able to use other diagnosis codes, such as motor apraxia, when referring the child with ADHD for occupational therapy treatment. This diagnosis may more accurately describe the neuromotor nature of the child's condition and may allow treatment to be covered under more insurance plans.

## Lifestyle/Lifespan

Since ADHD has a genetic component, some parents of children with ADHD may have the same issues, regardless of whether they have been diagnosed. Therefore, it may be difficult for parents to take suggestions about controlling their child's behavior or helping their child with organization. Many children with ADHD function better in a clearly structured routine. The occupational therapist may be able to educate parents on setting up a behavior plan to improve behavior, such as modeling, giving rewards, or making a consistent schedule for the child. In some situations, it may also be helpful to refer the parent to other professionals or support groups that can help them establish parenting skills.

Another important family consideration for helping the child with ADHD is establishing a home-based program for enhanced organization, improved behavior, and improved social–emotional functioning. This is consistent with the idea of providing a sensory diet for the child, as previously mentioned. When the child exhibits extreme regulatory and modulation difficulties, the occupational therapist should provide the family with sensory activities—consistent with family resources and routines—that are designed to enhance the child's ability to process tactile, proprioceptive, auditory, and vestibular input. For example, a touch- or pressure-based treatment protocol may be recommended 3 to 5 times per day to improve sensory processing and organizational or behavioral responses in the child with ADHD. Parents will be much more likely to follow the program if they are given concrete examples of how to build it into their daily routine. A concrete example may be to have the family perform the touch- or pressure-based protocol during every diaper change for the younger child with ADHD or during mealtimes and snack times for the older child. This type of concrete suggestion will likely help the child with ADHD progress more rapidly through use of his or her home-based program.

There is also growing information about prevention through testing for specific food allergies that can contribute to hyperactivity and impulsivity (Zavik & Thompson, 2002). An occupational therapist should be familiar with nutritional concepts, such as food sensitivities and allergies, and refer parents to a nutritionist when appropriate. As the child with ADHD grows, his or her needs for their home-based program may also. Dietary restrictions may change, as may the individual's need for specific sensory diet activities. For example, instead of a touch- or pressure-based protocol for enhanced organizational and behavioral skills, an auditory program may be suggested as a strategy during homework. In addition, the older child with ADHD may find it beneficial for his or her sensory diet to include broader suggestions, such as jogging, weight lifting, or a taking a karate class. These types of activities can help the individual with ADHD to move beyond the scope of direct occupational therapy treatment to a more consultative treatment approach.

## 🌿 Clinical Decision-Making Process

### Defining Focus for Intervention

The focus of occupational therapy treatment for the child with ADHD may vary depending on where services will be provided. Treatment will also vary depending on the frequency and duration of the service the funding source allows. For example, if the occupational therapist is working in a private practice setting in which Medicaid is the primary funding source, a child is allowed up to fourteen 15-minute units of occupational therapy per week, as long as the therapy is deemed medically necessary and approved by a physician. In this type of setting, with 14 units allowed per week, a therapist will be able to complete a thorough evaluation of the child's functioning. The SIPT may be the most appropriate assessment tool to define the child's underlying sensory processing and praxis deficits. However, this assessment would have to be completed in hourly increments on separate days to meet Medicaid guidelines.

Throughout the evaluation, the occupational therapist should gain information about primary parental concerns. These concerns should become the main focus of occupational therapy intervention once treatment is initiated. For example, if a parent's primary concerns are about self-grooming difficulties related to sensory defensiveness, then normalizing sensory processing should become the primary goal. If a child is referred for an occupational therapy evaluation but will not be able to attend therapy regularly because of funding issues, then establishing a home-based program is of primary importance.

The primary criterion for school-based occupational therapy is educational relevance. The focus of intervention might be fine motor control for handwriting, organizational skills for letter or number formation, postural control for better attention while seated in a desk, or self-regulation strategies for social interaction. In educational settings where inclusionary, rather than pullout, services are expected, occupational therapy services may be consultative and intervention strategies may be group, rather than individual, oriented. In that case, activity programs such as *How Does Your Engine Run?* (Williams & Shellenberger, 1996) and *Handwriting Without Tears* (Olsen, 2001) can be used to improve attention span and handwriting for a larger group.

### Establishing Goals for Intervention

Primary parental concerns should become goals within the private practice setting, whereas primary teacher concerns should become goals within the school setting. Since goals need to be functional and measurable, they should be worded clearly, with only one objective to be met per goal. It is also important to establish short-term goals that will ultimately allow the child to achieve his or her long-term goal, regardless of the practice setting.

If a child with ADHD is also developmentally delayed, it will be important to take into account the child's developmental status in order to make the goals attainable. For example, if the child is 5 years old but functioning at a 4-year-old level, it may not be appropriate to establish a goal that the child be able to tie his or her shoes independently. A child with ADHD frequently exhibits increased frustration. Therefore, goals should be broken down into small steps, giving the child several opportunities for success while working toward the major goal.

## Designing Theory-Based Intervention

The sensory integration frame of reference may be the most commonly used frame of reference when working with the child with ADHD. This frame of reference allows the therapist to evaluate the underlying neurological constructs that may be contributing to the child's developmental, social, or behavioral issues. Ayres (1991) defined *sensory integration* as the neurological process that organizes sensation from one's own body and from the environment and makes it possible to use the body effectively within the environment. According to this view, higher level organizational and learning abilities are dependent on the integrity of lower level brain centers that govern arousal levels and attention span (Ayres, 1979; Fisher & Murray, 1991). The therapist who uses a sensory integration frame of reference will design activities to remediate deficits in muscle tone, postural control, sensory defensiveness, and oculomotor control in order to achieve specific behavioral goals. Such goals include improved attention span, increased frustration tolerance, and better motor coordination.

## Evaluating Progress

Formal evaluations, such as the SIPT, the *Sensory Profile,* and the *Sensory Processing Measure* (Parham & Ecker, 2007), can provide quantitative data that can be used to monitor changes in function and provide feedback regarding the efficacy of treatment. They can be used at the outset of treatment and periodically throughout treatment. Qualitative data from clinical observation and the anecdotal reports of caregivers can be used to monitor changes in function and provide feedback regarding the effectiveness of treatment. Regulations regarding the frequency and form of progress documentation vary depending on the practice setting and funding source.

## Determining Change in or Termination of Treatment

The therapist should be able to determine when a change in treatment is warranted as the child progresses in therapy and improves his or her performance on the standardized tests and screening tools identified previously in this chapter. For example, the child may appear to have his or her behavior under control and be less impulsive and more aware of safety. At that point, the child may be ready to join a peer group or a small group of children in treatment, to address more social interaction concerns. It is also helpful to guide treatment changes based on information the parent or teacher provides. If the parent or teacher reports that the child is more organized, less impulsive, and able to attend for longer periods of time, it may be an appropriate time to introduce higher level intervention strategies, such as a handwriting group.

Termination of treatment is warranted once the child has met his or her established goals or if it appears that the child is not going to be able to meet the goals because of other circumstances (e.g., social concerns in the home). If the child has met his or her goals, the parent will likely appear much calmer about how the child is functioning. Before discharge, the family should be able to demonstrate proficiency in carrying out a home-based program. If transition to a new environment triggers additional organizational or behavioral challenges, the child may be referred to occupational therapy again. If the child appears unable to meet his or her expected goals secondary to other circumstances, then a referral to other professionals may be warranted. For example, family dynamics or other social–emotional pressures may exacerbate anxiety and impulsivity. In this situation, it may be appropriate to recommend that the family seek psychological counseling or additional social services.

## Case Study

### Description

CW is a 6-year-old boy with ADHD. He was referred to occupational therapy because of his parents' primary concerns about his academic difficulties. Specifically, teachers had reported poor handwriting, difficulty focusing/attending, poor organizational skills, and inappropriate social–emotional functioning. Other concerns included stubborn and defiant behavior, poor oculomotor (eye tracking) skills, and negative behaviors during grooming tasks (e.g., nail trimming, haircutting).

CW lives at home with his parents and younger sister. He attends a private school, where he is in a regular kindergarten classroom with eight children. Although he has exhibited other developmental delays, CW has never received any therapy services. Stimulant medication has been used with no significant effect on his ability to attend/focus. He is currently on no medications. Medical history is significant for strabismus in his right eye, which was surgically corrected.

Results of CW's SIPT indicated generalized sensory integrative dysfunction. Areas of severe dysfunction ($-3.00$ standard deviations [$SD$] below the norm) included Standing and Walking Balance, Localization of Tactile Stimuli, Graphesthesia, Praxis on Verbal Command, and Postural Praxis. His Postrotary Nystagmus score was $-2.82\ SD$ below the norm, and the Sequencing and Oral Praxis subtests indicated moderate dysfunction (between $-2.0$ and $-2.5\ SD$ below the norm). Visual perception scores (Space Visualization and Figure Ground) fell within the average range on the SIPT.

Results of the *Sensory Profile* indicated that CW demonstrated definite differences (−3.0 *SD* below the norm) with tactile, auditory, multisensory, and vestibular processing, sensory modulation deficits related to endurance/tone, sensory sensitivity, poor modulation of movement affecting activity level, and social–emotional responses at −2.0 *SD* below the norm. Results of clinical observations indicated that CW was unable to assume or maintain either prone extension or supine flexion postures. He also appeared to have decreased oculomotor control, poor convergence, difficulty planning smooth movements, decreased musculature contraction, and postural insecurity (i.e., fear of movement beyond his postural control).

Areas of strength reported during the evaluation include regular sleep patterns, good eating skills, independent toileting, and independent dressing. CW is a quiet child who does not play interactively with other children or toys and seems fearful of many new tasks. His favorite activities include playing with books and cars. It has been recommended that CW receive 2 hours of individual/direct therapy services per week in a private practice setting, in addition to a weekly consult with his kindergarten teacher.

## Long- and Short-Term Goals

The long-term goal of intervention for CW is to enable him to attend to a cognitive/fine motor activity for 15 minutes without requiring redirection. The short-term goals for CW are the following:

1. Maintain a supine flexion posture on the floor or over a large therapy ball for 10 seconds without compensation.
2. Maintain a prone extension posture for 5 minutes during a movement activity on suspended equipment.
3. Wheelbarrow walk for 10 feet while feet are held without falling to elbows.
4. Allow his nails to be trimmed by a primary caregiver without an aversive response.
5. Follow a two-step motor command 80% of the time without directions repeated.

## Therapist Goals and Strategies

The therapist's goals include the following:

1. Normalize sensory processing by reducing sensory defensiveness and enhancing body awareness.
2. Increase motor coordinative control through enhanced antigravity control and co-contraction.
3. Enhance motor planning through improved body awareness and vestibular processing.
4. Provide teacher education regarding strategies to enhance academic performance.

The therapist's strategies include the following:

1. Educate parents on implementing an intense touch/pressure program with the use of therapy brushes and a large muscle vibrator, to be performed 3 to 5 times per day.

2. Visit the home to instruct parents on sensory activities to enhance self-regulation and attention.

3. Educate school staff on the *How Does Your Engine Run?* program.

4. Provide opportunities in the clinic for enhanced tactile, proprioceptive, and vestibular processing, as well as oral motor and eye tracking activities.

5. Provide activities in the clinic incorporating play with peer and co-therapists, to enhance social functioning.

6. Educate parents on implementation of an auditory listening program 1 hour daily to enhance visual, vestibular, and auditory processing, and to improve postural control and motor planning.

7. Collaborate with other members of the professional team, such as the speech–language pathologist, the teacher, and the psychologist, on goal setting and implementation of strategies.

### Activity

CW will straddle a tire swing that is 12 to 18 inches off the ground and will pick up "fish" (stuffed beanbags) from the "ocean" (floor mats) without his feet touching the "water" while swinging. After a fish is successfully picked up, CW will throw each fish into a bucket with one hand without falling into the ocean.

### Treatment Objectives

CW will maintain adequate flexion posture on suspended equipment for 3 to 5 minutes while engaged in a dynamic upper extremity activity.

## Resources

ADHD News: www.adhdnews.com

American Occupational Therapy Association: www.aota.org

Children and Adults With Attention-Deficit/Hyperactivity Disorder: www.chadd.org

Conduct Disorders (parent support): www.conductdisorders.com

## References

American Psychiatric Association. (1994). *Diagnostic and statistical manual of mental disorders* (4th ed.). Washington, DC: Author.

Ayres, A. J. (1979). *Sensory integration and the child.* Los Angeles, CA: Western Psychological Services.

Ayres, A. J. (1991). *Sensory integration and praxis test.* Los Angeles, CA: Western Psychological Services.

Beery, K. E., Buktenica, N. A., & Beery, N. A. (2010). *Beery–Buktenica developmental test of visual–motor integration* (6th ed.). San Antonio, TX: Pearson Assessments.

Berry, C. A., Shaywitz, S. E., & Shaywitz, B. A. (1985). Girls with attention deficit disorder: A silent minority? A report on behavioral and cognitive characteristics. *Pediatrics, 76,* 801–809.

Bruininks, R. H., & Bruininks, B. D. (2005). *Bruininks–Oseretsky test of motor proficiency* (2nd ed.). San Antonio, TX: Pearson Assessments.

Burpee, J. D. (1994, March). *Developmental disabilities, dyspraxia, and sensory integration: A treatment process for pediatric therapists*. Paper presented at professional conference, Langhorne, PA.

Cermak, S. A. (1988a). The relationship between attention deficit and sensory integration disorders (Part 1). *Sensory Integration Special Interest Section Newsletter, 11*(2), 1–4.

Cermak, S. A. (1988b). The relationship between attention deficit and sensory integration disorders (Part 2). *Sensory Integration Special Interest Section Newsletter, 11*(3), 3–4.

Dunn, W. (1999). *Sensory profile*. San Antonio, TX: The Psychological Corporation.

Fisher, A. G., & Murray, E. A. (1991). Introduction to sensory integration theory. In A. G. Fisher, E. A. Murray, & A. C. Bundy (Eds.), *Sensory integration theory and practice* (pp. 3–26). Philadelphia, PA: FA Davis.

Folio, R., & Fewell, R. (2000). *Peabody developmental motor scales* (2nd ed). San Antonio, TX: The Psychological Corporation.

Furuno, S., O'Reilly, K., Inatsuka, T., Hosaka, C., Allman, T., & Zeisloft-Falbey, B. (1991). *Hawaii early learning profile* (Rev. ed.). Palo Alto, CA: VORT.

Greenspan, S. I. (1992). *Infancy and early childhood: The practice of clinical assessment and intervention with emotional and developmental challenges*. Madison, CT: International Universities Press.

Haley, S., Coster, W., Ludlow, L, Haltiwanger, J., & Andrellos, P. (1992). *Pediatric evaluation of disability inventory*. San Antonio, TX: The Psychological Corporation.

Hammill, D., Pearson, N., & Voress, J. (1993). *Developmental test of visual perception* (2nd ed.). Austin, TX: PRO-ED, Inc.

Hempel, K. (2003). *The Health Gazette*. Attention Deficit Hyperactivity Disorder, 6-1-03. www.tfn.net/HG/adhd.html

Huecker, G., & Kinnealey, M. (1998). Prevalence of sensory integrative disorders in children with attention deficit hyperactivity disorder: A descriptive study. *The Journal of Developmental and Learning Disorders, 2*(2), 265–292.

Individuals With Disabilities Education Act of 1990, 20 U.S.C. § 1400 *et seq.* (1990) (amended 1997).

Kimball, J. G. (1986). Prediction of methylphenidate (Ritalin) responsiveness through sensory integrative testing. *The American Journal of Occupational Therapy, 40*(4), 241–248.

Lane, S. J. (2002). Sensory modulation. In A. C. Bundy, S. J. Lane, & E. A. Murray, (Eds.), *Sensory integration theory and practice* (2nd ed., p. 103) Philadelphia, PA: F. A. Davis

Levine, M. D. (1985). *Pediatric examination of educational readiness in middle childhood*. Cambridge, MA: Educators Publishing Services.

Levine, M. D., & Schneider, E. A. (1983). *Pediatric examination of educational readiness*. Cambridge, MA: Educators Publishing Services.

Mailloux, Z. (1990). An overview of the Sensory Integration and Praxis Tests. *The American Journal of Occupational Therapy, 44*(7), 589–594.

Mangeot, S. D., Miller, L. J., McIntosh, D. N., McGrath-Clark, J., Simon, J., & Hagerman, R. J. (2001). Sensory modulation dysfunction in children with attention-deficit-hyperactivity disorder. *Developmental Medicine and Child Neurology, 43,* 399–406.

Martin, N. (2006). *Test of visual perceptual skills* (3rd ed.). Novato, CA: Academic Therapy.

Miller, L. J. (2006). *Miller function and participation scales.* San Antonio TX: Psychological Corporation.

Mutti, M., Martin, N. A., Sterling, H., & Spalding, N. V. (1988). *Quick neurological screening test* (Rev. ed.). Novato, CA: Academic Therapy.

Nass, R., & Bressman, S. (2002). Attention deficit hyperactivity disorder and Tourette syndrome. *Neurology, 58,* 523–524.

Oetter, P. (1986a). A sensory integrative approach to the treatment of attention deficit disorders. *Sensory Integration Special Interest Section Newsletter, 9*(2), 1–2.

Oetter, P. (1986b). Assessment: The child with attention deficit disorder. *Sensory Integration Special Interest Section Newsletter, 9*(1), 6–7.

Olsen, J. (2001). *Handwriting without tears.* Cabin John, MD: Handwriting Without Tears.

Parham, L. D., & Ecker, C. (2007). *Sensory Processing Measure manual.* Los Angeles, CA: Western Psychological Services.

Rehabilitation Act of 1973, 29 U.S.C. § 701 *et seq.* (1973) (amended 1986).

Reynolds, S., & Lane, S. (2009). Sensory overresponsivity and anxiety in children with ADHD. *The American Journal of Occupational Therapy, 63*(4), 433–440.

Royeen, C. B. (1985). Domain specifications of the construct tactile defensiveness. *The American Journal of Occupational Therapy, 39*(9), 596–599.

Shochat, T., Tzischinksy, O., & Engel-Yeger, B. (2009). Sensory hypersensitivity as a contributing factor in the relation between sleep and behavioral disorders in normal schoolchildren. *Behavioral Sleep Medicine, 7,* 53–62.

Silver, L. (1990). Attention deficit hyperactivity disorder: Is it a learning disability or a related disorder? *Journal of Learning Disabilities, 23*(7), 394–397.

Stahl, C. (1995). Solving the riddle of ADHD. *Advance for Occupational Therapists, 11*(7), 15–50.

Wilbarger, P., & Wilbarger, J. L. (1991). *Sensory defensiveness in children aged two to twelve: An intervention guide for parents and other caretakers.* Santa Barbara, CA: Avante Educational Programs.

Williams, M., & Shellenberger, S. (1996). *How does your engine run? A leader's guide to the Alert Program for Self-Regulation* (Rev. ed.). Albuquerque, NM: Therapy Works, Inc.

Yochman, A., Parush, S., & Ornoy, A. (2004). Responses of preschool children with and without ADHD to sensory events in daily life. *The American Journal of Occupational Therapy, 58*(3), 294–302.

Zavik, J., & Thompson, J. (2002). *Toxic food syndrome.* Fort Lauderdale, FL: Fun Publishing.

# Cerebral Palsy

*Meryl S. Cooperman*
*Roberta T. Ciocco*
*Deborah Humpl*

## 🦋 Synopsis of Clinical Condition

### Prevalence and Etiology

The term *cerebral palsy* is used to describe neuromuscular dysfunction associated with nonprogressive static encephalopathy. It occurs in 1.5 to 2.5 of every 1,000 births (Hirtz et al., 2007) and is the leading cause of disability that affects function and development in children (Thorogood, 2001). Low birth weight and lower gestational age are risk factors associated with cerebral palsy, and this condition is often diagnosed if a child does not meet expected motor milestones by 1 year of age. However, the initial insult to the brain may occur within the first 2 years of life and still be classified as cerebral palsy. Table 6.1 lists possible causes of cerebral palsy (Ratanawongsa, 2001; Thorogood, 2001). In order to offer timely and appropriate treatment, it is important to differentiate cerebral palsy from other conditions, such as the following:

- acid maltase deficiency myopathy
- acute poliomyelitis
- Becker muscular dystrophy
- Charcot–Marie–Tooth disease
- Kugelberg Welander spinal muscular atrophy
- lacunar stroke
- limb-girdle muscular dystrophy
- multiple sclerosis
- obstetric brachial plexus injuries
- postpolio syndrome
- posttraumatic syringomyelia
- spasticity

- pediatric stroke
- traumatic brain injury
- developmental coordination disorder
- mitochondrial disease
- chromosomal anomalies
- Angelman syndrome

## Common Characteristics and Symptoms

The status of muscle tone in the extremities is used to classify the type, distribution, and severity of cerebral palsy. Muscle tone, the state of the muscle during rest and movement, should vary according to activity. Children with cerebral palsy have difficulties with the degree of muscle activation at rest (increased or decreased tone), static (postural control), and dynamic tone (modulation of tone). The location of the brain lesion determines the type of tonal dysfunction and the type of cerebral palsy.

The three main types of cerebral palsy are spastic, dyskinetic, and ataxic. The fourth type is flaccid, or hypotonic, but this presentation is believed to be transient or a component of the other three types. The distribution of the motor dysfunction and the degree of involvement are used to further delineate the presentation of cerebral palsy (Gordon, Schanzenbacher, Case-Smith, & Carrasco, 1996; Ratanawongsa, 2001; Scherzer & Tscharnuter, 1982; Thorogood, 2001).

The distribution of the muscle tone ranges from involvement of the entire body to involvement of a single limb. *Quadriplegia* indicates involvement of the four extremities, trunk, and oral motor area. *Diplegia* refers to greater involvement of the lower extremities than of the upper extremities. *Hemiplegia* is used to describe involvement in one side of the body, with the upper extremity typically involved more than the lower extremity. Involvement of only one limb is called *monoplegia*.

**Table 6.1** Possible Causes of Cerebral Palsy

| Prenatal | Neonatal | Postnatal |
|---|---|---|
| Intrauterine infections | Prematurity (<32 weeks) | Trauma |
| Congenital malformations | Low birth weight (<2500 grams) | Infection |
| Toxic or teratogenic agents | Growth retardation | Intracranial hemorrhage |
| Multiple births | Periventricular-intracranial hemorrhage | Coagulopathies |
| Abdominal trauma (mother) | Trauma | |
| Maternal illness | Infection | |
| | Bradycardia and hypoxia | |
| | Seizures | |
| | Hyperbilirbinrmia | |
| | Abnormal birthing presentations | |

Cerebral palsy is further classified by the degree of involvement for each type. The terms *mild*, *moderate*, and *severe* are used to describe the amount of impairment. A child may be described as having severe spastic quadriplegia, mild ataxia, or moderate right hemiplegic athetosis. These descriptions help health care professionals target interventions appropriately, since the term *cerebral palsy* describes a broad array of conditions and functional levels.

Although cerebral palsy is defined based on motor dysfunction, a sensory impairment often coexists. The sensory impairment can be loss of the sensation from the area of brain damage; altered functioning of a sensory system, such as vision and hearing; sensory processing difficulties; or impaired sensory feedback from movement differences (Erhardt & Merrill, 1998).

Spastic cerebral palsy, the most common form of cerebral palsy, makes up 70% to 80% of the cases (Thorogood, 2001). The primary area of the lesion is in the cerebral cortex. The distribution can be quadriplegic, diplegic, hemiplegic, or monoplegic. Spastic cerebral palsy is characterized by increased tone in the extremities. The trunk can be either hypo- or hypertonic. The child has difficulty with the end ranges of movement and consequently only moves in the midranges. Postural control and stability is often diminished, and the child does not have sufficient proximal stability to maximize function of the extremities. Movements are slow, require effort, and incorporate synergistic movement patterns. The limited movement patterns and the midrange movement often lead to a loss of range of motion and contractures of joints (Bierman, 1991; Erhardt & Merrill, 1998; Gordon et al., 1996).

Dyskinetic (also known as athetoid or dystonic) cerebral palsy is caused by a lesion in the basal ganglia, and it makes up 10% to 15% of the cases of cerebral palsy. The distribution is most frequently quadriplegic with occasional hemiplegia. Dyskinesia with tonic spasms may also be present in a monoplegic distribution. Children with dyskinetic cerebral palsy move from one end range to another (full flexion to full extension) and are unable to sustain movement in midranges. They have difficulty with co-contraction for balance of muscle function around a joint and with postural control. They may use asymmetrical postures for stability (Boehme, 1987; Gordon et al., 1996).

Ataxia, which occurs when the lesion is in the cerebellar region, accounts for less than 5% of the cases of cerebral palsy. The distribution is quadriplegic. Ataxia is characterized by poor postural control and decreased tone of the trunk. Tremors are often observed distally (Boehme, 1987).

Children with flaccid tone present with poor postural control and increased mobility around joints (Boehme, 1994). The child has difficulty assuming and maintaining positions against gravity. Flaccidity often evolves into other forms of cerebral palsy or becomes part of a mixed form, such as athetosis with hypotonicity. Table 6.2 depicts some of the common characteristics of cerebral palsy by type. Children with milder forms may have less of the difficulties described in the table (Erhardt & Merrill, 1998; Gordon et al., 1996).

**Table 6.2** Characteristics of Cerebral Palsy

| Domain | Type of cerebral palsy | | |
| | Spastic | Dyskinetic | Flaccid |
|---|---|---|---|
| Movement | Moves in midranges | Moves in end ranges | Hypermobility |
| | More involved and increased risk of contractures/deformities | Decreased midrange control | Subluxation of joints |
| | Synergistic movement patterns | | |
| Reflexes and reactions | Reflexive movement patterns | Decreased equilibrium and righting reactions | Delays in protective, righting, and equilibrium reactions |
| Oral motor and respiration | Shallow respiration | Difficulties with volume of speech | Soft voice |
| | Decreased lip closure | | Decreased respiration |
| | Tongue thrust | Feeding difficulties | Drooling |
| | Difficult verbal communication | | Difficulties with facial expressions |
| | Feeding difficulties | | |
| Personality characteristics | Passive | Emotionally labile | Visually attentive |
| | Dependent | May get frustrated | Decreased motivation |

Cognitive limitations; visual deficits; hearing impairments; communication disorders; respiratory, feeding, digestive, and elimination difficulties; and seizures are conditions that may be associated with cerebral palsy (Gordon et al., 1996; see Table 6.3). Individuals with spastic quadriplegic, ataxic, or dyskinetic cerebral palsy are more likely to have a secondary condition. The more severe the cerebral palsy, the more likely the presence of other conditions. The Gross Motor Function Classification System has been found to be a helpful measurement instrument to identify individuals at risk for comorbidities (Shevell, Dagenais, & Hall, 2009).

In addition to the associated medical conditions of cerebral palsy, there are conditions resulting from the motoric deficit. Children with cerebral palsy often lack the variety of ways to move that are available to typical children because of weakness and lack of muscle tone. Since children want to move, limitations in the variety of movement patterns can lead to compensations, which become habits and may lead to contractures and, eventually, deformities (Alexander, Boehme, Cupps, & Kliebhan, 2009). The more severe the motoric deficit, the greater likelihood of abnormal motor development in the child with cerebral palsy.

## Target Areas for Intervention

Occupational therapists who work with children with cerebral palsy need to have an awareness of the interventions that are available across the different settings since the child may be receiving therapy and medical interventions in more than

**Table 6.3** Conditions Associated With Types of Cerebral Palsy

| Spastic | Dyskinetic | Ataxic | Flaccid |
|---|---|---|---|
| Seizures | Hearing loss | Nystagmus | Obesity |
| Cortical blindness | | Cognitive limitations | Sensory impairment |
| Deafness | | Sensory impairment | Prone to upper |
| Prone to upper respiratory infections | | Reliance on vision to assist with movement | respiratory infections |
| Cognitive limitations | | | |
| Imbalanced eye musculature | | | |
| Perceptual problems | | | |
| Learning disabilities | | | |
| Gastrointestinal difficulties | | | |

one setting. In the medical or rehabilitation setting, the occupational therapist may provide therapy as follow-up to medical intervention. Medical interventions for spasticity may include oral medication, botulinum toxin injection, or a surgically implanted intrathecal baclofen pump that releases medication in the body. A *rhizotomy* is a surgical procedure that reduces lower extremity spasticity and can facilitate lower extremity dressing, transfer skills, and postural control. Other surgical interventions include tendon releases, tendon transfers, osteotomies, and procedures to stabilize joints. Tendon releases and tendon transfers help to restore balance around a joint. An osteotomy changes the position of the bone alignment. Procedures to stabilize joints (arthrodesis) provide a fixed position for a joint. Other nontraditional medical interventions being explored by families include hyperbaric oxygen chambers and cord blood transplants. These interventions have not yet been scientifically proven to be effective and could pose a danger if not administered properly.

Rehabilitation-based interventions frequently include neurodevelopmental therapy and training in activities of daily living (ADL) skills. Other interventions that may be used in conjunction with neurodevelopmental therapy include dynamic splints or serial casting to improve range of motion (Yasukawa, 1992). Adaptive devices to help with mobility and daily living skills may also be the focus of treatment. Research is being conducted on the use of electrical stimulation at sensory levels and motor levels to determine its effectiveness with children with cerebral palsy. Treatments that were initially used for stroke rehabilitation are also being used for hemiplegia, including constraint-induced movement therapy (Facchin et al., 2009) and robotic therapy (Fasoli, Fragali-Pinkham, Hughes, Hogan, & Krebs, 2008). Kinesio Taping, TheraTogs, and dynamic Lycra suits may be incorporated into therapy programs. Equine-facilitated therapy (horseback riding), hydrotherapy, Interactive Metronome, yoga, and Pilates can also be used in the treatment of cerebral palsy.

In the preschool and school setting, the focus of treatment is on helping the child access an education in the least restrictive environment. The focus of occupational therapy intervention may include environmental accessibility, assistive technology, written communication, school-related self-care, seating, management of school supplies, and the development of home-based activity programs. Accessibility interventions may include an emergency evacuation plan or a recommendation for a wheelchair-accessible desk or table. Written communication skills may require accommodations ranging from low technology, such as a slant board, to high technology, such as a computer with specialty software. Occupational therapists employed in early intervention settings work within the family routines to promote the child's development of skills.

The occupational therapist has many opportunities to enhance the life of a person with cerebral palsy. ADL skills are a main focus for intervention. ADL skills need to be addressed over the lifetime of a client with cerebral palsy, progressing from basic dressing, mobility skills, and toileting issues, to more complex issues, such as driving and meal preparation. Accessibility should be considered along with ADL training. The occupational therapist can play an important part in educating the child and family about universal design and can provide resources to help them plan for current and future needs. Technology for seating and positioning, environmental control, and communication are areas that often need to be addressed with this population. Although some children ambulate with braces, they may have difficulty with navigating in the community. As these children get older and larger, ambulation may become less efficient as a primary means of mobility.

Children with cerebral palsy can exhibit delayed developmental skills. They often lack normal environmental opportunities that other children experience, in addition to the possible neurological causes of developmental delay. Perceptual skills, fine motor coordination, play skills, body awareness, and social skills are possible areas of weakness for children with cerebral palsy. They are also often at risk for low self-esteem and emotional problems.

# 🐾 Contextual Considerations
## Clinical

The clinical evaluation should include information regarding the sensorimotor status, musculoskeletal integrity, developmental status, and daily living skills of the child. A good understanding of the child's functional abilities helps to determine the type of intervention and equipment that may be needed and the level of impact that the child's disability has on the family.

The sensorimotor evaluation includes assessment of range of motion; muscle tone; and strength and sensation of the upper extremities, trunk, lower extremities, and oral musculature. The therapist needs to identify the area or areas most affected; differentiate between problems of spasticity, contracture, and dystonia, or distinguish hypotonia from weakness; evaluate balance reactions and postural control; and ascertain the level of reflex integration and determine its impact on functional performance. For example, a child who has not integrated the grasp reflex may have difficulty voluntarily releasing objects from the hand.

Sensory impairment is often associated with cerebral palsy and is frequently noted in persons with hemiplegia. The degree of sensory impairment is related to functional potential and spontaneity of use in the involved limb. Two-point discrimination and stereognosis are frequently used to evaluate sensation. It is important to evaluate sensation preoperatively if upper extremity surgical intervention is being considered.

The hemiplegic child poses a challenge for functional assessment because hemiplegia is a unilateral problem that typically affects the nondominant extremity. Many upper extremity assessments evaluate either dominant unilateral function or the accomplishment of a specific skill. It is helpful to evaluate the involved extremity for its functional use as an assist to the dominant extremity. The best way to assess functional use is by informal observation during functional activities and assessment of the various degrees of thumb and palm deformity, a problem often associated with cerebral palsy because of muscular imbalance around the thumb (House, Gwathmey, & Fidler, 1981). The *Assisting Hand Assessment* (Krumlinde-Sundholm, Holmefur, & Eliasson, 2007) is used to evaluate assistive hand function for children from ages 18 months to 12 years.

There are many developmental assessments available. A general developmental assessment, such as the *Peabody Developmental Motor Scales–Second Edition* (Folio & Fewell, 2000), the *Hawaii Early Learning Profile* (Furuno et al., 1991), or the *Learning Accomplishment Profile–Revised Edition* (Glover, Preminger, & Sanford, 1995), will provide information for the infant or preschool-age child. Modifications may be necessary for children with significant motor involvement, and, in some cases, some tests will not be able to be used at all. The *Carolina Curriculum for Handicapped Infants and Infants at Risk* (Johnson-Martin, Jens, Attermeier, & Hacker, 1991), the *INFANIB* (Ellison, 1994), the *Erhardt Developmental Prehension Assessment–Third Edition* (Erhardt, 1994), the *Erhardt Developmental Vision Assessment* (Erhardt, 1989), or the *Pediatric Evaluation of Disability Inventory* (Haley, Coster, Ludlow, Haltiwanger, & Andrellos, 1992) may be more appropriate for children with more significant motor impairment.

Children of school age can be evaluated using an assessment of visual–motor skills, perceptual skills, and fine and gross motor coordination. Common assessments include the *Beery–Buktenica Developmental Test of Visual–Motor Integration* (Beery, Buketnica, & Beery, 2010), the *Motor-Free Visual Perception Test–Third Edition* (Collarusso & Hammill, 2003), the *Test of Visual Perceptual Skills–Third Edition* (Martin, 2006), the *Jebsen Hand Function Test* (Jebsen, Taylor, Trieschmann, Trotter, & Howard, 1969), the *Melbourne Assessment of Unilateral Upper Limb Function–Revised* (Randall & Johnson, 1995), the *Quality of Upper Extremity Skills Test* (DeMatteo, Law, Russell, Pollack, Rosenbaum, & Walter, 1992), the *Bruininks–Oseretsky Test of Motor Proficiency–Second*

*Edition* (Bruininks & Bruininks, 2006), the *Gross Motor Function Measure* (Russell et al., 1989), the *Pediatric Evaluation of Disability Inventory* (Haley et al., 1992), and the *Miller Function and Participation Scales* (Miller, 2006). It may be necessary to modify or eliminate use of some of the evaluations of motor coordination for children with significant motor impairment.

A developmental ADL checklist can be helpful for children under the age of 3 years, but these assessments often do not accommodate the child with a physical limitation. A rehabilitation-based checklist may incorporate the use of adaptive equipment. The *Functional Independence Measure* (State University of New York, 1993) and the *Functional Independence Measure for Children* (Hamilton & Granger, 1991) provide information on many areas and are often used in research. This type of assessment groups many skills together, which can affect its sensitivity to discreet functional changes and its usefulness in short-term treatment. The *School Function Assessment* (Coster, Deeney, Haltiwanger, & Haley, 1998) is an interview-based instrument that is useful in the examination of ADL and school-related functional skills.

Since children with cerebral palsy often display oral motor impairment, any ADL assessment should address oral motor skills, such as lip closure, jaw and tongue control, and hand-to-mouth coordination. Feeding difficulties can be a major source of frustration and stress for families because feeding a child with significant oral motor impairment can be very time-consuming and emotionally draining. Seating and positioning of the child at mealtime has to be a prime consideration with this population. Various adaptive utensils may be used to increase success for self-feeding. Equipment such as coated spoons and cutout cups can also make a caregiver's job easier. When evaluating ADL skills by taking a caregiver report, the interviewer can also use the opportunity to establish rapport with the caregiver and gather data regarding other aspects of the family context, as discussed in the next section.

## Family

The family's values, priorities, and cultural preferences must always be considered. Information can be gathered using an informal interview. Open-ended questions may be more helpful than a yes/no checklist. This approach helps establish rapport with the family and may help the therapist gain information that might otherwise be overlooked. For example, "Tell me about a typical day," with supporting questions such as, "Does anybody help you get dressed?" or "What kinds of food do you like to eat?" can provide information on family routines in addition to ADL.

Families of children with cerebral palsy often express facing challenges coping with their own extended family and with community reactions to their child's disability. It is especially difficult for children and adolescents to deal with problems associated with oral motor dysfunction. Drooling, unclear speech, and difficulty chewing and swallowing can be difficult to accept in a public or community environment. Children with cerebral palsy may have very obvious gait deviations or may rely on adaptive devices, such as crutches, walkers, or wheelchairs, to get around in the community. This poses problems with accessibility and may limit their opportunities for interaction with nondisabled peers.

Children with cerebral palsy may have different needs for assistive devices during the transition from young childhood to school-age childhood, to adolescence, and to adulthood. The therapist needs to help the family and child determine what works best in each situation. The occupational therapist also needs to demonstrate sensitivity while gathering information about family resources, including medical coverage, formal and informal support groups, and information/educational resources. The occupational therapist can be a primary or secondary provider of information about coverage for medical expenses, support groups, special education, and rehabilitation laws. The information gathered may indicate that the family would like and benefit from referral to other professionals, agencies, or community programs for supportive help or additional resources.

The occupational therapist must be aware of future needs in order to provide the guidance necessary for addressing current needs. The family of the child who requires medical equipment such as wheelchairs, positioning equipment, orthotics, and splints must be made aware of reimbursement issues for medical equipment. Many third-party payers (e.g., insurance, medical assistance) will provide services on a limited basis, provide one-per-lifetime coverage, or not cover durable medical equipment. The occupational therapist providing services individually or as part of a team can help select the appropriate equipment. The family may need information on alternate funding sources to help with expenses not covered by the family's insurance plan.

## Practice Setting

Individuals with cerebral palsy often require occupational therapy in acute care hospitals, rehabilitation hospitals, rehabilitation outpatient facilities, early intervention (such as home day care) settings, preschools, and school-based settings. In all of these settings, the occupational therapist functions as a member of a multidisciplinary team composed of professionals from disciplines such as developmental neurology, orthopedic medicine, nursing, physical therapy, social work, psychology, therapeutic recreation, speech–language pathology, and special education. Family members and other primary caregivers are important team members. Parents may be confused about the roles of the various professionals involved in their child's care, and that confusion may be compounded if the child is receiving services from different settings simultaneously. It is important to establish and maintain communication between therapists, family, and other members of the team to ensure consistency of care and facilitate transitions between service settings as the child matures.

The acute care therapist may first encounter the individual with cerebral palsy in the neonatal nursery or through the high-risk follow-up programs. The parents should be provided with education and information about arranging therapy assistance in the community. The occupational therapist must work with other professionals to assist the family with coping with and preparing for a child with special needs. Positioning and handling techniques are important for caregivers to know in order to reduce spasticity and facilitate functional ability. *Finnie's Handling the Young Child With Cerebral Palsy at Home* (Bower, 2009) is an excellent resource. These children may also be prone to oral motor difficulties that impair feeding abilities. The therapist should have special training or knowledge to provide intervention related to oral motor skills. Oral motor intervention often falls within the purview of speech therapy. Occupational therapy intervention may focus on facilitating strength in trunk and upper extremity musculature, postural control, and adapted positioning.

The rehabilitation hospital–based occupational therapist often provides therapy services for a specific period of time following a surgical procedure or pharmacological intervention, or for specific rehabilitation goals. The child may have a rehabilitation admission for postoperative rehabilitation, ADL training, or adaptive equipment training. Occupational therapists and other members of the rehabilitation team would provide coordinated intervention for the identified needs based on support of the surgical or pharmacological intervention. For example, a child whose status post surgery requires hamstring releases and hip adductor muscle releases will usually have difficulty donning pants while sitting or in a long sit. The therapy goals and treatment can be tailored to facilitate stretching the hamstrings and hip adductors while teaching the child to reach to feet for socks or pants while sitting in a corner to support compromised balance. A clinical follow-up program may be based at the rehabilitation hospital. Periodic follow-up is important for children with cerebral palsy. As they grow and develop, there is potential for problems associated with joint contractures and deformity from muscle imbalances. The clinic-based therapist in the rehabilitation hospital should also be able to assist the child and family with transitioning to an adult setting for needed services.

The outpatient-based occupational therapist often provides ongoing services to help the child develop gross motor, fine motor, perceptual, visual–motor, social, play, sensory processing, ADL, and oral motor skills. The therapist may also make recommendations and facilitate the acquisition of special equipment. Since the child is often seen only once a week, the development of home programs that are designed to be implemented by parents and caregivers is essential for the child's ongoing developmental progress.

Occupational therapists working in an early intervention program may provide home-based and/or community-based services. The focus of intervention would be working in partnership with the family to foster skills that enable the child to participate in typical family routines and in their community. The therapist works with the family to enhance gross and fine motor skills, visual–motor and perceptual skills, play skills, sensory processing skills, oral motor skills, and

ADL skills, which impact the child's daily routines and school readiness. Therapists in this setting may also be involved with seating and positioning issues and with using assistive technology to facilitate communication and environmental access.

The school-based therapist provides therapy with an emphasis on the skills needed in the school environment. The school therapist can work collaboratively with the rehabilitation or outpatient-based therapist as well as the classroom teacher in order to establish educationally relevant intervention plans. The focus of the school therapist, in accordance with the Individuals With Disabilities Education Act (IDEA, 1997), is to be a supportive service to enable full participation in the school program and successful transition to adulthood. The child with cerebral palsy may experience perceptual and visual–motor delays, as well as sensory processing problems. These may interfere with mobility, social skills, self-care, and the ability to manage school-related tools and supplies. For the child to participate in all aspects of the educational process with nondisabled peers, a variety of assistive technologies may be required. Therapists need to collaborate with technological support personnel and other members of the team in the development of high-tech and low-tech strategies for proper seating and positioning, environmental access, mobility, and written communication.

## Sociopolitical

There are three primary laws that relate to children with cerebral palsy. These laws relate to education, rehabilitation, and accessibility. The Individuals With Disabilities Education Act (IDEA, 1997) mandates that all children are entitled to a free and appropriate education in the least restrictive environment. The Rehabilitation Act (1973) ensures the equal rights of individuals with disabilities in all institutions, agencies, or organizations that receive federal funding or financial assistance. The Americans With Disabilities Act (ADA) guarantees equal opportunities for employment, accessibility, transportation, and government services. Additional legislation includes the Technology Act and the Vocational Rehabilitation Service Act (Technology Related Assistance for Individuals With Disabilities Act, 1988; Vocational Rehabilitation Service Act, 1973).

The child with cerebral palsy has a legal right to be educated with his nondisabled peers. He has the right to appropriate technology to help him benefit from his education, with the goal of participating in the mainstream of society following completion of his educational program. IDEA mandates the development of a plan that facilitates the transition from school to work when the child is 16 years old. The school-based transition plan encompasses community living, employment, and socialization and is informed by the abilities, interests, needs, and goals of the student. Vocational rehabilitation services mandated by the Vocational Rehabilitation Service Act assist the child with cerebral palsy in entering the world of work after completing school.

**Table 6.4** Lifestyle/Lifespan Factors

| Accessibility | Financial | Medical | Family | Social |
|---|---|---|---|---|
| Home<br>School<br>Community<br>Driving/<br>transportation | Daily supplies and medicine<br>Home modifications<br>Durable medical equipment<br>Special driving/<br>transportation equipment or needs | Surgery to enhance function or prevent or correct deformity<br>Require periodic follow-up for issues of growth and new equipment<br>Medications to manage muscle tone | Increased time for daily care<br>Coping<br>Sibling relationships<br>Care of caregivers | Interaction with peers<br>Adaptive sports<br>Leisure activities |

## Lifestyle/Lifespan

It is important to make the individual and the family aware of issues that the individual with cerebral palsy will face throughout his or her lifetime. These issues may relate to accessibility or to the financial, medical, family, and social aspects of life. Table 6.4 highlights the issues discussed in this section. Although the issues are discussed separately, there is often overlap.

Accessibility issues for home modifications for a child with a cerebral palsy often include assistive devices to maximize function. For example, a buttonhook, a tub transfer bench, positioning equipment, or a wheelchair may facilitate independence. Extensive home modifications may be necessary for a child with significant motor impairment. Specialized evaluation, training, and adaptations may be needed for driving. Some adolescents or young adults may not have the potential for driving and may require special equipment, such as a van with a wheelchair lift, for transport.

Financial issues will vary depending on the family's economic resources. Insurance may not cover the cost of some supplies, and this will affect household budgets. It is important to remember that families generally meet needs based on priorities for survival, with food and shelter being first on the list. Clothing and daily medical equipment may come next. Insurance reimbursement often has limitations, and money for medical equipment, adaptive equipment, and orthosis may have to be found. The occupational therapist needs to be aware of resources for the family and about equipment that can "grow" with the child to promote maximum use during the child's growing years. The focus of the needs of children with cerebral palsy may also change as they grow. It is important to recognize that the use of equipment may vary over the lifetime of the child.

The child with mild cerebral palsy is often able to participate in typical community programs with minimal adaptations. Encouragement to participate in sports will be beneficial to the child for physical fitness and peer relationship reasons. Children with more severe involvement may require specialized programs or accommodations to participate in sports or other community activities.

Teenagers and young adults with cerebral palsy may also have enough cognitive and motor capability to participate in some type of prevocational training

**Table 6.5** Functional Impact of Performance Components on the Client Trying to Obtain a Career

| Skill area | Considerations |
|---|---|
| Gross motor skills and transfers | Can the client reach for supplies overhead and on the ground and move from point A to point B independently while carrying items? |
| Fine motor skills | Can the client assemble small parts, type, utilize a checklist inventory form, or operate phone systems? |
| Self-care | Is an aide needed for toileting and lunch breaks? Does the client have awareness of appropriate work attire |
| Cognitive skills | Can the client recall all steps to a new task, or will he or she need visual or auditory aides? Can the client get to work independently? |
| Perceptual skills | Can the client see and process all of the task items and place them in the appropriate places? |
| Social skills | Does the client have appropriate customer service skills and general politeness? Does he or she know how to discuss issues at the workplace? |
| Instrumental ADL skills | Has the client followed a routine of preparing a lunch and doing chores? |

program, if they are not headed to college after high school. These programs, which are designed to prepare students to join the workforce, may start as programming in the local high school or as a transition program with the guidance counselor at a local vocational rehabilitation office. It is important for the therapist to guide the client toward a career that will lead to the most success (see Table 6.5 for some considerations).

# Clinical Decision-Making Process

## Defining Focus for Intervention

The practice setting helps to determine the focus of intervention. For example, the child in a school setting may require intervention for the development of visual perceptual skills, handwriting, fine motor and bilateral hand coordination, and self-care skills related to the school environment. Activity programs—based on an assessment of ADL status, range of motion, strength, motor coordination, cognitive abilities, perceptual status, social skills, and adaptive equipment requirements—that are designed for home-based intervention may need to be continued during a child's hospitalizations. Children with cerebral palsy may benefit from short rehabilitation admissions or outpatient services to work on ADL skills. These admissions may be required periodically as the child is developmentally able to take on more responsibility for self-care. Transfers, wheelchair mobility, dressing, and bathing are some of the skills that are typical targets for intervention.

The age and developmental level of the child indicate the nature of the intervention services required. Family education and support, with a focus on the developmental and physical needs of the child, is paramount for the infant newly diagnosed with cerebral palsy. In the preschool years, environmental exploration and mobility issues often need to be addressed. Independent mobility, with or without assistive devices, has a positive impact on a disabled child's cognitive and emotional well-being. As noted above, the school-age child may need intervention related to learning difficulties or visual perceptual impairment. Self-care skills usually need ongoing attention across the lifespan.

The advent of adolescence presents physical, social, and emotional challenges for the child with cerebral palsy. Weight gain and growth can exacerbate mobility problems. Individuals who have ambulated with lower extremity braces as young children may find that they are unable to continue as functional community ambulators and may need to use a wheelchair. Unless appropriate adaptations are made, children with cerebral palsy may have fewer opportunities for interaction with the community. The adolescent with cerebral palsy is at risk of becoming isolated and demoralized at the stage where the development of peer networks and feelings of personal competence are crucial. Successful transition to adulthood may depend on the development of competence in home management skills, community mobility, and peer interactions. Strategies such as adapting a van for transportation, engaging in pet-assisted living, and initiating involvement in church and community and/or special interest groups may facilitate the transition to adulthood. Advances in technology are creating new opportunities for many individuals with disabilities through online resources.

## Establishing Goals for Intervention

The setting in which services are being delivered often dictates the amount of time available for service provision and defines the scope of intervention. The chronological and developmental age of the child also influences the goals that are established. It is important to consider the normal developmental progression, the functional level of the child when establishing goals, and the needs and interests of the child and the family. The neuromuscular and physical data from the evaluation, combined with information on cognitive and perceptual skills, will help to define treatment goals. For example, a child with moderate cerebral palsy and minimal cognitive deficits may learn to use a power wheelchair for independent mobility; however, a child with moderate cerebral palsy and severe cognitive limitations may be dependent on a caregiver for transport in a manual wheelchair. Family attitudes, cultural practices, and values need to be considered. The physical environment is also an important consideration. Accessibility issues may influence the priority of a goal or dictate the level of independence that is realistic to expect. For example, if the child uses a wheelchair for mobility and is unable to access the bathroom, independent toothbrushing may not be possible. Sociopolitical factors and lifestyle implications may also influence treatment goals. Reimbursement issues and relevant legislation may dictate the length or frequency of treatment and the consequent prioritization of treatment goals.

Goals are also based on the medical intervention that the child receives. The child may have surgical intervention to improve range of motion and balance and surgically create muscle balance around a joint to enhance function. An example would be lengthening or release of a muscle such as the adductor pollicus brevis and transfer of the flexor carpi ulnaris to the extensor carpi radialus brevis to facilitate thumb and wrist extension to enhance the grasp of objects. Postoperative management would include scar management, splinting, range of motion, muscle strengthening, muscle reeducation, and functional skill training.

## Designing Theory-Based Intervention

There are many theoretical frameworks in occupational therapy that can be used to provide services for children with cerebral palsy. Theory selection should be guided by the use of evidence-based practice and the World Health Organization's International Classification of Functioning, Disability, and Health. The following descriptions and examples of how different theories might be applied should not be considered an all-inclusive list.

Many treatment approaches are influenced by the model of human occupation (Kielhofner, 2008), which focuses on the development and maintenance of the roles and behaviors associated with daily routines, consistent with the values of the individual. This approach assists the therapist in developing intervention strategies that are relevant to, and facilitative of, the child's myriad role requirements—as sibling, student, son, daughter, worker, and/or community member.

Developmental theories and/or frames of reference focus on the patterns of skill acquisition as progressive and predictable. Children with cerebral palsy face many obstacles and interruptions in the development of skills related to the primary motor problems and secondary associated conditions. The therapist employs an understanding of normal development to assist the child in the design of treatment programs that provide for the progressive acquisition of the skills that are the substrate for functional activity. Other useful approaches include neurodevelopmental therapy and sensory integration. Neurodevelopmental treatment is a sensorimotor approach that is often the approach of choice for the child with cerebral palsy, although studies have not firmly established its effectiveness (Sharkey, 2002). Handling techniques and positioning principles are used to influence the sensorimotor system and foster the development of postural control, equilibrium and righting reactions, and a larger repertoire of movement patterns. In this approach, sensory input is used to prepare the body for the movement, facilitate the use of weak muscles, inhibit muscles with increased tone, and increase the variety of movement patterns. Examples of sensory input include tapping for facilitation of a muscle, weight bearing for co-contraction, and neutral warmth for inhibition of a muscle. Neurodevelopmental techniques are used to facilitate the development of motor skills in the child and to help a caregiver position the child to complete daily care needs.

Sensory integration is another theoretical approach that may be helpful when working with this population. These children may display sensory processing problems, sensory registration and modulation problems, and sensory defensiveness. Sensory integration treatment principles are often helpful when combined with neurodevelopmental therapy techniques.

Children with cerebral palsy also may benefit from treatment based on the rehabilitation or biomechanical frame of reference as a part of their therapy program. The rehabilitation frame of reference focuses on the performance of ADL skills using compensatory methods, technology, and environmental adaptations (Dutton, 1995). Occupational therapy intervention may include the use of splints and serial casting to improve range of motion and mitigate limitations of motor function. It may also include adaptive techniques and assistive devices, such as pencil grips, soap holders, and adapted eating utensils, to compensate for these limitations. The biomechanical frame of reference considers how range of motion, muscle strength, and endurance are related to the completion of purposeful activities (Dutton, 1995). These approaches are helpful in addressing the physical limitations presented by children with cerebral palsy and should be used in combination with other approaches that consider the other sensory and motor impairments that often coexist in these children.

Motor learning theories are also used in treatment approaches for children with cerebral palsy. Treatment is based on structured practice and feedback, fostering the development and refinement of specific motoric patterns, such as grasp patterns. This treatment may also help develop motor behaviors, such as writing, which incorporate clusters of motor patterns.

Learning theory and rehabilitation theory are often combined to teach ADL skills to the child with cerebral palsy. For example, it may be necessary to break a task such as buttoning into small steps that are taught sequentially and to use an assistive device to achieve independence with buttoning.

In conclusion, treatment should be based on several theories that foster the development of roles and occupations, motor skills, and functional skills, as well as developmental and learning principles. A treatment session may begin with handling techniques from neurodevelopmental therapy to prepare for movement that increases range of motion. The biomechanical frame of reference may then be employed through the use of strengthening strategies to support postural control and increase the variety of movement patterns. Once postural control is established, reaching into a shirtsleeve (for the development of ADL skills from the rehabilitation frame of reference) may be the first step to donning a pullover shirt. The activity may be approached using learning perspectives to introduce the task in small parts. Learning to don a shirt and complete ADL is a role/occupation of a growing child and part of the occupational behavioral theoretical models.

## Evaluating Progress

Meeting established goals (usually annual long-term and short-term objectives) is the most tangible method of evaluating progress. Measurable goals typically focus on improving motor abilities and enhancing developmental skills, including self-care and the integration and use of appropriate equipment or technology in the child's daily life. In the clinic setting, repeated measures such as the *Functional Independence Measure for Children* (Hamilton & Granger, 1991) or the *Pediatric Evaluation of Disability Inventory* (Haley et al., 1992) will help to monitor the changes that occur over time. Video recording can be a powerful tool to evaluate subtle progress that is not measurable on standardized tests. Family members and caregivers can also provide insight into significant or less significant improvements by reporting changes in the child's behavior or accomplishments at home. For example, positive changes in the child's mood or temperament, increases in incidents of successful coping behaviors, or the increased ease with which a parent can dress a child may be indicative of improvement.

## Determining Change in or Termination of Treatment

Change in or termination of treatment is warranted when the child does not appear to be capable of meeting an established goal or when the child has met an established goal. In either event, the therapist needs to reevaluate the situation to determine whether the goals should be modified or replaced. The new goal could reflect a change of focus or an adjustment in the expected outcome. Sometimes a particular treatment technique doesn't work for a child. For example, using a therapy ball to develop balance and righting reactions and to help inhibit or facilitate muscle tone and movement patterns is a very common practice. If a child happens to be gravitationally and posturally insecure, he or she may be terrified of being on the ball, and another method of treatment may need to be found, or the treatment of sensory processing issues may need to proceed before work can be done with balance and righting reactions. Discharge from therapy may occur when the child has reached a maximum level of independence for his or her age and has acquired a sufficient level of foundational skills to promote independent problem solving and future skills acquisition.

Occupational therapy may be episodic during the child's lifetime. Occupational therapy may be reinstated when the child is old enough to learn a new skill or to learn the use of new or different technology. Times of transition or change in a child's life may also require therapy services to be modified or techniques to be changed.

## Case Study

### Description

MH is a 5-year-old with cerebral palsy, presenting with moderate left spastic hemiplegia. He ambulates independently with a molded ankle foot orthosis (MAFO) and an abnormal gait. MH has a history of febrile seizures. He was the product of a full-term pregnancy with a complicated delivery. He has a night splint for wrist, thumb, and finger extension and a day splint for wrist extension. The left upper extremity is used as a gross active assist for task-specific activities. Protective reactions on the left are delayed, and righting and equilibrium reactions are impaired. Passive range of motion is limited in the end ranges of thumb abduction, supination, and elbow extension. Active range of motion is limited for shoulder external rotation, shoulder abduction and flexion, elbow extension, wrist extension, supination, and thumb extension. He can grossly extend his fingers to grasp and release an object with a weak grasp and demonstrates poor active assistance. Sensation is difficult to assess because of his age; however, it appears to be diminished. A flexor synergy posture is observed and intensifies with energy and emotion.

MH is in a preschool program and will transition into a school-based kindergarten program next fall. He is doing well, with visual–motor and visual perceptual skill development scores in the 25th percentile on the *Beery–Buktenica Developmental Test of Visual–Motor Integration* (Beery, Buktenica, & Beery, 2010). Fine motor skills are limited for bilateral tasks. He has difficulty with the use of scissors, buttons, and zippers.

MH lives with his mother, father, and younger sister in a two-story house. MH is able to ascend and descend the stairs using a nonreciprocal gait pattern. MH has friends in the neighborhood and tries to participate in typical preschool activities, but he has difficulty with bicycle riding and ball activities.

MH requires assistance for dressing. He has difficulty manipulating fasteners and putting on and removing a pullover shirt, socks, and his MAFO. He is able to put on and remove his pants and shoes. MH receives outpatient occupational therapy services once a week.

### Long- and Short-Term Goals

The long-term goal of intervention for MH is to improve left upper extremity active range of motion and strength in preparation for use as a functional assist for bilateral fine motor activities and self-care skills. This will be accomplished by focusing on the following intervention planning:

1. Increase independence with self-care, in keeping with his peers.
2. Improve passive and active range of motion and strength of the left upper extremity to enhance participation in self-care and home activities.
3. Foster the development of bilateral hand skills with or without assistive devices to use age-appropriate tools, such as scissors.
4. Facilitate socializing and play with neighborhood friends.

The short-term goals of intervention for MH are as follows:

1. Independently put on and take off a pullover shirt, socks, and MAFO splints.
2. Put on and take off a light jacket using an over-the-head method, including zipping and unzipping using a large zipper pull.
3. Cut across a piece of paper on a target line.

### Therapist Goals and Strategies

The therapist's goals include the following:

1. Improve range of motion in the left upper extremity.
2. Improve grasp and release in the left upper extremity.
3. Explore and expand opportunities to play with neighborhood children.

The therapist's strategies include the following:

1. Improve alignment of shoulder girdle and trunk with positioning and handling techniques to reduce muscle tone.
2. Engage in activities that facilitate righting reactions, equilibrium reactions, and weight shift in upper and lower extremities.
3. Work and discuss strategies with caregivers to increase socializing with peers in ways that do not involve balls or bikes.
4. On an ongoing basis, evaluate the effects of splint usage.
5. Provide opportunities for carryover to the home and community environments.
6. Break down new tasks into small parts for learning, and teach this approach to caretakers.
7. Incorporate assistive devices as needed for environmental mastery, communication, and socialization.

*Activity: Theraplast Ice Cream Cones*

Theraputty will be rolled into large balls using both hands. The balls will be placed on top of a cone held like an ice cream cone in the left hand. The right hand will add the "sprinkles" pegs while the left hand holds the cone. The Theraplast ice cream cones will be made by MH and offered to the therapist, to MH's sister, and to his mother. Plans for carryover include MH helping to organize and work at the ice cream table at the block party being planned in the neighborhood.

*Treatment Objective*

MH will sustain grasp on an object with his left hand while manipulating the object with his dominant, right hand.

# Resources

Alliance for Technology Access: www.ataccess.org

American Academy for Cerebral Palsy and Developmental Medicine: www.aacpdm.org

American Occupational Therapy Association: www.aota.org

National Dissemination Center for Children With Disabilities: http://nichcy.org

National Institute of Neurological Disorders and Stroke: www.ninds.nih.gov

Neuro-Developmental Treatment Association (NDTA): www.ndta.org

United Cerebral Palsy: www.ucp.org

# References

Alexander, R., Boehme, R., Cupps, B., & Kliebhan, L. (2009). Motor development in cerebral palsy. In R. Boehm (Ed.), *Approach to treatment of the baby* (pp. 5–14). Milwaukee, WI: Boehm Workshops.

Americans With Disabilities Act of 1990, 42 U.S.C. § 12101 *et seq.* (1990).

Beery, K. E., Buktenica, N. A., & Beery, N. A. (2010). *Beery–Buktenica developmental test of visual–motor integration* (6th ed.). San Antonio, TX: Pearson Assessments.

Bierman, J. (1991). *8-week pediatric NDT certification course* [Lecture notes]. Augusta, GA.

Boehme, R. (1987). *Developing mid range control and function in children with fluctuating muscle tone.* Milwaukee, WI: Boehm Workshops.

Boehme, R. (1994). *The hypotonic child: Treatment for postural control, endurance, strength, and sensory organization.* Milwaukee, WI: Boehm Workshops.

Bower, E. (2009). *Finnie's handling the young cerebral palsied child at home* (4th ed.). Philadelphia, PA: Elsever Mosby/Saunders.

Bruininks, R. H. (2006). *Bruininks–Oseretsky test of motor proficiency* (2nd ed.). San Antonio, TX: Pearson Assessments.

Callarusso, R. P., & Hammill, D. D. (2003). *Motor-free visual perception test* (3rd ed.). Novato, CA: Academic Therapy Publications.

Coster, W., Deeney, T., Haltiwanger, J., & Haley, S. (1998). *School function assessment.* San Antonio, TX: The Psychological Corporation.

DeMatteo, C., Law, M., Russell, D., Pollack, N., Rosenbaum, P., & Walter, S. (1992). *QUEST: Quality of upper extremity skills test.* Hamilton, Ontario, Canada: McMaster University, Neurodevelopmental Clinical Research Unit.

Dutton, R. (1995). *Clinical reasoning in physical disabilities.* Philadelphia, PA: Lippincott, Williams & Wilkins.

Ellison, P. H. (1994). *The INFANIB: A reliable method for the neuromotor assessment of infants.* San Antonio, TX: The Psychological Corporation.

Erhardt, R. P. (1989). *Erhardt developmental vision assessment* (2nd ed.). Maplewood, MN: Erhardt Developmental Products.

Erhardt, R. P. (1994) *Erhardt developmental prehension assessment* (3rd ed.) Maplewood, MN: Erhardt Developmental Products.

Erhardt, R. P., & Merrill, S. C. (1998). Neurological dysfunction in children. In M. E. Neistadt & E. B. Crepeau (Eds.), *Occupational therapy* (9th ed., pp. 582–608). Philadelphia, PA: Lippincott, Williams & Wilkins.

Facchin, P., Rosa-Rizzotto, M., Turconi, A., Pagliano, E., Fazzi, E., Stortini, M., & Fedrizzi, E. (2009). Multisite trial on efficacy of constraint-induced movement therapy in children with hemiplegia: Study design and methodology. *American Journal of Physical Medicine and Rehabilitation, 88*(3), 216–230.

Fasoli, S., Fragali-Pinkham, M., Hughes, R., Hogan, N., & Krebs, H. (2008). Upper limb robotic therapy for children with hemiplegia. *Journal of Physical Medicine and Rehabilitation, 87,* 929–936.

Folio, R., & Fewell, R. (2000). *Peabody developmental motor scales* (2nd ed.). San Antonio, TX: The Psychological Corporation.

Furuno, S., O'Reilly, K. A., Inatsuka, T., Hosaka, C. M., Allman, T. L., & Zeisloft-Fabley, B. (1991). *Hawaii early learning profile.* Palo Alto, CA: VORT.

Glover, M. E., Preminger, J. L., & Sanford, A. R. (1997). *Early learning accomplishments profile for developmentally young children: Birth to 36 months.* New York, NY: Kaplan Press.

Gordon, C. Y., Schanzenbacher, K. E., Case-Smith, J., & Carrasco, R. C. (1996). Diagnostic problems in pediatrics. In J. Case-Smith, A. S. Allen, & P. N. Pratt (Eds.), *Occupational therapy for children* (3rd ed., pp.113–162). St. Louis, MO: Mosby.

Haley, S., Coster, W., Ludlow, L., Haltiwanger, J., & Andrellos, P. (1992). *Pediatric evaluation of disability inventory*. San Antonio, TX: The Psychological Corporation.

Hamilton, B. B., & Granger, C. U. (1991). *Functional independence measure for children (Wee-FIM)*. Buffalo, NY: Research Foundation of the State University of New York.

Hirtz, D., Thurman, D. J., Gwin-Hardy, K., Mohamed, M., Chaudhuri, A. R., & Zalutsky, R. (2007). How common are the "common" neurological disorders? *Neurology, 68,* 326–337.

House, J. H., Gwathmey, F. W., & Fidler, M. O. (1981). A dynamic approach to the thumb-in-palm deformity in cerebral palsy. *Journal of Bone and Joint Surgery, 63A,* 216–225.

Individuals With Disabilities Education Act of 1997, 20 U.S.C. § 1400 *et seq.* (1997).

Jebsen, R. H., Taylor, N., Trieschmann, R. B., Trotter, M. J., & Howard, L. A. (1969). An objective and standardized test of hand function. *Archives of Physical Medicine and Rehabilitation, 50,* 311–319.

Johnson-Martin, N., Jens, K. G., Attermeier, S. M., & Hacker, B. (1991). *The Carolina curriculum for handicapped infants and infants at risk*. Baltimore, MD: Paul H. Brookes.

Kielhofner, G. (2008). *Model of human occupation* (4th ed.). Baltimore, MD: Lippincott, Williams & Wilkins.

Krumlinde-Sundholm, L., Holmefur, M., & Eliasson, A. (2007). *Manual: The Assisting Hand Assessment* (Version 4.4). Stockholm, Sweden: Wily Blackwell.

Martin, N. (2006). *The test of visual perceptual skills* (3rd ed.). Navato, CA: Academic Therapy.

Miller, L. J. (2006). *The Miller function and participation scales*. San Antonio, TX: The Psychological Corporation.

Randall, M., & Johnson, L. (1995). *The Melbourne assessment of unilateral upper limb function–Revised*. Victoria, Australia: Royal Children's Hospital.

Ratanawongsa, B. (2001). *Cerebral palsy*. Retrieved from http://www.emedicine.com/neuro/topic533.htm

Rehabilitation Act of 1973, 29 U.S.C. § 701 *et seq.* (amended 1986).

Russell, D. J., Rosenbaum, P. L., Cadman, D. T., Gowland, C., Hardy, S., & Jarvis, S. (1989). The Gross Motor Function Measure: A means to evaluate the efforts of physical therapy. *Developmental Medicine and Child Neurology, 31,* 341–352.

Scherzer, A. L., & Tscharnuter, I. (1982). *Early diagnosis and therapy in cerebral palsy*. New York, NY: Marcel Dekker, Inc.

Sharkey, M. A. (2002). The debate: NDTA & AACPDM. Neuro-developmental treatment for cerebral palsy: Is it effective? *NDTA Network Newsletter, 9*(5), 1–9.

Shevell, M. I., Dagenais, L., & Hall, N. (2009). Comorbidities in cerebral palsy and their relationship to neurological subtype and GMFCS level. *Neurology, 72,* 2090–2096.

State University of New York. (1993). *Functional independence measure*. Buffalo, NY: Author.

Technology Related Assistance for Individuals With Disabilities Act of 1988. Public Law 100–407, 29 U.S.C. § 2201 *et seq.* (1988).

Thorogood, C. (2001). *Physical medicine and rehabilitation for cerebral palsy.* Retrieved from http://www.emedicine.com/pmr/topic24.htm

U.S. Department of Education. (n.d.). *Building the legacy: IDEA 2004.* Retrieved from http://idea.ed.gov/explore/home

Vocational Rehabilitation Service Act of 1973. Public Law 93–112, 29 U.S.C. §§ 31–42 (1973).

Yasukawa, A. (1992). Upper extremity casting: Adjunct treatment of the child with cerebral palsy. In P. Case-Smith & C. Pehoski (Eds.), *Development of hand skills in the child* (pp. 111–123). Bethesda, MD: AOTA.

# Spina Bifida

*Meryl S. Cooperman*
*Roberta T. Ciocco*
*Deborah Humpl*

## 🌿 Synopsis of Clinical Condition

### Prevalence and Etiology

*Spina bifida* (literally, "cleft spine") is a neural tube defect that occurs in utero as a result of an incomplete closure of the spinal column. The defect occurs during the first trimester of the pregnancy and is associated with maternal folic acid deficiency. According to the Association of Spina Bifida and Hydrocephalus (2002), there are three types of spina bifida:

1. *Spina bifida occulta*, in which there is bony abnormality of the vertebrae with no damage to the spinal cord. This type is usually undetected and poses no clinical problems.

2. *Meningocele*, in which the meninges (the protective covering of the spinal cord) have been pushed through the vertebral defect in a sac called the *meningocele*. In this condition, the spinal cord remains intact. Repair can result in little or no damage to the nerve pathways. Functional results for this group are very favorable.

3. *Myelomeningocele* is the most severe form of spina bifida. In this form, the spinal cord itself protrudes through the vertebral defect. In some cases, the resulting sac is covered with skin, but sometimes the tissues and nerves are exposed. Surgery to close a newborn's back is usually performed within 24 hours of birth to minimize the risk of infection. In this population, there is certain paralysis, but the degree of functional impairment varies according to the level and severity of the defect.

The latter two conditions are considered *spina bifida manifesta* and are the focus of this discussion.

Spina bifida occurs in approximately 1 in every 1,000 live births. Within this group, there is a 96% incidence of myelomeningocele and only a 4% incidence of meningocele (National Information Center for Children and Youth With Disabilities, Spina Bifida, 2002).

Research is currently being conducted in the United States to try and minimize the loss of function through intrauterine surgery to correct the *cele*, or protrusion. The preliminary results of these studies suggest that children with spina bifida will have fewer secondary medical complications, although there is concern about the surgical risks. Researchers worldwide are exploring different surgical techniques to minimize the complications of intrauterine surgery, and this could be a deciding factor for many families and doctors when weighing treatment options (Chescheir, 2009).

## Common Characteristics and Symptoms

Spina bifida can be present at the thoracic, lumbar, or sacral level of the spinal cord. The higher the level of the cele, the greater the physical loss of muscle function and the greater the risk of neurological and orthopedic disorders (Rowe & Jadhav, 2008). The functional effects of spina bifida include weakness and/or paralysis of muscles, loss of sensation, loss of bowel and bladder control, and possible associated neurological conditions. Some of the information in this chapter may also be applied to the pediatric spinal cord population. Although they do not share the associated neurological problems, they do have many commonalities with regard to physical, self-care, and environmental needs. The level of paralysis or weakness is determined by the level of the lesion and can be considered static. The secondary neurological conditions can be progressive and can result in loss of skills and orthopedic deformities (Rowe & Jadhav, 2008).

Frequently, a condition known as *hydrocephalus* is associated with spina bifida. Hydrocephalus is a buildup of fluid in the brain that, if left untreated, can cause brain damage, seizures, or blindness. This condition is treated by a procedure called *ventriculoperitonial shunting*, in which a drain is implanted to divert the excess ventricular fluid to the abdominal cavity. It is common for children with a shunt to undergo multiple surgical revisions to keep the shunt functioning properly as they grow and develop. Some children with spina bifida may also have seizure disorders that require treatment with medication.

*Arnold–Chiari malformation type II* (ACM II) is a neurological deformity that is associated with spina bifida. ACM II is characterized by a downward herniation of the cerebellar tonsils and the fourth ventricle at the formen magnum. Approximately half of all children with ACM II may also have a kink in the medulla, which can cause brainstem or cervical cord compression. ACM II requires surgical intervention, which usually consists of decompression by removing part of the cervical vertebra and the lower part of the skull, shunt placement, and reconstruction of the posterior fossa. Symptoms of ACM II may be serious.

Other neurological conditions that may occur with spina bifida include tethered cord syndrome and hydromyella. *Tethered cord syndrome* occurs when the spinal cord is stretched as the result of attachments that restrict movement. *Hydromyella* are cysts in the spinal cord. The neurological sequela has a significant influence on the lives of children with spina bifida in addition to the physical level of skills. Orthopedic conditions associated with spina bifida include hip dislocation, knee contractures, foot deformities, scoliosis, and kyphosis (Rowe & Jadhav, 2008).

Children with spina bifida and hydrocephalus often experience learning difficulties, low levels of motivation, and visual perception impairment. Nonverbal learning disorders (NLDs) are frequently seen in these children. A child with an NLD presents with a specific cluster of neuropsychological, academic, and social–emotional characteristics. The primary deficit is in nonverbal reasoning. These children often present with weak visual–spatial and visual discrimination abilities, poor organizational skills, difficulty with abstract and mathematical reasoning, and decreased social competence (Spina Bifida Association of America, 2002). Many children with spina bifida can also exhibit behaviors associated with attention-deficit/hyperactivity disorder (ADHD), specifically the inattention subtype. Communication disorders may be present. For instance, the child may use "cocktail speech," or the mimicry of sophisticated language patterns, without comprehension.

Children with spina bifida are prone to latex allergies. This may be due to their increased exposure to latex products from use of catheters and other medical products. Medical suppliers are now producing latex-free products for people who are susceptible to latex allergies. Care should be taken when treating someone with spina bifida to avoid using anything with latex, such as balloons, elastic bandages, and pacifiers.

Children with spina bifida can exhibit various orthopedic problems. Sometimes this is due to their vertebral instability and muscle paralysis. Kyphosis and scoliosis, a rounding or curving of the spine, are often secondary complications of spina bifida. Hip dysplasia and other lower extremity deformities can also occur from muscle imbalances resulting from partial paralysis. As the child gets older, upper extremity tendonitis is sometimes an associated problem caused by the stress and strain put on the upper extremities for mobility and transfers. These children can also be more prone to injury and fracture of their lower extremities because of their lack of sensation and poor body awareness. Sensory loss can also pose other problems for children with spina bifida. They can develop decubitus ulcers, especially as they reach adolescence, when weight gain and hormonal changes cause increased pressure over their bony prominences. It is important that these children are aware of safety precautions to avoid burns and abrasions of insensate areas.

Obesity is another frequent problem that children with spina bifida face due to their sedentary lifestyle. Children with spina bifida need to be encouraged to participate in physical activity whenever possible because they lack the benefit of burning calories in the kind of physical play activities that their able-bodied peers enjoy. Urinary tract infections are another common problem for those children who have to rely on self-catheterization. Children and adolescents with spina bifida are at risk for low self-esteem and emotional problems (DiCianno, Gaines, Collins, & Lee, 2009). They also tend to have poor social skills and motivational

**Table 7.1** Possible Symptoms of and Conditions Associated With Spina Bifida

| Systemic/autonomic | Sensory | Cognitive | Motor |
|---|---|---|---|
| Apnea | Sensory impairment | Learning disorders | Paralysis |
| Dysphagia | Visual blurring | Language comprehension problems | Ataxia |
| Gastroesophogeal reflux | Sensory processing difficulties | Attention difficulties | Upper extremity muscle weakness |
| Latex allergy | | | Decreased fine motor coordination |
| Seizures | | | Lower extremity joint contractures |
| Obesity | | | Scoliosis |
| Bowel and bladder incontinence | | | Skin integrity issues (decubitus ulcers) |

problems. Table 7.1 summarizes some of the symptoms and associated conditions that may occur.

## Target Areas for Intervention

The occupational therapist has many opportunities to enhance the life of a child, adolescent, or adult with spina bifida. Activities of daily living (ADL) skills and instrumental activities of daily living (IADL) skills are a main focus for intervention. Daily living skills need to be addressed in a developmental progression over the lifetime of a client with spina bifida, starting with basic dressing and mobility skills and progressing to more complex tasks, such as bowel and bladder management, and then on to independent living skills, such as driving and meal preparation. Accessibility should be considered along with ADL training. The occupational therapist can play an important part in educating the child and the family about universal design and providing resource information to help them plan for current and future needs. Seating and positioning are also areas that often need to be addressed. Although some children do ambulate with braces, they are often unable to be functional as community ambulators. As these children get older and larger, ambulation usually becomes less efficient as a primary means of mobility.

Children with spina bifida can exhibit delayed developmental skills due to neurological causes and diminished opportunities for environmental exploration. They are at risk for difficulties with visual–motor coordination, body awareness, self-esteem, and social–emotional adjustment.

## 🐾 Contextual Considerations

### Clinical

The clinical evaluation must incorporate information regarding the integrity of the musculoskeletal system and developmental skills acquisition, including ADL.

The musculoskeletal integrity, in concert with developmental ability, determines whether the child may be capable of performing life tasks independently, either with adaptive techniques or equipment or with varying degrees of caregiver assistance. Since children with spina bifida often have accompanying developmental difficulties associated with hydrocephaly in addition to physical limitations, it is important to combine the knowledge of the musculoskeletal status with developmental skills.

The physiological evaluation includes information on the range of motion, muscle strength, and sensation of the upper and lower extremities. The physical therapist on the intervention team can provide detailed information regarding lower extremity status. Lower extremity status is relevant for dressing the lower extremities, bowel and bladder care, skin management, bath and bathing, and transfer techniques.

There are many developmental assessments available. A general developmental assessment, such as the *Peabody Developmental Motor Scales–Second Edition* (Folio & Fewell, 2000), the *Hawaii Early Learning Profile* (Furuno et al., 1991), or the *Pediatric Evaluation of Disability Inventory* (Haley, Coster, Ludlow, Haltiwanger, & Andrellos, 1992), will provide information for the preschool-age child.

Children of school age can be evaluated using an assessment of visual–motor skills, perceptual skills, and fine motor coordination. Common assessments include the *Beery–Buktenica Developmental Test of Visual–Motor Integration* (Beery, Buktenica, & Beery, 2010), the *Test of Visual Motor Skills–Third Edition* (Martin, 2006a) the *Test of Visual Perceptual Skills: Non-Motor–Third Edition* (Martin, 2006b), the *Jebsen Hand Function Test* (Jebsen, Taylor, Trieschmann, Trotter, & Howard, 1969), and the *Bruininks–Oseretsky Test of Motor Proficiency–Second Edition* (Bruininks, 2006). It may be necessary to modify some of the evaluations of motor coordination to accommodate the child's physical limitations.

A thorough evaluation of ADL skills needs to incorporate skin checks and self-management of the bowel and bladder, in addition to the areas of dressing, feeding, hygiene, and grooming. A developmental ADL checklist can be helpful for young children (under 3 years of age). However, these assessments often do not accommodate children with physical limitations. An adult rehabilitation checklist may incorporate transfer skills, skin checks, and the use of adaptive equipment. The *Functional Independence Measure* (Hamilton & Granger, 1991a) and the *Functional Independence Measure for Children* (Hamilton & Granger, 1991b) provide information on many areas and are often used in research. These assessments group many skills together, which make them insensitive to smaller changes when used for short durations and for goal setting. When evaluating ADL skills by caregiver report or self-report, the interview should be structured to help establish a rapport and learn more about the family, as discussed in the following section.

The occupational therapist may also complete an evaluation related to pre-vocational and vocational skills for teenagers and young adults with spina bifida. The evaluation would incorporate assessment of gross and fine motor skills, upper extremity strength, transfers, self-care, cognitive and perceptual skills, social skills, and IADL skills. In addition, the following standardized assessments can be used to gather information on vocational skills: the *Lowenstein Occupational Therapy Cognitive Assessment* (Katz, Itzkovich, Averbuch, & Elaszer, 1989), the *Kitchen Task Assessment* (Baum & Edwards, 1993), and the *Canadian Occupational Performance Measure* (Law et al., 2005). A more career-specific assessment is the *Career Orientation Placement and Evaluation Survey* (Knapp, Knapp, & Knapp-Lee, 1995), which is a questionnaire that helps the individual become more self-aware regarding career choice. According to Knapp et al., effective career development programs are based on their efforts toward increasing individuals' self-awareness of their individual, personal characteristics as they relate to the type of work in which they are interested. The *COPS Interest Inventory* (Knapp & Knapp, 1995) is also a questionnaire that helps guide the individual in some type of career decision in 14 areas, including outdoor, science and technology, business, clerical, arts, and service careers.

## Family

Family values, priorities, and cultural preferences must be considered. It is often possible to gather information using an informal interview with a few key questions. Open-ended questions may be more helpful than a yes/no checklist and help to establish rapport. For example, "Tell me about a typical day," with supporting questions such as, "What time do you wake up?" or "Does anybody help you get dressed?" or "What do you usually eat for breakfast/lunch/dinner?," can provide information on family routines in addition to ADL skills.

The occupational therapist needs to demonstrate sensitivity while gathering information about family resources, including medical coverage, formal and informal support groups, and information or educational resources. The occupational therapist can be a primary or secondary provider of information about coverage for medical expenses, special education and rehabilitation laws, and care of the caregivers. The information gathered may indicate the need for a social service referral to assist in accessing counseling services and other forms of support in the community.

The occupational therapist must be aware of future needs in order to provide the guidance necessary for addressing current needs. The occupational therapist can help select a wheelchair that can grow with the child, to minimize costs for the family. The family of the child who requires medical equipment, such as wheelchairs or shower/bath chairs, must be made aware of the criteria for reimbursement. Many third-party payers will reimburse services on a limited basis but will not cover durable medical equipment. Medical assistance often covers this type of equipment with very specific guidelines. The family may need information on medical assistance to help with expenses not covered by the family's insurance plan.

It is important for the occupational therapist to support the concept of back care and proper positioning or lifting techniques for the caregiver. Families with young children may need to prepare themselves as their child grows and requires more assistance with transfers and ADL skills. Families with school-age and older children with spina bifida may need guidance on using adaptive equipment and incorporating improved body mechanics into their care routines.

## Practice Setting

Individuals with spina bifida require occupational therapy services throughout their lifetimes, in various settings. Occupational therapists may provide services in an acute hospital, a rehabilitation hospital, a rehabilitation outpatient facility, an early intervention center, and school-based settings. The occupational therapist functions as a member of a multidisciplinary team that is often composed of professionals from disciplines such as neurology, orthopedic medicine, nursing, physical therapy, social work, psychology, therapeutic recreation, speech–language pathology, and special education. The team also includes family members and other primary caregivers. Parents may be confused about the roles of the various professionals involved in their child's care, and that confusion may be compounded if the child is receiving services in different settings simultaneously. It is important to establish and maintain communication among therapists and other members of the team to ensure consistency of care and facilitate transitions between service settings as the child matures.

The acute care therapist may first encounter the individual with spina bifida in the neonatal intensive care unit. The child usually requires surgical intervention for the cele and hydrocephaly (if present). Initial care may be limited to assisting with positioning and feeding issues. The parents should be provided with education and information about arranging therapy upon discharge. The occupational therapist must work with other professionals to assist the family with coping and preparing for having a child with special needs.

The rehabilitation hospital–based occupational therapist often provides therapy services for a specific period after a surgical procedure or for specific rehabilitation goals. For example, a child may have a rehabilitation admission for ambulation issues, ADL skills, bowel and bladder management, and treatment of skin breakdowns. Occupational therapy intervention would focus on environmental adaptation to accommodate compromised ambulation skills, adaptive seating, personal hygiene aids, and training regarding the prevention and care of skin breakdowns.

The occupational therapist who works in outpatient settings often provides services to facilitate the ongoing development of fine motor, perceptual, visual–motor, social, play, and ADL skills. Parent education is an important aspect of the intervention plan since the therapist often sees the child on a weekly or monthly basis.

Occupational therapists working in an early intervention program may provide home-based and/or community-based services focused on the development of gross and fine motor skills, hand skills, perceptual skills, visual–motor skills, play skills, and ADL skills within the context of natural environments. The occupational therapist, in concert with other members of the intervention team, including the family, addresses environmental modifications, ergonomic seating, handling and positioning strategies, and planning for future needs.

The school-based therapist provides therapy with a focus on skills needed to be successful throughout the school day. The school therapist can work collaboratively with the rehabilitation or outpatient therapist. The focus of the school-based therapist, in accordance with the Individuals With Disabilities Education Act (IDEA, 1997), is to provide a supportive service that enables full participation in the school program. The child with spina bifida may experience accessibility issues with stairs or table and desk heights, or he or she may have problems with accessibility in the school lunchroom, in the school classroom, and on the playground, all of which may affect participation in school activities. Perceptual issues may affect written communication and other learning skills. The child may also have difficulty with social skills. Dressing issues associated with managing outer garments and clothing for toileting and hygiene associated with toileting may also require intervention.

## Sociopolitical

Three primary laws relate to children with spina bifida. The Individuals With Disabilities Education Act (IDEA, 1997) entitled all children to a free and appropriate education in the least restrictive environment and, whenever possible, with nondisabled peers (IDEA, 1997). The Rehabilitation Act (1973) ensures the civil rights of individuals with disabilities in all institutions, agencies, or organizations that receive federal funding or financial assistance. The Americans With Disabilities Act (1991) guarantees equal opportunities for employment, accessibility, transportation, and government services. Additional legislation includes the Technology-Related Assistance for Individuals With Disabilities Act (1988) and the Vocational Rehabilitation Service Act (VRSA, 1973).

As a result of this legislation, a child with disabilities may receive occupational therapy and other related services—including supporting technology—in order to be educated with nondisabled peers, with the goal of preparation for life in the mainstream of society. IDEA mandates the development of a plan that facilitates the transition from school to life after school when the child is 16 years old. The school-based transition plan addresses community living, employment, and socialization. It is informed by the abilities, interests, needs, and goals of the student. Vocational rehabilitation services mandated by the VRSA help the child with spina bifida to enter the world of work after completing school.

Federal, state, and local government programs—as well as private agencies—may provide financial resources for individuals with spina bifida. Children with spina bifida may qualify for medical assistance based on their disability, not the financial resources of the family. Social Security Income may also be available for the child and the family. Home modifications may be supported through programs ranging from Habitat for Humanity to local agencies. Some automobile manufacturers will pay a limited amount for modifications if a new vehicle is purchased. The VRSA will help fund home and vehicle modifications if they are necessary for the individual's employment.

## Lifestyle/Lifespan

It is important to help the individual and the family become aware of the issues that an individual with spina bifida will face throughout life. These include accessibility, financial, medical, family, and social issues. Table 7.2 highlights the issues discussed in this section.

Many families will learn about accessibility issues in the home and community by encountering obstacles with their child. Individuals with spina bifida often locomote with crutches or a wheelchair. Speed, endurance, management of stairs and curbs, and climbing into and out of family vehicles will be some of the obstacles with which families will need to cope. The needs of the child may change as he or she grows and becomes heavier and needs larger equipment. Families often cope with accessibility issues for young children easily because managing a stroller is a common occurrence. However, as the child with spina bifida grows, the family will have to continue to cope with accessibility beyond the preschool years. The family with a young child with spina bifida may be able to carry the child up and down stairs to a second story bathroom or to enter or exit the family home. As the child grows, if he or she is dependent on mobility devices, the family may need to consider home modifications or relocating to an accessible home.

Financial concerns will vary depending on the family's economic resources and the availability of private insurance and government assistance programs. Insurance may not cover the cost of some supplies, and this will affect household budgets. Diapers may be a routine expense that families anticipate with young

**Table 7.2** Lifestyle/Lifespan Factors

| Accessibility | Financial | Medical | Family | Social |
|---|---|---|---|---|
| Home School Community | Daily supplies for medicine and bowel and bladder issues Durable medical equipment Home modification Living arrangements for the future | Latex allergy Shunt care Skin management | Increased time for daily care Coping with ongoing medical needs Sibling relationships Care of the caregivers | Interaction with peers Adaptive sports |

children, but the child with spina bifida may require diapers for many years. Diapers and other bowel and bladder supplies are often not covered by insurance. Day care services, babysitters, and other elements of family life may be more costly. Insurance reimbursement often has limitations, so that the cost of walkers, crutches, wheelchairs, lifts, adapted vans, and home modifications may not be covered. It is important to recognize that the use of equipment may vary over time, depending on the needs and interests of the child and family. The occupational therapist needs to be aware of resources for the family, the cost effectiveness of equipment, and environmental modifications that can "grow" with the child.

Medical issues will need to be addressed beyond the cost factors often associated with medical needs. Individuals with spina bifida and their families need to be diligent about health-related issues in order to receive timely treatment that will minimize or prevent the functional loss of skills (Rowe & Jadhav, 2008). Coping with the need for hospitalizations related to a shunt or orthopedic deformities will impact the life of the child and the family. Work schedules and family routines will need to be readjusted. If siblings are present, planning requirements will increase.

Latex allergies often result in lifestyle changes for the entire family. A common latex object is the balloon. Parents will need to learn what toys and objects contain latex and be advocates for their young children. It can be challenging to limit or restrict exposure to latex in the community since it is present in many commonly used objects. The older child with spina bifida and a latex allergy will need to be educated on avoiding and dealing with exposure.

Skin integrity is a very important issue. Young children with spina bifida generally are able to tolerate many positions and often do not experience skin breakdowns. As the child grows, several factors increase the risk for skin breakdowns. The child may need to learn to perform skin checks, practice pressure relief, and make other lifestyle changes. The onset of puberty results in increased sweat glands and weight changes that translate into an increased risk of skin breakdowns. The child with spina bifida and his or her family must cope with these changes, in addition to the emotions associated with puberty. Occupational therapists could provide resources for community programs or counseling to help with the adjustment to adolescents.

As caregivers age, it may become challenging to perform some of the daily care tasks of children who do not independently perform ADL. Caregivers may require training to alleviate or prevent back strain and pain. Parents also may need to engage in long-term planning in the event that they are no longer able to provide care. Siblings may assume some or all of the primary caregiver role as adults or teenagers. When designing home programs for parents, the occupational therapist should consider the importance of balancing the daily needs of the child with spina bifida with those of siblings. Play activities that engage siblings can help to promote positive family relationships.

Social experience with peer groups in the community is often disrupted because of physical limitations and learning or social differences. Encouragement to participate in adaptive sports will be beneficial to the child for physical fitness and peer relationships.

## ✐ Clinical Decision-Making Process

### Defining Focus for Intervention

Visual perceptual skills, cognitive abilities, handwriting, fine motor and bilateral hand coordination, school-related self-care, accessibility issues, prevocational issues, and social skills related to the academic environment are often the focus of school-based occupational therapy intervention. ADL status, range of motion, strength, motor coordination, environmental accessibility, skin integrity, adaptive equipment, and prevocational issues may be the focus of hospital-based and rehabilitation intervention. Transfers, wheelchair mobility, dressing, bathing, self-catheterization, and IADL skills are typically addressed in short-term rehabilitation admissions or outpatient services.

The other major consideration is the child's age or the timing of intervention. Early in the child's life, parent education, assessment, and facilitation of developmental skills are paramount. Assisting the child in achieving independent mobility takes precedence in the preschool years and impacts the child's feelings of self-efficacy and emotional well-being. Most children are capable of independent wheelchair mobility by 2 years of age. The school-age child may need intervention related to learning difficulties or visual perceptual impairment. Self-care skills are usually in need of ongoing attention. Putting on lower extremity braces, tying shoelaces, and self-catheterizing can be quite challenging for the spina bifida child with perceptual problems and/or fine motor coordination deficits.

Adolescence brings some additional challenges for the child with spina bifida. Even though ambulation may be effective in the confines of the elementary school or home setting, the middle and high school experience often requires the child to adapt to the use of a wheelchair to interact with peers in a variety of educational and social activities and thus reduce the risk of social isolation. Although increased mobility may afford many opportunities, prolonged sitting can foster weight gain and skin lesions. Driver education with adapted vehicles, self-care, home management, and prevocational skills are target areas for intervention that will foster self-efficacy and independence and prepare the child for the transition to adulthood. The occupational therapist also must consider the family's and child's interests and needs, in addition to environmental problems and limitations or opportunities that may be guided by regulatory, legislative, or reimbursement situations.

### Establishing Goals for Intervention

Depending on the chronological age, developmental age, and functional abilities of the child; the practice setting; and the needs and interests of the primary caregivers, the therapist may consider goals that compensate, remediate, or prevent disability. Although most children learn to tie their shoes around the age of 5 years, a child with significant visual perception impairment may require the use of Velcro closures to achieve independence in this skill at the expected age. The biomechanical and physical data from your evaluation may help guide goal development. Some children will present with a higher thoracic level cele. These children usually have no sensory or motor preservation in the lower extremities and trunk and tend to have greater orthopedic deformity (e.g., kyphosis, scoliosis, hip dislocation). Goals for independent mobility are geared toward wheelchair use with a complex seating system to address orthopedic deformities and diminished trunk control. Lower lumbar level celes will indicate little functional impairment of the lower extremities, and goals would relate to independent management of orthotics.

Accessibility issues may influence the priority of a goal or dictate the level of achievable independence. For example, if the child's wheelchair does not fit through the cafeteria line, then a goal for the child to be independent in buying his or her lunch and negotiating the cafeteria line may not be appropriate. But engaging the child in preparing his or her own lunch and bringing it to school might be an appropriate and viable solution—one that will develop independence and prevent social isolation. Environmental limitations can provide great opportunities for engaging parents, children, and other involved parties, such as teachers and classroom aides, to develop relevant and viable treatment goals. The prioritization of goals may be dictated by legislative and reimbursement criteria that establish the focus and frequency of treatment.

## Designing Theory-Based Intervention

This population presents with a variety of problems; therefore, several theoretical models are applicable. The rehabilitation frame of reference focuses on acquiring ADL skills using compensatory methods, technology, and environmental adaptations (Dutton, 1995). This framework might be used in combination with principles of learning theory when teaching a child who has significant lower extremity paralysis to put on pants. The activity would be broken down into several steps, such as putting the pants over the feet, pulling them up to the knees, lying down and rolling side to side to pull them up in the back, and buttoning and zippering. These steps might be introduced to the therapy session one or two at a time. Techniques may be modified, and/or adaptive equipment may need to be introduced at various steps. Trial-and-error problem solving is often used to refine the process. Afterward, practice to reinforce the skill would be indicated.

The biomechanical frame of reference (Dutton, 1995) is used with individuals with neuromuscular or musculoskeletal problems. This frame of reference is based on principles of physics, physiology, neuroscience, and kinesiology and is often used in combination with the rehabilitation frame of reference when adaptive equipment is necessary. For example, a complicated seating system may be indicated to provide a child with enough trunk stability and upper extremity use for functional activities. The final seating system design depends on an understanding and application of biomechanical and physiological concepts inherent to joint position, movement, and fixed deformities.

The developmental frame of reference is certainly relevant to any pediatric population. Children with spina bifida face many obstacles and interruptions in the normal progression or acquisition of skills. The occupational therapist must have a good understanding of normal development in order to devise interventions that remediate or prevent disruption in the progression of developmental skill.

Neurodevelopmental treatment (NDT) is a sensorimotor approach that is used primarily with neurological and motor control problems. Although this approach is widely used with the child with cerebral palsy, handling techniques and positioning principles may be applicable to children with spina bifida. An example of an appropriate use of this frame of reference might be the case of a child who has poor head control. Frequently, children with spina bifida have hydrocephalus and therefore have difficulty gaining stability because of lower limb and trunk paralysis. NDT handling techniques and positioning principles foster the development of efficient postural adjustments and distal limb movement on a firm base of central trunk stability.

Sensory integration is another theoretical approach that may be applicable to this population. Because of neurological involvement, these children often experience sensory processing problems. Problems with sensory registration and modulation, as well as sensory defensiveness, can be exhibited by these children.

The model of human occupation (Kielhofner, 2002) focuses on the development and maintenance of roles and associated daily routines. This approach assists in the development of intervention strategies that are relevant to and facilitative of the child's evolving role expectations and the ability to benefit from his or her education and lead a productive and fulfilling life.

## Evaluating Progress

Meeting established goals (usually annual long-term goals and short-term objectives) is the most tangible method of evaluating progress. Readministration of testing may be necessary to evaluate progress in some areas, such as visual perception and visual–motor integration. Interviews with the child and family can also provide a measure of progress. Parents usually take notice of new skills that their child is able to demonstrate in the home or community environment. Another measure of progress that is less objective is the child's and family's adaptation to and coping with the disability. Even if the child has not reached a goal of independence with bowel care, for instance, the family may have established a routine that is more comfortable for the child and the caregiver. Another example would be if a child with spina bifida who is not yet independent with transfers becomes able to request assistance and provide instruction to the person helping with the transfer.

## Determining Change in or Termination of Treatment

Change in or termination of treatment is warranted when the child does not meet the goals established or has met all the goals established. In either event, the therapist needs to reevaluate to see if new goals are appropriate. The new goals could represent a change of focus or expectations of higher levels of independence and function. Discharge from therapy may occur when the child has reached a maximum level of independence for his or her age and has acquired a sufficient level of foundational skills to promote independent problem solving and future skill acquisition. Therapy may also be terminated when the child has reached a plateau of progress.

Occupational therapy may be episodic during the child's lifetime. Occupational therapy may be reinstated when the child is old enough to learn new skills. For example, therapy may be indicated when the child is old enough to learn bowel and bladder management and deal with skin integrity issues or when he or she transitions from a school to a work environment. Occupational therapy in the elementary school may be discontinued and reinstated when the child transitions to a new school and has new expectations, such as using a locker and dressing and undressing for gym class.

### Case Study

*Description*

TC is an 8-year-old female with spina bifida. Her motor and sensory level is thoracic 10. She ambulates for exercise with only HKAFO (hip–knee–ankle–foot orthosis). She is currently not using her braces because she has a small open sore on her right lateral malleolus. TC's main means of mobility is her lightweight wheelchair. TC has a 30-degree thoracic scoliosis. She has worn a body jacket in the past, but she has recently been noncompliant with the brace because it restricts her mobility. Her orthopedic surgeon has agreed to let her try going without the brace for part of the day if her seating system can be redesigned to offer her more support. She currently has a planar seating system that consists of a solid seat and back with lateral trunk supports that are always loose and out of position.

TC has a shunt for hydrocephalus. She has undergone six surgical revisions. TC is in the second grade with part-time learning support in a resource room because she has trouble with math and reading. She is functioning at a beginning first-grade level in both areas. TC also has visual–motor and visual perceptual difficulties. She scored in the 16th percentile on the *Beery–Buktenica Developmental Test of Visual–Motor Integration.* She has difficulty drawing diagonal lines and frequently reverses her letters and numbers. On the *Test of Visual Perceptual Skills* she scored in the 25th percentile. Her lowest scores were on the subtests that involved visual memory, spatial relations, figure–ground, and visual closure.

TC lives with her mom, dad, and younger sister. They live in an older two-story house with wheelchair accessibility problems. The bathroom presents the biggest problem. Mom or Dad has to carry TC into the bathroom and lift her into the tub because the wheelchair doesn't fit into the bathroom. Mom has recently been experiencing back pain. The family has a car for transportation, but they are considering the purchase of a minivan because it is difficult to fit TC's equipment into the car with everyone. TC's mom is also having difficulty lifting the wheelchair in and out of the trunk. TC has a few friends in the neighborhood and school with whom she occasionally plays. Most of her free time is spent playing with her younger sister. She is a very bubbly and engaging child.

TC is independent in upper extremity dressing. She requires moderate assistance for lower extremity dressing and bathing. She is independent in level-surface transfers, and she is dependent with bowel and bladder care. TC is being admitted to a pediatric rehabilitation center for an intense 3-week rehabilitation stay.

### Long- and Short-Term Goals

The immediate goals of TC's admission are as follows:

1. Increase TC's independence with self-care.
2. Complete a seating evaluation and make the appropriate modifications to TC's seating system.
3. Address TC's skin issues.
4. Evaluate the home and make recommendations to improve accessibility.

The long-term goal of intervention for TC is to enable her to increase her independence with ADL from a current level of dependence for all lower extremity activities to a level of partial dependence for lower body care.

The short-term goals of intervention for TC are as follows:

1. TC will use modifications and/or adaptive equipment to don and doff lower extremity garments with independence.
2. TC will use modifications and/or adaptive equipment to don and doff socks and shoes with independence.
3. When provided with setup, TC will participate in self-catherization activities to the level of partial physical assistance by the caregiver.
4. During transfer activities using a tub bench, TC will transfer to the level of contact guard by the caregiver.
5. During bathing activities, TC will wash her entire body and perform hair care using modifications and adaptive equipment to the level of supervision by the caregiver.
6. During skin checks, TC will use adaptive equipment to perform the skin check to the level of supervision by the caregiver.

### Therapist Goals and Strategies

The therapist's goals include the following:

1. Provide recommendations and funding resource information for adaptive equipment.

2. Assist with evaluation and ordering of the new wheelchair seating system.

3. Assist with educating the child and family in independent skin checks.

The therapist's strategies include the following:

1. Provide opportunities to explore adaptive equipment to facilitate independence.

2. Try different adaptive techniques for positioning TC's body for dressing activities.

3. Explore different teaching styles and task analyses (such as pictures, verbal cues, lists, and props) to compensate for perceptual deficits.

4. Provide opportunities for repetition and practice.

5. Evaluate the home (in person or through interviews).

6. Instruct the caregivers regarding the home program.

### Activity: The Dressing Relay

TC will navigate through an obstacle course. Skills such as rolling, picking up garments, getting into and out of her wheelchair, transferring to a tub bench, tying shoelaces, and putting on and taking off articles of clothing (from the dress-up bin) will be incorporated into the course. This activity can be graded over time. Initially, TC would start with a few simple tasks, and, eventually, more stations with increased complexity would be added. Different skills, such as perceptual–motor skills and upper extremity strengthening, could also be incorporated. Techniques will be taught to the mother for carryover into daily routines.

### Treatment Objectives

Treatment session objectives may include TC putting on her pants independently using modifications and/or adaptive equipment with the correct orientation.

## Resources

American Occupational Therapy Association: www.aota.org

Council for Exceptional Children: www.cec.sped.org

National Dissemination Center for Children With Disabilities: www.nichcy.org

Spina Bifida Association: www.spinabifidaassociation.org

## References

Americans With Disabilities Act of 1990, 42 U.S.C. § 12101 *et seq.* (1990).

Association for Spina Bifida and Hydrocephalus. (2002). *What is spina bifida?* Retrieved from http://www.asbah.org/whatissb.html

Beery, K. E., Buktenica, N. A., & Beery, N. A. (2010). *Beery–Buktenica developmental test of visual–motor integration* (6th ed.). San Antonio, TX: Pearson Assessments.

Bruininks, R. H. (2006). *Bruininks–Oseretsky test of motor proficiency* (2nd ed.). San Antonio, TX: Pearson Assessments.

Chescheir, N. C. (2009). Maternal-fetal surgery: Where are we and how did we get here? *Obstetrics & Gynecology, 113*(3), 717–731.

DiCianno, B. E., Gaines, A., Collins, D. M., & Lee, S. (2009). Mobility, assistive technology use, and social integration among adults with spina bifida. *American Journal of Physical Medicine and Rehabilitation, 88*(7), 533–541.

Dutton, R. (1995). *Clinical reasoning in physical disabilities.* Philadelphia, PA: Lippincott, Williams & Wilkins.

Folio, R., & Fewell, R. (2000). *Peabody developmental motor scales* (2nd ed.). Austin, TX: PRO-ED, Inc.

Furuno, S., O'Reilly, K., Inatsuka, T., Hosaka, C., Allman, T., & Zeisloft-Falbey, B. (1991). *Hawaii early learning profile.* Palo Alto, CA: VORT.

Haley, S. M., Coster, W. J., Ludlow, L. H., Haltiwanger, J. T., & Andrellos, P. J. (1992). *Pediatric evaluation of disability inventory.* San Antonio, TX: The Psychological Corporation.

Hamilton, B. B., & Granger, C. U. (1991a). *Functional independence measure.* Buffalo, NY: Research Foundation of the State University of New York.

Hamilton, B. B., & Granger, C. U. (1991b). *Functional independence measure for children.* Buffalo, NY: Research Foundation of the State University of New York.

Individuals With Disabilities Education Improvement Act of 2004, 20 U.S.C § 1400 *et seq.* (2004).

Jebsen, R. H., Taylor, N., Trieschmann, R. B., Trotter, M. J., & Howard, L. A. (1969). *Jebsen–Taylor test of hand function.* Bolingbrook, IL: Sammons Preston.

Kielhofner, G. (2002). *Model of human occupation.* Baltimore, MD: Lippincott, Williams & Wilkins.

Knapp, R. R., Knapp, L., & Knapp-Lee, L. (1995). *Career orientation placement and evaluation survey.* San Diego, CA: EdITS.

Knapp-Lee, L., Knapp, R. R., & Knapp, L. (1982). *COPS system.* University of Toronto Press Guidance Centre.

Law, M., Baptiste, S., Carswell, A., McColl, M. A., Polatajko, H., & Pollack, N. (2005). *Canadian occupational performance measure* (4th ed.). Ottawa, Ontario, Canada: CAOT Press.

Martin, N. (2006a). *Test of visual motor skills* (3rd ed.). Novato, CA: Academic Therapy Publications.

Martin, N., (2006b). *Test of visual perceptual skills—Non-motor* (3rd ed.). Novato, CA: Academic Therapy Publications.

Rehabilitation Act of 1973, 29 U.S.C. § 701 *et seq.* (1973).

Rowe, D. E., & Jadhav, A. L. (2008). Care of the adolescent with spina bifida. *Pediatric Clinics of North America, 55*, 1359–1374.

Technology Related Assistance for Individuals with Disabilities Act of 1988. Public Law 100-407, 29 U.S.C. § 2201 *et seq.* (1988).

Vocational Rehabilitation Service Act of 1973. Public Law 93-112, 20 U.S.C. § 701 *et seq.* (1973).

# Genetic Conditions

*Fern Silverman*

## ✿ Synopsis of Clinical Condition

### Prevalence and Etiology

Our genetic code has been called "the secret of life" (Watson & Berry, 2003), a secret that scientists have now deciphered. An international team of researchers has successfully sequenced and mapped the human genome, which is made up of 30,000 to 40,000 human genes. This information can be thought of as a basic set of inheritable "instructions" for the development and function of a human be- ing (National Human Genome Research Institute, 2011). Humans have 23 pairs of chromosomes, including 22 identical pairs of autosomes and one pair of sex chromosomes. The sex chromosomes are identical (XX) if the human is female and disparate (XY) if the human is male.

When our genetic code is altered in some way, a genetic disorder may result. Risks that lead to genetic conditions include abnormalities in the chromosomes, single-gene mutations that produce genetic diseases and conditions, and more complex, multifactorial disorders. It is estimated that 2% to 3% of newborns have a major genetic defect (Blackman, 1997). These include Down syndrome, muscular dystrophies, cystic fibrosis, fragile X syndrome, sickle cell anemia, and Tay–Sachs disease, among others.

Incidence rates for genetic disorders vary according to the specific condition. The prevalence of genetic conditions in newborns is tracked as a vital statistic, as are infant mortality and birth weight. For example, in *National Vital Statis- tics Reports* (Martin, Hamilton, Ventura, Menacker, & Park, 2002), the inci- dence rate of Down syndrome is listed as 46.9 per 100,000 live births. Compare this to a much more rare condition, Hurler syndrome, which has a rate of 1 per

---

The editors gratefully acknowledge the contributions of Kristie P. Koenig to earlier versions of this chapter.

100,000. A thorough understanding of all genetic disorders is outside the scope of this chapter, as a multitude of conditions have their origins in the genetic map. However, many genetic conditions lead to disability and/or decreased ability to fully participate in all aspects of daily living. Therefore, a basic understanding of incidence, inheritance patterns, and common genetic conditions that the occupational therapist may encounter is necessary for best practice.

Genetic causes can be classified as (a) chromosomal abnormalities, meaning an error in the number or structure of chromosomes present; (b) single-gene disorders, where there is there is an alteration in the genetic material within the chromosomes on one gene; and (c) multifactorial disorders, which are caused by an interplay of genetic and environmental factors. The latter are the most prevalent.

An example of a chromosomal abnormality would be trisomy 21, or Down syndrome, where there is an extra chromosome 21. In this case, too much genetic material is present; in other chromosomal conditions, genetic material is missing. Chromosomal abnormalities can also reflect a problem with chromosomal structure. An example is Ewing's sarcoma, a bone cancer found in children and young adults. In Ewing's sarcoma, the chromosomal abnormality is caused by a chromosomal translocation, in which a small piece of one chromosome switches places with a small piece of another chromosome. Chromosomal irregularities can be identified through karotyping. This diagnostic process examines the number and structure of chromosomes in a sample of cells from a tissue specimen.

A single-gene disorder can be an alteration in a single gene or a pair of genes on either the autosomes or the sex chromosomes. The inheritance pattern can be recessive or dominant in nature and causes such conditions as cystic fibrosis, fragile X syndrome, tuberous sclerosis, and Duchenne and Becker muscular dystrophies. The defective condition can be an autosomal dominant or recessive condition or an X-linked dominant or recessive condition.

Autosomal recessive inheritance indicates that an abnormal gene must be in a paired condition (i.e., both parents have the gene) in order for the child to inherit the disease. For each pregnancy, there is a 25% chance that the child will have the paired genes and the condition will be expressed. In autosomal recessive inheritance patterns, there is also a 50% chance that the child will become a carrier for the condition. Males and females are at equal risk. The risk of an unaffected offspring being a carrier is 66%, with a 33% chance of being an unaffected noncarrier. Typically, both parents are carriers but have no symptoms of the condition. For many conditions, these carrier states can be identified through early diagnostic testing. There are several common genetic conditions that are caused by autosomal recessive inheritance, including cystic fibrosis in the European American population, Tay–Sachs disease in the Ashkenazi Jewish population, and sickle cell disease in the African American population.

Autosomal dominant conditions indicate that the abnormal gene is present on one of the non-sex chromosomes. There is no carrier state for autosomal dominant conditions. If the gene is present, the child will have the condition. For each pregnancy, there is a 50% chance that the child will have the condition. Huntington's chorea is an example of an autosomal dominant condition. Genetic counseling accompanies the prenatal screening that identifies carrier and affected states.

X-linked inheritance disorders may be recessive or dominant. X-linked dominant diseases are considered very rare and are usually lethal if a male inherits the gene, since he only has one X chromosome. This is why fathers cannot pass the trait to their sons, since fathers provide the Y that determines that the sex of the child will be male. A mother can be a carrier, and there are differential risks for male as compared to female offspring. Each time the carrier mother becomes pregnant with a boy, the child has a 50% chance of being affected. Since the female is XX, each time the carrier mother becomes pregnant with a girl, the child has a 50% chance of being a carrier (Schopmeyer & Lowe, 1992).

Multifactorial, or polygenic, disorders have a more complex causal pattern and can include cardiac malformations, cleft lip and palate, and myelomeningocele (Blackman, 1997). Multifactorial conditions suggest a more complex interplay between the genetic material and environmental factors. In these cases, genes do not have a direct impact on whether an individual has a genetic condition. Instead, there may be more subtle influences in combination with other genetic and environmental influences.

## Common Characteristics and Symptoms

Some genetic conditions are nonprogressive. Two well-known nonprogressive genetic conditions, Down syndrome and fragile X syndrome, are the most common causes of developmental disabilities and mental retardation in the general population (Schopmeyer & Lowe, 1992). Down syndrome has a higher incidence rate (4 to 5 per 1,000 births) and is seen more commonly than fragile X syndrome. However, fragile X syndrome, with its X-linked recessive pattern, is the most common inherited cause of mental retardation in males, with an estimated incidence of 1 per 4,000 (Bailey, Hatton, Tassone, Skinner, & Taylor, 2001). Down syndrome is not an inherited genetic condition but rather a chromosomal abnormality. These two conditions have similarities and differences but are frequently seen in pediatric occupational therapy practice.

Fragile X syndrome is a single-gene disorder carried on the X chromosome. The disorder can be passed through several generations in the carrier state, with each generation at higher risk of having the gene that causes the syndrome (Bailey, Skinner, Hatton, & Roberts, 2000). Typically, this gene is transmitted stably from parent to child. However, in individuals with fragile X syndrome, there is a mutation and expansion in one end of the gene that does not allow the FMR1 gene to be expressed, so no FMR1 protein is made. The production of this protein is believed to be essential for normal brain functioning (Bailey et al., 2001). Both males and females can have this syndrome; however, males are usually more severely affected than females. Individuals with fragile X syndrome may experience delays in all areas of development, especially in the areas of cognition and communication. In contrast to children born with Down syndrome, children with fragile X may look and behave normally at birth. Males may develop distinguishing physical features that include an elongated face, large ears, hypotonia, and hyper-extensibility at the finger joints (Schopmeyer & Lowe, 1992). Behaviorally, children with fragile X syndrome may demonstrate hyperactivity, tactile defensiveness, and other sensitivities to sensory stimulation. They may also demonstrate autistic-like behaviors, such as hand flapping and avoidance of eye contact. Miller et al. (1999) found that children with fragile X syndrome manifested the most severe sensory processing disorders of all the clinical groups studied (i.e., autism and attention-deficit/hyperactivity disorder). The sensory processing deficits can have an impact on occupational performance. Baranek et al. (2002) found that children with fragile X syndrome who avoided sensory experiences had lower levels of school participation, self-care, and play skills than did children with fragile X who did not avoid sensory experiences. It is often these behaviors that result in a child being referred to occupational therapy, even before a diagnosis of fragile X syndrome.

Down syndrome (also called *trisomy 21*) is the most common chromosomal abnormality, with an overall incidence rate from 1 per 600 to 1 per 800 (National Down Syndrome Society [NDSS], 2011). As the name *trisomy 21* indicates, the condition involves a triplication of genetic material. Although Down syndrome has an unknown etiology, the age of the mother is a documented risk factor. If a mother is under the age of 25, she has a 1 per 1,600 chance of having a child with Down syndrome. At 35 years of age, the risk increases to 1 per 340. If the mother is over the age of 43, the risk increases dramatically to 1 per 40 (National Dissemination Center for Children With Disabilities, 2010). The primary genetic cause of Down syndrome is an error in genetic cell division called *nondisjunction*, resulting in a triplication at chromosome 21. Translocation and mosaicism are two additional chromosomal abnormalities that result in Down syndrome, but at a significantly lower rate than nondisjunction (NDSS, n.d.).

At birth, the characteristic physical features are usually identifiable, including a flattened nasal bridge, minimal space in the oral cavity with resulting tongue protrusion, short hands with short fingers, a palmar simian crease, hypotonia, hyperextensibility at the joints, and decreased or inefficient sucking patterns (Case-Smith, 2005). Children with Down syndrome exhibit motor and developmental delays that impair occupational performance and frequently trigger an evaluation for occupational therapy services. In addition, there are specific medical concerns associated with a diagnosis of Down syndrome, including possible cardiac abnormalities that require surgical repair, an increased risk for leukemia, increased risk of respiratory infections, and atlantoaxial dislocation of the vertebra (Case-Smith, 2005).

Unlike Down syndrome and fragile X, other genetic conditions have a progressive course of increasing decline or disability. Cystic fibrosis, Tay–Sachs disease, sickle cell anemia, and muscular dystrophy are examples. These conditions are more likely to result in premature death; only approximately 50% of patients with sickle cell anemia survive beyond the fifth decade (Platt et al., 1994), and children with Tay–Sachs disease experience a rapid deterioration of neuromotor and cognitive function and generally have a life expectancy of 4 years (National Institute of Neurological Disorders and Stroke, 2007).

Two progressive genetic conditions that are most often seen by occupational therapists are cystic fibrosis and muscular dystrophy. Cystic fibrosis is one of the most common life-threatening autosomal recessive conditions affecting European Americans, with approximately 30,000 children and adults affected in the United States and 70,000 worldwide. Average life expectancy is 37.4 years (Cystic Fibrosis Foundation, 2008). Affected individuals will have two copies—one inherited from each parent—of the mutated CFTR gene, which carries the codes for a protein called the *cystic fibrosis transmembrane conductance regulator*. Carriers will have one normal and one mutated gene, and their health will not be affected. However, carriers have the potential to pass on the gene to their offspring. The condition may first be suspected when a child has a history of unexplained breathing or digestive problems, chronic lung infections, chronic sinusitis, or poor growth. As the condition progresses, thick, sticky mucus is produced, clogging the lungs and leading to life-threatening lung infections. The mucus also obstructs the pancreas, which stops natural enzymes from helping the body break down and absorb food. Children with cystic fibrosis may be small in stature and have gastrointestinal and breathing difficulties.

Muscular dystrophies are genetic disorders characterized by progressive muscle wasting and weakness that begin with microscopic changes in the muscle. As muscles degenerate over time, the person's muscle strength declines. There are more than 30 types of muscular dystrophy, which fall into three different patterns of inheritance. The two most common types, Duchenne and Becker muscular dystrophy, are X-linked recessive. This means that they are carried on one of the two paired genes on the X chromosome of the mother, who passes it on to an offspring. If the affected gene on the X chromosome is passed on to a male child, he will develop the disease.

The frequency of Duchenne muscular dystrophy (DMD) is 1 in every 3,500 live male births in the general population (Cleveland Clinic, 2009). DMD occurs when a particular gene on the X chromosome fails to make the protein dystrophin in the muscles. Many boys with DMD follow a normal pattern of development during their first few years of life. Between ages 3 and 5 years, symptoms such as stumbling, difficulty going up stairs, and toe walking begin to appear. A child may start to struggle to get up from a sitting position (Gowers' sign) or have a hard time pushing things, like a wagon or a tricycle. One common clinical sign is hypertrophy of the calf muscles, as muscle tissue is replaced by fat and calves appear enlarged. Typically, boys with DMD use a wheelchair for locomotion by adolescence. The disease gradually weakens the skeletal muscles, especially those in the arms, legs, and trunk. By the early teens or even earlier, the boy's heart and respiratory muscles also may be affected. About a third of boys with DMD have some degree of learning disability.

Becker muscular dystrophy (BMD) is a less common and much milder version of the condition. Its onset is usually in the teens or early adulthood. As with

DMD, the pattern of muscle loss in BMD usually begins with the hips and pelvic area and later affects the shoulders as well. In BMD, the rate of muscle degeneration varies a great deal from one person to another. Some men require wheelchairs by their 30s, while some manage for many years with aids such as canes. As in boys with DMD, children with BMD may have learning problems, often in attention focusing, verbal learning and memory, and emotional interaction.

## Target Areas for Intervention

Common to both fragile X syndrome and Down syndrome are developmental delays that typically cross several areas of development, including motor, language, social, adaptive behavior, functional independence, play skills, sensory processing, and cognitive skills. The child with Down syndrome typically experiences delays in reaching most developmental milestones, including motor, language, learning, and adaptive skills. Postural and fine motor skills are typically decreased, affecting independence in activities of daily living (ADL), including functional mobility, self-feeding, dressing, and tool use. Children with fragile X syndrome might have learning problems and difficulties with social interactions. There may be sensory processing and integration issues in children with Down syndrome or fragile X syndrome, resulting in defensive behavior or a failure to register sensory input. Children with Down syndrome have a higher than normal incidence of visual acuity deficits requiring correction, and children with fragile X syndrome may have strabismis or acuity problems as well. The occupational therapist plays a vital role on the treatment team, addressing the myriad issues associated with a diagnosis of either Down syndrome or fragile X syndrome.

Children with progressive genetic disorders will need increasing amounts of support in multiple performance areas, such as ADL, communication, education, and play. Technology may play a major part in adapting the non-human environment to enhance these children's ability to participate meaningfully in purposeful activities. Mental health issues, such as depression or anxiety, might also be addressed by the occupational therapist as the child continually readjusts to his or her changed level of functioning. Each progressive genetic disorder is different; for example, a young child with Tay–Sachs disease will rapidly exhibit declining mental function, while a child with cystic fibrosis will not. Therefore, treatment must also be aligned with normal developmental needs and expectations to the greatest degree possible, since some areas, such as motor capacity or bodily functions, may be in decline, while other areas, such as cognitive skills, may be advancing in a typical developmental sequence.

# 🌿 Contextual Considerations

## Clinical

The clinical evaluation of the child with a genetic disorder can be varied as a result of the differential nature of genetic conditions, but there are some common elements that should be addressed. The clinical evaluation is dependent on the service delivery setting, the age of the child, and the reason for referral. In general, the purpose of the occupational therapy assessment with a child with a genetic condition is to assess strengths and weaknesses in broad areas of development, including gross and fine motor skills, cognitive skills, and sensory processing, and adaptive functioning in the areas of ADL, play, education, and work, as framed by the *Occupational Therapy Practice Framework* (American Occupational Therapy Association [AOTA], 2008).

Since children with genetic conditions often present with delays in many areas of development, evaluation data that provide a broad perspective of developmental functioning is beneficial. Standardized and criterion-based assessments, such as the *Bayley Scales of Infant Development–Second Edition* (Bayley, 1993), the *Battelle Developmental Inventory–Second Edition* (Newborg, 2005), the *Miller Assessment for Preschoolers* (Miller, 1988), and the *Hawaii Early Learning Profile* (Furuno et al., 1991), provide data in a broad number of developmental areas. These can include motor, cognitive, language, and social skills, as well as adaptive skills related to dressing, bathing, play, and feeding.

Feeding can be an issue, especially in children with Down syndrome. Many nonstandardized procedures are used to assess a child's oral–motor and feeding skills, including control and praxis of oral–motor structures, oral sensitivity, a comprehensive feeding history, and (for the older child) an observation of self-feeding skills.

Children with genetic conditions are frequently delayed in their attainment of motor milestones. Data from criterion-referenced and standardized tests, including the *Peabody Developmental Motor Scales–Second Edition* (Folio & Fewell, 2000), the *Bruininks–Oseretsky Test of Motor Proficiency–Second Edition* (Bruininks, 2006), and the *Erhardt Developmental Prehension Assessment* (Erhardt, 1994), will provide the therapist with information on how the child's gross motor and fine motor skills compare to a developmental norm. But test results should be supplemented by clinical observations related to functional gross and fine motor skills (e.g., climbing stairs, getting on or off a bus, tool use in the classroom). For children with declining motor skills, assessment can monitor and document the rate and impact of change so that the therapist can plan adaptations and accommodations accordingly.

Children with genetic conditions may have sensory defensiveness that can impact their engagement with and participation in life activities. The *Sensory Profile* (Dunn, 1999) is a standardized assessment based on caregiver interviews that provides information on the child's ability to process and respond to a variety of sensory information in a variety of settings. The *Sensory Profile School Companion* (Dunn, 2006) allows the therapist to gain critical sensory information about the child that specifically relates to the school environment.

Functional assessments that look at developmental skills within context include the *School Function Assessment* (SFA), which evaluates a child's (K–6) performance, level of participation, and need for assistance in school activities, including physical, cognitive, and behavioral tasks (Coster, Deeney, Haltiwanger, &

Haley, 1998). The *Vineland Adaptive Behavior Scales–Second Edition* measures communication, daily living skills, socialization, and motor skills with a behavioral rating scale (Sparrow, Cicchetti, & Balla, 2005). An important component to these functional assessments is to consider the child's cognitive abilities and level of mental retardation, which, for children with genetic conditions, can range from mild to severe.

Cases of intellectual disability, specifically for those whose IQ is less than 70, can be classified into ranges of mild, moderate, severe, or profound. Individuals with mild impairment can acquire basic math and reading skills and work in semiskilled jobs with vocational training. Individuals with moderate impairment may be able to learn basic skills that will help them with community integration, such as writing a legal signature, reading for safety, using public transportation, managing money, and working with the help of a job coach and supervision. Individuals who fall in the "severe" category typically need programs that focus on basic self-care skills and structured prevocational skills. Children classified with profound intellectual disability have delays in many functional areas and are usually dependent for all areas of basic self-care skills, including feeding, dressing, and toileting. Children with profound impairment typically have severe central nervous system impairment and often require family support and respite programs because they are dependent on the caregiver. Within each classification of impairment, there can be a wide range of adaptive functioning and cognitive skills.

Cognitive abilities, as they relate to functional occupational performance, include the ability to attend and follow directions, memory skills, general knowledge of basic concepts, judgment and self-awareness, and problem solving. In addition to looking at the classification system and standardized intelligence testing as a guide, these abilities should be informally evaluated within the context of functional occupational performance. For example, when out in the community, does the adolescent with Down syndrome have the cognitive ability to independently purchase an item from a retail store? These types of naturalistic observations will provide data on areas that may require direct intervention in order for the individual to be successful, or will help determine levels of assistance that may be required.

Assistive technology and environmental assessments can yield important information with regard to promoting function and successful participation for children with progressive or nonprogressive genetic conditions. The Compass Access Assessment is a software evaluation that can help the occupational therapist determine the child's speed and accuracy of computer skills. Compass assesses three broad categories of computer usage: pointing, scanning, and text entry. This can be important for measuring progress and identifying aspects of computer use that need to be adapted. Another evaluative tool that surveys students' assistive technology needs is the Wisconsin Assistive Technology Initiative's *Assessing Students' Need for Assistive Technology*. This publication contains observational assistive technology checklists for a wide variety of clinical needs. There are descriptions of devices included that can assist the communication needs of children with Down syndrome, who frequently have speech and language delays. There are also descriptions of software for the computer that assists with the motor process of keyboarding, as well as with the cognitive processes of spelling, grammar, and so forth. Children with Down syndrome and fragile X syndrome have learning difficulties that can be addressed through computer software design. This resource also allows the therapist to examine the need for assistive technology adaptations for feeding, dressing, and other ADL skills that might be useful for children with a variety of genetic disorders.

Children with muscular dystrophy experience a severe decline in motor skills in childhood and adolescence and benefit dramatically from assistive technology. They frequently use a power wheelchair and need a ventilator as their condition progresses. They might also require computer adaptations or environmental control units to help them access their environment. Some children with genetic disorders such as Canavan disease are significantly compromised in voluntary movements and might benefit from switch technology for interacting with their environment. An evaluative tool that assesses the need and type of switch that would be beneficial for a client is the Switch Assessment and Planning Framework, from the United Kingdom (http://www.ace-north.org.uk/pages/resources/documents/SwAssessmentFramework.pdf). All assistive technology evaluations should involve a hands-on component when different equipment is tried with the student. Most states have a resource center where assistive technology items can be borrowed and tried before purchase.

## Family

Families that have a child with a genetic condition may be very aware of the nature of the condition either before the child is born or at the child's birth. Prenatally, there are screening tests that assess the risk of having a child with a genetic condition and diagnostic testing that tells whether the fetus has the condition. To detect Down syndrome, for example, two screening blood tests are available, the triple screen and the alpha-fetoprotein plus, which are used in conjunction with a sonogram and the age of the mother to assess risk (NDSS, n.d.). These screenings accurately detect 60% of fetuses with Down syndrome, but many women get false-positive results and others get false-negative results. A prenatal diagnosis of Down syndrome can be made with chorionic villus sampling at 8 to 12 weeks gestation, amniocentesis at 12 to 20 weeks, and percutaneous umbilical blood sampling after 20 weeks gestation (NDSS, n.d.). All of these procedures carry a small risk of miscarriage but are 98% to 99% accurate in confirming a diagnosis of Down syndrome. Many other genetic conditions are also detectable prenatally, but screenings may only be conducted on high-risk groups.

Genetic counseling is given in conjunction with prenatal genetic testing. If the pregnancy continues, the early diagnosis often puts the family in touch with support groups, early intervention services, and a wealth of Internet resources related to the specific conditions. The early diagnosis does not negate the need to focus on family-centered care, which takes into account the priorities, values, goals, and culture of the family. The child with Down syndrome or fragile X syndrome is not going to "grow out of it" or be cured. A genetic condition is lifelong and, if inherited, has implications for subsequent pregnancies.

The family's routines, habits, and priorities will be altered rapidly with the birth of a child with an identified genetic condition such as Down syndrome or Tay–Sachs disease. At all times, the therapist needs to be culturally sensitive to the experiences, values, and beliefs of the family through this process. Additionally, the primary caregiver's bond with the baby can be affected by the clinical characteristics of the genetic condition. For example, feeding a child with Down syndrome may be prolonged and more difficult for the caregiver, impairing the basic satisfaction a parent feels when nourishing his or her baby. This can be due to low tone and a weak suck–swallow pattern. Another factor that can affect the process of attachment is the separation of mother and child at birth because of the baby's need to be in the neonatal intensive care unit (NICU). Additionally, aspects of the baby's genetic disorder may keep him or her from responding in a way that fosters attachment. For example, the child may have an immature sensory system that is overly sensitive to touch, creating a situation where the parent cannot hold and comfort him or her successfully. The child may also have an impaired visual system, diminishing ability to sustain eye contact and gaze with his or her parent. An occupational therapist can help a parent learn to hold and feed the baby, accommodate sensory and postural needs, and encourage kangaroo care (Ludington-Hoe, 2006) and other bonding strategies when medically permissible.

For other families, the process of recognizing and identifying their child's genetic disorder may be extended and convoluted. A parent may suspect that something is wrong with his or her child's development but may not get a diagnosis for several years. For children with muscular dystrophy, for example, parents might notice early symptoms in the first year of life, such as a delay of motor milestones, including sitting and standing independently. The mean age for walking in boys with DMD is 18 months. Soon after, in early childhood, calf muscles typically enlarge and are replaced with fat and connective tissue (pseudohypertrophy). A clinical diagnosis may be made when a boy has progressive symmetrical muscle weakness, his symptoms present before age 5 years, and he has extremely elevated creatine kinase blood levels. A muscle biopsy for dystrophin studies is done to look for abnormal levels of dystrophin in the muscle. Genetic testing can help confirm the diagnosis. The parents of a child with muscular dystrophy who are coping with a new diagnosis or their child's decline in function will need support from professionals. Caregivers of a child with muscular dystrophy have been shown to be more likely than the general population to suffer a major depressive episode (Daoud, Dooley, & Gordon, 2004).

Fragile X is similarly not usually diagnosed at birth, and families may have numerous concerns before their child's condition is identified. The first clinical clue in children often is delayed attainment of one or more developmental milestones.

On average, boys with fragile X syndrome sit without support at 10 months of age and walk and talk at 20 months (Wattendorf & Muenke, 2005). The average age of fragile X syndrome diagnosis currently is 32 months (Bailey, Skinner, & Sparkman, 2003; Wattendorf & Muenke, 2005). Families report barriers to discovering fragile X syndrome and frustration with the process, such as initial dismissal of concerns by pediatricians and the need for multiple visits to professionals before genetic testing is suggested (Bailey et al., 2003). In a study of 460 families with a child with fragile X syndrome, over one third of the parents reported that more than 10 office visits were required before a recommendation for fragile X syndrome testing was made (Bailey et al., 2003).

Occupational therapy can be equally instrumental in helping these families who have children with suspected genetic conditions but no diagnosis. These children, like their diagnosed counterparts, generally exhibit difficulties with performance areas and components of rest and sleep, feeding, bonding, and meeting developmental milestones. Parents need support to consistently nurture and connect with their baby throughout the diagnostic process. Without a correct diagnosis, parents may not be able to easily access the appropriate medical, community, therapeutic, and personal supports suited to their child's needs.

It is vital to keep in communication with the family on an informal basis, as well as conducting structured interviews, to get a sense of the family's typical day, the areas of family functioning that are being impacted, and parental stress levels around routines and daily habits. The therapist can offer suggestions and adaptive equipment that may make feeding and self-care skills easier. Many times, close communication with the family is a focus of early intervention services but decreases dramatically when the child enters school. By scheduling time to maintain communication with the family via logs or phone calls, in addition to face-to-face contact at Individualized Education Program (IEP) meetings, the therapist can also educate the family about the role of intervention and how service delivery models may change as the child goes through formal schooling. The occupational therapist has an important role in stressing advocacy for the family and providing resources for the family of a child with a genetic condition. This may include "futuring," or finding out what the family's vision is for their child, to determine when occupational therapy services are most appropriate and what the focus of intervention should be, based on the relevant occupations of the child within the context of the family.

## Practice Setting

Children with genetic conditions interface with medical, educational, and community-based practice settings. Most children with genetic conditions would be seen primarily in early intervention centers, school-based settings, and private practice. The determination of practice setting is largely based on the child's age. From birth to age 5 years, services can be delivered in the NICU, the acute or rehabilitation hospital, and private practice, or services can be community based, including early intervention that is home and/or center based. Infants with Down syndrome often have medical complications, including feeding and respiratory difficulties and congenital heart defects that require the services of the NICU. The therapist will focus on positioning, strategies to improve feeding, and facilitation of developmental milestones. If a child with Down syndrome requires cardiac surgery to correct a heart defect, a therapist may deliver services in the acute and rehabilitation stages of the child's recovery, including positioning to decrease swelling and promote postural drainage immediately after surgery and intervention to improve endurance to activity. During the rehabilitation phase of intervention, goals would be associated with returning the child to postsurgery levels of functioning and communicating with family and community-based therapists.

Early intervention services are provided within the natural environment from birth to age 3 years, which often means home-based services or services that are delivered in a primary day care setting. Therapists providing early intervention for children with Down syndrome and fragile X syndrome typically work as part of a treatment team because of the multiple areas of developmental delay. From the ages of 3 to 5 years, children with Down syndrome and fragile X syndrome may continue to be seen in the home but are often transitioned to center-based programs, such as regular day care programs or preschools, where they are integrated with children without disabilities. The transition to school-based services is then made, with the majority of therapy services received during the course of the school day. The therapist works with the child to ensure that he or she can benefit from special education programming, focusing on developing fine motor skills, social skills, ADL skills, and prevocational and vocational readiness skills. School-based services, as required under the Individuals With Disabilities Education Improvement Act (IDEIA, 2004), should be delivered within inclusive settings to the greatest degree possible. During the transition from school to adulthood, the therapist may deliver services in a variety of community-based programs that service individuals with developmental disabilities such as Down syndrome and fragile X syndrome. These settings include (but are not limited to) institutional programs, group homes, supported employment, and sheltered workshops. Practice settings may also include adult day care programs and long-term care facilities that provide services for adults with developmental disabilities.

## Sociopolitical

The laws concerning services and education for children with disabilities also apply to children with genetic conditions. Specifically, the Individuals With Disabilities Education Improvement Act (IDEIA, 2004) entitles all children with disabilities to a free and appropriate public education and related services. In addition, many children with genetic defects are diagnosed at birth and qualify for early intervention services. Under Part C of IDEIA, which outlines services for children from birth to age 3 years, Down syndrome and fragile X syndrome are classified as an established risk factor, which includes conditions that have a high probability of resulting in developmental delay (IDEIA, 2004). Occupational therapists offer family-centered care in natural environments and are considered direct service providers for children from birth to 3 years of age.

IDEIA (2004) mandated special education services in schools for children from 3 to 21 years of age who are identified and coded with a disability. Most children with a genetic condition that affects development would be classified to receive special education services. Occupational therapy is a related or supportive service that is utilized when a child needs occupational therapy to benefit from his or her education program. School-based occupational therapy services may also be provided under the Rehabilitation Act of 1973 with a 504 Plan, which ensures that students with disabilities are given equal access to school activities and that reasonable accommodations are made to allow students to access these activities. Children with Down syndrome and fragile X syndrome, for example, would be classified and coded with a condition that would entitle them to education services under IDEIA and provide for occupational therapy services as a related service if necessary for the child to benefit from his or her program.

IDEIA also strengthened the legislative mandate for transition planning, education, and vocational services for individuals with disabilities. Through this reauthorization, transition planning and programming must be in place by the time the child is 16 years of age, to focus on success and participation in society after 21 years of age. Often, students with Down syndrome and fragile X syndrome will begin to explore vocational options, engage in prevocational tasks to build foundational skills, practice instrumental ADL, and engage in community-based activities.

IDEIA provides more due process guarantees for parents, unifies IEP goals across service providers, and requires research-based intervention strategies delivered by highly qualified professionals. One change from IDEA to IDEIA that is specifically relevant to the occupational therapist is a greater emphasis on appropriate assistive technology for students as needed (IDEIA, 2004, § 300.105). IDEIA has been worded to clearly state that for all children, the multidisciplinary team must consider the need for assistive technology devices and services. Children with both progressive and nonprogressive genetic disorders can benefit greatly from this provision, since the appropriate use of assistive technology by the occupational therapist can help them access their environment and their educational program.

IDEIA also more vigorously requires inclusion of students with disabilities in typical classrooms (the least restrictive environment [LRE]) alongside their peers. Under IDEIA, each state must establish LRE targets that are both rigorous and measurable and report such progress toward these targets annually to the U.S. Department of Education and to the public. The presumption is that IEP teams begin placement discussions with a consideration of the general education classroom and the supplementary aids and services that are needed to enable a student with a disability to benefit from educational services. The occupational therapist can be part of a Response to Intervention (RTI) service delivery model that supports students academically by differentiating instruction within general education before they are referred to special education (Barnett, Daly, Jones, & Lentz, 2004). They can also contribute to the positive behavioral supports (sensory processing needs, for example) that address the mental health and social needs of children in typical classrooms before a special education referral takes place.

When a child does qualify for occupational therapy as a related service, the renewed focus on the LRE provision of IDEIA has prompted more occupational therapy interventions to occur within natural settings in the school, such as the classroom, the cafeteria, or the playground. The use of segregated education settings must be explained and justified. Delayed developmental skills can impact a child's ability to participate in educational and play activities with typical peers, but so can poor social skills, which also create major barriers to successful inclusion. Occupational therapists who work with children with genetic disorders are challenged to enhance their skills in all areas and adapt the environment in ways that promote inclusion in schools.

## Lifestyle/Lifespan

Depending on the specific genetic condition, there will be a variety of lifestyle and lifespan issues to consider. For example, individuals with Down syndrome can lead productive lives, live independently or with minimal supervision, have a diverse and rich social life, and become gainfully employed. The level of success in the community is dependent on the severity of the disability, the availability of community resources and supports, and whether there is a focus on independent functioning and quality of life from the outset. The key to success in the community is often related to the level of the individual's adaptive skills, and this should be the focus throughout the lifespan and during times of transition (e.g., elementary to middle school, school to work).

Individuals with genetic conditions may have a reduced life expectancy or a higher incidence of medical complications. Individuals with Down syndrome have a life expectancy of approximately 50 years, with a higher incidence of dementia and Alzheimer's disease, an increased risk of mortality from specific causes like leukemia, and an elevated risk of other cancers (Hill et al., 2003).

## 🌿 Clinical Decision-Making Process

### Defining Focus for Intervention

The revised *Occupational Therapy Practice Framework* (AOTA, 2008) serves as the primary vehicle with which to describe the child's functioning and identify the focus for intervention within the occupational therapist's domain of practice. The *Practice Framework* outlines the areas of the child's functioning to be addressed. For children with genetic disorders, all areas of occupation may be impacted. Children with Down syndrome, for example, may have difficulties in education and social participation. Children with DMD will need adaptations to participate in work settings and leisure activities. Rest and sleep might be an issue for children with cystic fibrosis. Performance skills need to be carefully assessed to set goals and areas for intervention. The occupational therapist must have specific knowledge of the child's abilities in the areas of motor and praxis skills, sensory perception, emotional regulation, cognition, and communication and social skills. The therapist must also consider the client factors, especially body functions and structures that may be affected by the genetic condition. The age of the client, for example, will determine whether the focus of occupational therapy intervention should be on developing foundational skills, compensating for a lack of skill that may not develop, modifying the environment, adapting the task, or a combination of several of these methods. By analyzing the context and environment as well as the activity demands, the occupational therapist will be able to design an effective treatment plan that enhances opportunities for meaningful participation.

## Establishing Goals for Intervention

Just as there are key elements that determine the focus of intervention, there are specific elements that assist in the establishment of goals for intervention. The *Practice Framework* guides the therapist through the clinical reasoning that leads to appropriate goal setting and effective intervention by examining evaluation, intervention, and outcomes. The *Practice Framework* describes the occupation and client-centered process used in the delivery of occupational therapy services. For a child with a genetic disorder, the evaluation phase of the *Practice Framework* will yield key information to frame treatment. Through a careful occupational profile, the occupational therapist can learn about the child's occupational status and the child's and family's priorities. This is then followed by standard and nonstandardized evaluative tools to establish baseline data for goal setting. The intervention plan includes theory- and evidence-based approaches and specific, measurable goals with a defined time frame. The nature of the genetic disorder will determine the approach chosen. For example, a child with a progressive condition may benefit more from an approach that focuses on modifications rather than establishing or restoring skills. Treatment is implemented and continually reviewed for modifications as needed. As the educational context and developmental expectations change, a different occupational therapy service delivery model may be required.

Goals should be directly related to the age of the child, client factors that influence the potential for independence, and the setting where services are delivered. They should also be grounded in the priorities of the family and/or caregivers. Services that are delivered in the schools must have goals directly related to the child's ability to benefit from his or her educational program, while considering the curriculum context. Services delivered in a hospital, home, or private clinic may focus more on functional goals that relate to ADL.

The time frame for meeting long-term goals is dependent on the practice setting. In schools, a long-term goal is typically for the duration of a school year, but this may be changing in some states. The delivery of one-to-one direct services in schools may be decreasing, with an increased utilization of group treatment and indirect interventions such as monitoring and periodic technical assistance for environmental adaptations or assistive devices. In rehabilitation hospital settings, the duration is shorter, typically 1 to 2 months. Short-term goals (also referred to as *behavioral objectives*) are steps to meet the long-term goal. Short-term goals should have measurable criteria so that progress can be evaluated. Goals for children with Down syndrome and fragile X syndrome should be grounded in adaptive skills, since those are instrumental to successful participation in the community. Goals for children with progressive genetic disorders may center on environmental adaptations and assistive technology.

## Designing Theory-Based Intervention

As discussed, children with genetic conditions typically have developmental delays in several areas, including motor, cognitive, language, sensory, play, and ADL. The occupational therapist may use several frames of reference, theories, and models applicable to this population to guide assessment and treatment.

Developmental theories, such as those developed by Erickson, Piaget, Freud, and Havinghurst, shape the therapist's conceptualization and knowledge of normal development, which is essential to pediatric practice. Developmental theories guide the intervention initially, to build necessary foundational skills in an expected developmental sequence. For example, the therapist would try to develop postural stability and mobility skills with a child with Down syndrome in prone and supine positions before working in a quadruped or sitting position. Having a solid understanding of normal development and the theories that explain expected progressions will help the therapist recognize deviations in development that may need compensation.

The model of human occupation (Kielhofner, 2008) is essential to frame intervention with this population. Different occupations that provide meaning and purpose to the individual are engaged in throughout the life cycle. The child with Down syndrome will not be in a student role forever, and therapy must focus on this shift in roles and expectations. By using an occupation-based perspective, the therapist can frame interventions that will facilitate successful engagement using the abilities the individual possesses. For example, it may not be necessary to continue to work on handwriting legibility and spacing if the child or adolescent can write and sign his or her name. This may be the highest level of functioning in this area that the individual can obtain. Time may be better spent looking at other performance skills he or she may need to be successful in the role of student or family member, or in the future role of employee. Inherent in the model of human occupation is an examination of the roles, routines, habits, and volitions of the child and family members, as well as the environmental context. This framework is essential to practice with any population.

Sensory integration is a theoretical framework that can be used to improve sensory integration and processing. Children with fragile X syndrome are often hypersensitive to sensory stimulation, which can lead to behavioral responses that include avoidance and withdrawal, nonadaptability, and a need to control the amount of stimulation that is received. A therapist can use the principles of sensory integration theory to influence how a child responds to sensory stimuli and to reduce extremes in behavioral response patterns (e.g., increase accepted foods, eliminate hitting during grooming activities, impact sleep patterns).

## Evaluating Progress

Measurable outcomes have become increasingly important in occupational therapy as a means of demonstrating the utility of therapy to the client. Supporting health and participation in the engagement in occupation is the intended outcome of the occupational therapy intervention process (AOTA, 2008). Outcomes, as described in the *Practice Framework*, fall into nine categories: occupational performance, adaptation, participation, health and wellness, prevention, quality of life, role competence, self-advocacy, and occupational justice. Each of these has special significance to children with genetic disorders. In terms of occupational performance, adaptation, and participation, children with genetic conditions may work toward therapy outcomes that will facilitate meaningful inclusion and engagement. For example, a child with Down syndrome might successfully use a communication device that increases his social interactions, a child with fragile X syndrome might complete an assignment using computer software that helps her organize her thoughts in social studies, or a child with muscular dystrophy might be able to use a bathroom adaptation to be able to bathe safely with less assistance. Occupational therapy outcomes can also focus on health and wellness and prevention. A teen with cystic fibrosis, for example, may learn to manage her medical devices well enough to be able to be included in school field trips. Her independence at this task may prevent a hospitalization or school absences. Outcomes can include quality of life and role competence issues. The child's view of life satisfaction relates to his sense of control, choice, and mastery. By facilitating successful participation in important occupations, quality of life and role fulfillment will be enhanced. Finally, occupational therapy outcomes can promote self-advocacy and occupational justice. Children with genetic conditions can be helped to understand their self-worth and advocate for themselves among their peers, in their schools, and in their communities. A child who explains his genetic condition to a neighbor can reduce social barriers. A student with fragile X syndrome who can ask a teacher to repeat directions might do better on an exam. A teenager who raises money for cystic fibrosis research may feel a greater sense of control over her circumstances. Concrete outcomes provide a means for the efficacy of occupational therapy services to become apparent.

In an increasingly litigious and economically stressed society, accountability in terms of specific therapy outcomes is an essential piece of therapy. Children with genetic conditions may require therapy services for an extended period of time because of the chronicity or progression of their disorder. Therefore, the occupational therapist must be able to clearly justify and document the attainment of functional treatment objectives that are of value to the child, the family, the school or health care system, and society at large.

Progress is assessed based on the specific goals and benchmarks that were established. Goal attainment warrants a revision of the goals to continue with progress or a determination of whether services are no longer indicated. Outcomes, as outlined by the *Practice Framework*, should be functional and based on the child's or adolescent's occupational role performance. Is he or she succeeding in participating and engaging in occupations that are relevant to the age, the diagnosis, and the practice setting? A review of established goals, formal reevaluation, and interviews with parents and teachers are the best ways to evaluate progress.

## Determining Change in or Termination of Treatment

Occupational therapy services should be utilized intensively upon the diagnosis of a genetic condition, to work with the child and family to maximize functioning in delayed areas and impact the ability to participate in occupational roles. The focus of intervention should change as the child develops, as should expectations for participation in different activities. As these expectations shift, the occupational therapist can provide intervention to enhance specific skills, habits, or behaviors; adapt or change the context; or work as a consultant with the child's caregivers or other adults who are frequently with the child to enable participation in activities. Termination of services is appropriate when the child or adolescent is functioning at his or her maximal level and/or has reached a plateau. In many cases, it may be best to reduce service amounts or intensity gradually rather than abruptly. This ensures that the child is maintaining new skills or use of adaptations and allows the family to adjust to a change in service delivery support.

Treatment should take place in natural contexts as much as possible. If the treatment sessions are given in an isolated setting, it is imperative that the occupational therapist communicate with family members and other professionals to make sure goals and interventions are relevant to functional needs. Sometimes services are terminated and then resumed. Occupational therapy in context implies that services may be terminated in one context, but as the context changes, services may be required in order to achieve maximum functioning in the individual's occupational roles. A resumption of therapy services may also be indicated if a child's skills decline, as in the case of some progressive genetic disorders.

## Case Study

### Description

AK is a 14-year-old boy with Down syndrome. AK has received early intervention services and special education services throughout his schooling. He is in the first year of high school, in a full inclusion class with a one-to-one aide, and he participates in special education programming for half of his school day. AK has mild to moderate cognitive impairment and good receptive language skills but limited expressive language skills. He uses a picture exchange communication system and simple sign language to supplement his limited vocabulary. He becomes easily frustrated and angry when he is not understood. Socially, AK doesn't initiate interaction with his peers, but he enjoys social interaction if initiated by his classmates. Because AK is 16 years of age, transition planning services are being developed and implemented. His curriculum currently consists of exploring potential areas of employment and focuses on a life skills approach.

A multidisciplinary team, which includes AK, his parents, his aide, both his special education and his general education teachers, an occupational therapist, a speech–language pathologist, and the school psychologist, has met to formulate a transition plan. The plan uses AK's strengths and interests to begin to explore vocational activities in which he might be the most successful. AK has identified an interest in working with papers and having an office. He has always liked having his own task that he can try to see through to completion, versus working collaboratively with a group of individuals. AK can be easily distracted when there are increased auditory stimuli in the environment. A review of his IEP and his most recent 3-year evaluation results made the team members aware of his strengths and weaknesses and of teaching strategies that have worked with AK in the past. He appears to have some relative strength with visual–motor skills.

In transition planning, critical considerations include the client's priorities, goals, and interests. These must intersect with the abilities and potential skills that the team has identified. AK has identified an interest in working with papers and has documented strengths in the area of visual perceptual skills. The team chose a real-world sorting activity that lets him work independently, uses his strengths, and could potentially lead to vocational work if he is successful. The task was broken down into key elements in order to have AK achieve a sense of mastery and task completion.

### Long- and Short-Term Goals

The long-term goal of intervention for AK is to enable him to independently sort incoming mail for 30 minutes on 3 consecutive days with 100% accuracy. The short-term goals of intervention for AK are as follows:

1. Match 10 names to the correct mailbox with 80% accuracy.
2. Complete a sorting and matching task with no more than two verbal reminders to remain on task.

### Therapist Goals and Strategies

The therapist's goals include the following:

1. Improve AK's on-task behavior.
2. Enhance AK's visual discrimination and matching abilities.
3. Improve AK's motor speed.

The therapist's strategies include the following:

1. Use visual cuing with colors to improve task orientation and focusing.
2. Provide opportunities for repetition, practice, verbal cuing, and reward.

3. Conduct task analysis to gain understanding of potential strengths and weaknesses.

4. Upgrade the activity to include the time, speed, and accuracy necessary to perform the job in a real-world context.

### Activity: Last Name First

AK will be given a green highlighter and an initial template of envelopes that show several ways a last name can appear. For example, "Mr. Smith," "Mr. James Smith," "The Smiths," "The Smith Family," and "To the parents of Thomas Smith." AK will be required to initially scan each envelope and locate the last name on the envelope. If correct, he will be required to highlight the last name and put in the "done" box. If incorrect, AK will be verbally cued to put the envelope aside and continue. After the activity is completed, AK will count the number of correct pieces of mail and give himself a score. Each incorrect piece of mail will be reviewed with AK in a teach-and-learn process.

### Treatment Objective

AK will correctly highlight the last name on 15 random pieces of mail without verbal cuing.

## Resources

### Internet Resources

Council for Exceptional Children: www.cec.sped.org

National Dissemination Center for Children With Disabilities: www.nichcy.org

National Down Syndrome Society: www.ndss.org

National Fragile X Foundation: www.fragilex.org

National Human Genome Research Institute: www.genome.gov

National Institutes of Health, Office of Rare Diseases Research: www.rarediseases.info .nih.gov

### Print Resources

Compass-Access Assessment Software, Version 2, by Koester Performance Research Spectronics Australia, P.O. Box 88, Rochedale, Queensland 4123, Australia

Switch Assessment and Planning Framework: http://www.ace-north.org.uk/pages/ resources/documents/SwAssessmentFramework.pdf

Wisconsin Assistive Technology Initiative: Assessing Students' Need for Assistive Technology: http://www.wati.org/WatiMaterials
http://www.wati.org/content/supports/free/pdf/ASNAT4thEditionDec08.pdf

## References

American Occupational Therapy Association. (2008). Occupational therapy practice framework: Domain and process (2nd ed.). *American Journal of Occupational Therapy, 62,* 625–683.

American Psychiatric Association. (2000). *Diagnostic and statistical manual of mental disorders* (4th ed., text revision). Washington, DC: Author.

Bailey, D. B., Hatton, D. D., Tassone, F., Skinner, M., & Taylor, A. K. (2001). FMRP and early development in fragile X syndrome. *American Journal of Mental Retardation, 106,* 16–27.

Bailey, D. B., Skinner, D., Hatton, D., & Roberts, J. (2000). Family experiences and factors associated with diagnosis of fragile X syndrome. *Journal of Developmental and Behavioral Pediatrics, 21*(5), 315–321.

Bailey, D. B., Skinner, D., & Sparkman, K. (2003). Discovering fragile X syndrome: Family experiences and perceptions. *Pediatrics, 111,* 407–416.

Baranek, G. T., Chin, Y. K., Greiss Hess, L. M., Yankee, J. G., Hatton, D. D., & Hooper, S. R. (2002). Sensory processing correlates of occupational performance in children with fragile X syndrome: Preliminary findings. *American Journal of Occupational Therapy, 56,* 538–546.

Barnett, D., Daly, E., Jones, K., & Lentz, F. (2004). Response to intervention: Empirically based special services decisions from single case designs of increasing and decreasing intensity. *The Journal of Special Education, 38* (2), 66–79.

Bayley, N. (1993). *Bayley scales of infant development* (2nd ed.). San Antonio, TX: The Psychological Corporation.

Blackman, J. A. (1997). *Medical aspects of developmental disabilities in children birth to three* (3rd ed.). Gaithersburg, MD: Aspen.

Bruininks, R. H., & Bruininks, B. D. (2005). *Bruininks–Oseretsky test of motor proficiency* (2nd ed.). San Antonio, TX: Pearson Assessments.

Case-Smith, J. (2005). *Occupational therapy for children* (5th ed.). Philadelphia, PA: Mosby.

Cleveland Clinic. (2009). *Muscular dystrophy.* Retrieved from http://my.clevelandclinic .org/disorders/muscular_dystrophy/hic_musculardystrophy.aspx

Coster, W., Deeney, T., Haltiwanger, J., & Haley, S. (1998). *School function assessment (SFA).* San Antonio, TX: The Psychological Corporation.

Cystic Fibrosis Foundation. (2008). *About CF.* Retrieved from http://www.cff.org/

Daoud, M. A., Dooley, J., & Gordon, K. (2004). Depression in parents of children with Duchenne muscular dystrophy. *Pediatric Neurology, 31*(1), 16–19.

Dunn, W. (1999). *Sensory Profile user's manual.* San Antonio, TX: The Psychological Corporation.

Dunn, W. (2006). *Sensory profile school companion.* San Antonio, TX: Pearson Assessments.

Erhardt, R. P. (1994). *Erhardt developmental prehension assessment* (Rev. ed.). San Antonio, TX: The Psychological Corporation.

Folio, R., & Fewell, R. (2000). *Peabody developmental motor scales* (2nd ed.). Austin, TX: PRO-ED, Inc.

Furuno, S., O'Reilly, K., Inatsuka, T., Hosaka, C. M., Allman, T., & Zeisloft-Falbey, B. (1991). *The Hawaii early learning profile.* Palo Alto, CA: VORT.

Hill, D. A., Gridley, G., Cnattingius, S., Mellemkjaer, L., Linet, M., Adami, H. O., . . . Fraumeni, J. F. Jr. (2003). Mortality and cancer incidence among individuals with Down syndrome. *Archives of Internal Medicine, 163,* 705–711.

Individuals With Disabilities Education Act of 1990, 20 U.S.C. § 1400 *et seq.* (1990) (amended 1997).

Individuals With Disabilities Education Improvement Act of 2004, 20 U.S.C. §1400 *et seq.* (2004).

Kielhofner, G. (2008). *Model of human occupation theory and application* (4th ed.). Baltimore, MD: Lippincott, Williams & Wilkins.

Ludington-Hoe, S. (2006). Developmental aspects of kangaroo care. *Journal of Obstetric, Gynocologic, & Neonatal Nursing, 25*(8), 691–703.

Martin, J. A., Hamilton, B. E., Ventura, S. J., Menacker, F., & Park, M. M. (2002). Maternal demographic characteristics. *National Vital Statistics Reports, 50*(5), 1–102.

Miller, L. J. (1988). *Miller assessment for preschoolers.* San Antonio, TX: The Psychological Corporation.

Miller, L. J., McIntosh, D. N., McGrath, J., Shyu, V., Lampe, M., Taylor, A. K., . . . Hagerman, R. (1999). Electrodermal responses to sensory stimuli in individuals with fragile X syndrome: A preliminary report. *American Journal of Medical Genetics, 83,* 268–279.

National Dissemination Center for Children With Disabilities. (2010). *Down syndrome fact sheet* (NICHCY Disability Fact Sheet No. 4). Retrieved from http://nichcy.org/disability/specific/downsyndrome

National Down Syndrome Society. (2011). *What causes Down syndrome?* Retrieved from http://www.ndss.org

National Human Genome Research Institute. (2011). *Specific genetic disorders.* Retrieved from http://www.genome.gov

National Institute of Neurological Disorders and Stroke. (2007). *NINDS Tay-Sachs disease information page.* Retrieved from http://www.ninds.nih.gov/disorders/taysachs/taysachs.htm

Newborg, J. (2005). *Battelle developmental inventory* (2nd ed.). Rolling Meadows, IL: Riverside.

Platt, O. S., Brambilla, D. J., Rosse, W. F., Milner, P. F., Castro, O., Steinberg, M. H., & Klug, P. P. (1994). Mortality in sickle cell disease—Life expectancy and risk factors for early death. *New England Journal of Medicine, 330,* 1639–1644.

Reed, P., & Lahm, E. (Eds.). (2004). *Assessing students' needs for assistive technology: A resource manual for school district teams* (4th ed.). Milton, WI: Wisconsin Assistive Technology Initiative.

Rehabilitation Act of 1973, 29 U.S.C. § 701 *et seq.* (1973).

Schopmeyer, B. B., & Lowe, F. (1992). *The fragile X child.* San Diego, CA: Singular Publishing Group, Inc.

Sparrow, S. S., Cicchetti, D. V., & Balla, D. A. (2005). *The Vineland adaptive behavior scales* (2nd ed.). San Antonio, TX: Pearson Assessments.

Watson, J., & Berry, A. (2003). *The secret of life.* New York, NY: Knopf.

Wattendorf, D., & Muenke, M. (2005). Diagnosis and management of fragile X syndrome. *American Family Physician, 72*(1), 111–113.

# Pediatric Upper Limb Conditions

*Roberta T. Ciocco*
*Meryl S. Cooperman*
*Deborah Humpl*

## Synopsis of Clinical Condition

### Prevalence and Etiology

Pediatric upper limb conditions make up a very broad diagnostic group. This chapter will refer to two different groups within this category: those with anatomical or structural anomalies (congenital limb deficiencies) and those without structural deformity (obstetrical brachial plexus injuries). Within these broad categories, there are many different manifestations of structural deformities.

Upper limb conditions with structural anomalies include congenital and acquired transverse upper limb deficiencies, which are decreased or absent long bones of the upper extremity. According to Gover and McIvor (1992), there are five categories of transverse deficiencies:

- *Phocomelia*, a congenital deformity where the limbs are very short. In some cases, the hand is directly attached to the trunk.
- *Radial deficiency*, a congenital deformity where the radial side of the forearm and hand is missing or partially absent. Presentation may result in a very short radius, hyperradial deviation of the wrist, and very little to no thumb.
- *Ulnar deficiency*, a congenital deformity where the ulnar side of the hand is missing or partially absent. This presentation may include very short or absent ulna, hyperulnar deviation of the wrist, and very short or absent little finger.
- *Central deficiency*, a deformity where one or more central digits of the hand are deficient or absent. It may present as a lobster-claw hand, cleft hand, or syndactyly.
- *Hypoplasia*, a deformity or underdevelopment of the thumb and/or other digits.

Upper limb conditions without structural anomalies include the following obstetrical brachial plexus injuries:

- Erb's palsy
- Klumpke's palsy
- global plexus palsy

The development of the limbs takes place between 3 and 8 weeks gestation. The type of limb deformity that occurs will be dictated by the time of insult. Three causes, or sequences, are generally attributed to problems with limb development. The first is a malformation sequence. This means that there is a malformation in the embryo that already exists at the time of limb development. The second possibility is a deformation sequence. In this case, an abnormal external mechanical or structural force causes the deformity. The third possibility is a disruption sequence. In this situation, the healthy embryological tissue is subjected to injury or breakdown by an infection, such as rubella, or a drug-induced deformity.

Congenital deformities affect 1% to 2% of newborns, and 10% of these cases involve the upper extremities. Congenital upper limb deformities are the second most prevalent deformity, with congenital heart deformities being the most prevalent. Some of the less severe problems, such as syndactyly, are reported to occur at a rate of 1 in 600 births (Kozin, 2007). Other, more severe deformities are reported to occur at a rate of 1 in 100,000 births (Glynn, 2002; McDonnell, Scott, & McKay, 1988). Congenital or obstetrical brachial plexus injuries are not associated with structural deformity and are typically caused by a traction injury to all or part of the brachial plexus at the time of delivery. The incidence of obstetrical palsies is reported to be between .04 and 2.5 cases per 1,000 live births (Skirven, Callahan, Osterman, Schneider, & Hunter, 2002). This problem is almost always unilateral.

## Common Characteristics and Symptoms

Limb deficiencies are classified by the type and degree of structural impairment. The following classification system, which was developed by Swanson (1976), is used today by hand surgeons and physicians to label the various types of deformity.

- Type I–Failure of formation: transverse arrest (amputations), longitudinal arrest, preaxial (radial deficiency), central (cleft hand), postaxial (ulnar deficiency), intercalated longitudinal arrest (phocomelia)
- Type II–Failure of differentiation: soft tissue (arthrogryposis), skeletal (delta phalanx), tumorous conditions
- Type III–Duplication (polydactyly)
- Type IV–Overgrowth (macrodactyly)
- Type V–Undergrowth (hypoplasia)
- Type VI–Constriction band syndromes
- Type VII–Generalized anomalies and syndromes

Children with congenital upper limb deformities may also present with cardiac problems, blood disorders, visceral problems, and/or lower extremity involvement. The involved extremity is frequently smaller in size and/or malformed. This discrepancy often contributes to difficulties with bilateral hand function and is often the cause of self-consciousness and social–emotional distress. Frequently, multiple surgical procedures are performed for cosmetic as well as functional

**Table 9.1** Typical Surgical Interventions

| Diagnosis | Functional/structural problem | Surgical procedure |
|---|---|---|
| Radial deficiency | Significant wrist radial deviation | Centralization procedure; use of an external fixator to gradually realign hand on wrist |
| | Absence of thumb | Pollicization (surgical rotation of index finger into position of thumb) |
| | Elbow flexion contracture | Soft tissue release |
| Transverse deficiency at metacarpal or phalangeal level | Shortened digits, making grasp of large objects difficult | Web space deepening<br>Bone distraction |
| | Poor or absent thumb | Toe-to-thumb transfer |
| Syndactyly | Two or more fingers joined together; may be just soft tissue or may involve bony fusion | Digit separation—method of skin coverage may vary (flaps, z-plasty, or skin graft) |
| | | Correction of bony deformity |
| Arthrogryposis | Recurring wrist flexor contractures with no available motors for transfer, requires full-time use of orthotic to keep wrist at neutral position | Arthrodesis of wrist when skeletally mature (may also require proximal row carpectomy) |
| | Lack of active elbow flexion with good passive range | Flexorplasty using the triceps, latissimus, or pectoralis muscles |
| | Decreased passive elbow or wrist motion | Joint release or tendon lengthening |

reasons. Alternative treatment options may include the use of orthotic or prosthetic devices and/or use of adaptive equipment and techniques for functional tasks. For example, some compensatory strategies may include using the crook of the elbow to hold objects, stabilizing objects against the body, or using the mouth as a substitute for an assist hand. Surgical and mechanical interventions are primarily focused on the achievement of hand-to-mouth and grasp-and-release movements, although cosmesis is usually a secondary gain of surgical intervention. Regardless of the treatment course, regular long-term contact with a medical facility that specializes in upper limb orthopedic treatment is necessary. Table 9.1 lists the most typical surgical interventions for some of these diagnoses (Glynn, 2002).

Obstetrical brachial plexus injuries are seen most frequently in children of large birth weight. The three types of injury that can occur at the time of birth include a stretch, a tear, or an avulsion of the nerves at the level of the brachial plexus. A stretch injury is the least damaging injury and often will repair itself. A tear is the next level of injury and can affect part or all of the nerve. An avulsion is the most serious and occurs when the nerves are torn from the spinal cord.

There are three classifications of obstetrical brachial plexus injury. The first is an upper plexus injury, which is referred to as *Erb's palsy*. In this case, the C-5 and C-6 musculature and sensation are most affected. There is very poor shoulder control and often some weakness at the elbow. The second, and less common, type of injury is the lower plexus, known as *Klumpke's palsy*. In this case, the

**Table 9.2** Surgical Options for Shoulder and Elbow

| Involved joint | Functional problem | Surgical procedure |
|---|---|---|
| Shoulder | Lack of external rotation | Latissimus-to-infraspinatus transfer |
| | | Derotational osteotomy of the humerous |
| | Lack of shoulder abduction | Transfer of the trapezius to the lateral aspect of the humerus |
| | | Bipolar latissimus dorsi transfer |
| | Severe shoulder dysfunction without possible motor donors | Shoulder arthrodesis |
| Elbow | Lack of elbow flexion | Flexorplasty using the latissimus, pectoralis major, triceps, or flexor–pronator muscles |
| | | Free muscle (gracilis) transfer |
| | Lack of extension | Latissimus-to-triceps transfer |
| | | Biceps-to-triceps transfer |

C-7 and C-8 muscles and distal sensation are usually affected. A child with this condition would present with good proximal strength but very weak wrist and hand musculature.

Although it is rare, in the last type, *global obstetrical palsy*, both the upper and lower plexus can be injured, resulting in total arm paralysis and sensory impairment. Children who have obstetrical brachial plexus injuries may also present with dystocia or fractures of the clavicle. Horner's sign (eye ptosis and myosis) is sometimes seen with severe brachial plexus injury (Mackinnon, 2002).

Frequently, children with obstetrical brachial plexus palsy have some degree of spontaneous recovery within 3 to 5 months. Children who do not demonstrate bicep function within that time period are often considered for a nerve graft or nerve transfer. The results of nerve grafting are variable, and improvement may be seen within 6 months of surgery. However, despite a successful graft, there may still be residual deficits. Over time, muscle imbalances due to partial paralysis can cause deformity. Another consequence of brachial plexus palsy is a difference in the size of the involved extremity. The extremity is often smaller in size. The most common functional problems resulting from muscle imbalances are elbow flexion and internal rotation deformities. Surgery may be indicated to prevent future deformity, improve function, or release contractures prior to tendon transfers. Tendon transfers are often used to improve the function and appearance of the arm. An evaluation conducted by the entire intervention team (including the occupational therapist, the physical therapist, the nurse, the pediatric physiatrist, and the hand surgeon) must ascertain muscle strength, sensation, functional skills, and any other medical or social complications before surgical intervention. Table 9.2 summarizes possible surgical options for the shoulder and elbow (Skirven, Callahan, Osterman, Schneider, & Hunter, 2002).

Tendon transfers are less common in lower plexus injuries because there are usually fewer options for donor muscles to transfer in the wrist and hand. An evaluation conducted by the entire intervention team, including the occupational therapist, the physical therapist, and the surgeon, must ascertain muscle strength, sensation, and functional skills before surgical intervention. Social and family situations must be evaluated to assure that postoperative management is optimized. Longer hospitalization or different postoperative decisions may be necessary, depending on the family compliance and reliability history.

## Target Areas for Intervention

The occupational therapist can provide the family and child with education, guidance, and support throughout the various stages of development. Children with upper limb conditions often require direct intervention in infancy and periodic intervention throughout childhood and adolescence for splinting, range of motion, adaptive equipment, functional skills training, and prosthetic training, if necessary. Optimally, the child would be followed by a multidisciplinary clinic group that has experience and special knowledge in the area of limb deficiencies. Local community therapists can follow through with recommendations and serve as a resource to clinic staff by providing more detailed information of functional abilities and deficit areas. Those children who require surgical intervention will often require occupational therapy services for postoperative rehabilitation.

## 🌿 Contextual Considerations

### Clinical

The clinical evaluation for limb conditions both with and without structural deformity must incorporate information about sensorimotor and developmental status and activities of daily living (ADL). An ADL evaluation provides information regarding the skills that the child may be capable of completing independently or with the assistance of adaptive equipment and provides insight into the coping strategies of the child and family. The sensorimotor evaluation yields information on the range of motion, muscle strength, and sensation of the upper extremities. In infants and young children, an accurate sensory test may be challenging, so trying to elicit a wrinkle response from the skin with prolonged immersion in water may be helpful. If the skin on the hand wrinkles after being in water 20 to 30 minutes, then it is assumed that there is some sensation at the dermatome. This can be accomplished by a long bath or aquatic therapy with the occupational therapist. Upper limb conditions with structural anomalies pose a challenge for testing because landmarks may be absent or in an alternative position. This is because the bone structure may be incomplete or absent. If prosthetic options, specially designed orthoses, or other technologies are being considered, it is important to be knowledgeable about the skills needed to support and operate the device. For example, a conventional body-powered prosthetic is operated by scapular protraction and retraction. In addition to considering functional need and cultural and emotional factors, evaluations of proximal muscle strength and the amount of scapular excursion available are needed to assess the appropriateness of such a device.

Children with brachial plexus injury or other forms of paralysis often use patterns of substitution for weak or paralyzed muscles. A few common substitutions include using lateral trunk flexion to assist with shoulder abduction and using shoulder abduction to assist with elbow flexion. If formalized manual muscle testing is a challenge for the child, then the therapist must find some type of functional marker to measure strength. For example, wheelbarrow walking can be graded by how much support the child needs (ankle, knee, or pelvic support), the distance walked, and how much trunk or arm compensation there is with the walking task.

Many upper limb conditions are unilateral, and the involved extremity is typically the nondominant extremity. This poses a challenge for assessment because most assessments evaluate either unilateral function or the accomplishment of a specific skill. It is helpful to evaluate the involved extremity for its functional use as an assist to the dominant extremity. The *University of New Brunswick Test of Prosthetic Function* (UNB; Sanderson & Scott, 1985) is a standardized test for the use of a below-elbow prosthesis as an assist to an intact extremity. A clinical assessment using the format of the UNB is helpful to determine the effectiveness of intervention for many unilateral limb conditions. The *Prosthetic Upper Extremity Functional Index* (PUFI) is a questionnaire that helps to quantify the extent of use and the perceived usefulness of a prosthetic device. The *Child Amputee Prosthetics Projects Functional Status Instruments* (1996) is another questionnaire that looks at the use and effectiveness of prosthetic devices in daily and developmental activities. The *Assisting Hand Assessment* (Krumlinde-Sundholm, Holmefur, & Eliasson, 2007) may also be useful for both children with brachial plexus injury and those with structural deficiency. This assessment is designed to evaluate nondominant-hand function in children ages 18 months to 12 years.

Children with upper limb deficiencies also pose a challenge for evaluation because fine motor assessments are based on an intact structure. A child with an absent thumb will not be able to perform a pincer grasp without surgical intervention. A child with paralysis of the wrist extensors will not be able to demonstrate a mature grasp pattern with wrist extension. Therefore, the therapist must be able to extrapolate information and focus on the accomplishment of functional skills.

There are many developmental assessments available. A general developmental assessment, such as the *Peabody Developmental Motor Scales–Second Edition* (Folio & Fewell, 2000), the *Hawaii Early Learning Profile* (Furuno et al., 1991), the *Miller Function and Participation Scales* (Miller, 2006), or the *Pediatric Evaluation of Developmental Inventory* (Haley, Coster, Ludlow, Haltiwanger, & Andrellos, 1992), will provide information for the preschool-age child. A developmental ADL checklist can be useful for children under the age of 3 years; however, many of these assessments are not sensitive to unilateral physical limitations. Credit is usually given for task completion, and the quality or efficiency of movement is not considered in the scoring.

Children of school age can be evaluated using an assessment of visual–motor skills, perceptual skills, and fine motor coordination. Common assessments include the *Beery-Buktenica Developmental Test of Visual Motor Integration* (Beery, Buktenica, & Beery, 2010), the *Test of Visual Perceptual Skills–Third Edition* (Martin, 2006), the *Jebsen Hand Function Test* (Jebsen, Taylor, Trieschmann, Trotter, & Howard, 1969), and the *Bruininks–Oseretsky Test of Motor Proficiency–Second Edition* (Bruininks & Bruininks, 2005). It may be necessary to modify some of the evaluations of motor coordination to accommodate physical limitations. In addition, the therapist may find it useful to take short video clips using a digital camera during assessment to better document and describe the quality of movement of the affected limb.

An adult rehabilitation–based checklist may incorporate the use of adaptive equipment. The *Functional Independence Measure* (Uniform Data System for Medical Rehabilitation, 1993) and the *Functional Independence Measure for Children* (Hamilton & Granger, 1991) provide information on many areas and are often used in research, but these evaluations are usually not sensitive enough for this population. These assessments group many skills together, which make them less sensitive to incremental changes if used for short-term goal setting. When evaluating ADL skills through parent report, the interview should be structured to help establish rapport and learn more about the family.

## Family

The family's values, priorities, and cultural preferences must be considered. It is often possible to gather information using an informal interview with a few key questions. Open-ended questions may be more helpful than a yes/no checklist and help to establish rapport. For example, "Tell me about a typical day" with supportive questions such as, "What time do you wake up?" "Does anybody help you get dressed?" and "What do you usually eat for breakfast/lunch/dinner?," can provide information on family routines in addition to ADL.

Families of children with a limb condition often express challenges coping with their extended family and community reactions to the presence of the limb condition. As the child grows, he or she may become more self-conscious of the limb condition. The occupational therapist needs to be aware of the social-communication function of the upper extremity and be sensitive to interventions that influence this role. There will be times when function is a priority over cosmesis and other times when cosmesis will be the primary concern.

Children with limb deficiencies vary in their choice of assistive devices during the transition from young child to school-age child, to adolescent, and to adult. It may be difficult for the family to accept the desires of the child if the child chooses to use devices that are different from the family's expectations. It is the responsibility of the therapist to ensure that the child has the most successful experience possible with an assistive device in order for the child and his or her family to make an informed decision. The therapist may need to help the family understand why a child prefers different options.

The occupational therapist needs to demonstrate sensitivity while gathering information about family resources, including medical coverage, formal and informal support groups, and information and educational resources. The occupational therapist can be a primary or secondary provider of information about coverage for medical expenses, support groups, special education, and rehabilitation laws. The information gathered may indicate the need to refer the family to a social worker to help with contacting agencies and receiving supportive counseling.

The occupational therapist must be aware of the potential equipment needs of an individual in order to guide the selection of devices. The family of the child who requires medical equipment such as prosthetics and splints must be made aware of reimbursement issues for medical equipment. Many third-party payers (e.g., insurance, medical assistance) will provide services on a limited basis, provide one-per-lifetime coverage, or not cover durable medical equipment. The occupational therapist providing services individually or as part of a team, which includes prosthetists, can help with selecting prosthetic components and aspects of a functional splint. The family may need information on medical assistance to help with expenses not covered by the family's insurance plan.

## Practice Setting

Individuals with limb deformities often receive occupational therapy in acute care hospitals, early intervention programs, rehabilitation hospitals or outpatient facilities, and school-based settings. A child with an upper limb condition may receive occupational therapy service at a variety of settings simultaneously and/or over time. Parents may be confused about the role of occupational therapy as the child transitions from community-based early intervention settings to school-based settings. It is important to establish communication between settings to ensure program consistency. The therapist with limited knowledge of these conditions should seek clinical mentorship from a colleague or institution that has experience in treating these conditions. Many of the available treatment options are time sensitive, and these children can present with unique and complex issues that are best handled by experienced practitioners.

The acute care therapist may first encounter the individual with an upper limb condition in the nursery. The occupational therapist must work with other professionals to assist the family by providing education regarding the child's special needs and information about community resources.

The rehabilitation hospital–based occupational therapist often provides therapy services for a specific period of time after a surgical procedure or for specific rehabilitation goals. Occupational therapy and other members of the rehabilitation team would provide intervention in the form of prosthetics, adaptive equipment, or splint training and clinical follow-up programs

Occupational therapists based in early intervention and outpatient programs provide ongoing home- and community-based services to help the child develop fine motor, perceptual, visual–motor, social, play, and ADL skills, and to help the child refine the use of assistive devices.

The focus of school-based therapy is the development of educationally relevant skills that will facilitate maximum levels of participation in the school program. The management of school-related tools and supplies, peer socialization, and dressing and hygiene related to toileting are frequently identified areas for intervention.

## Sociopolitical

Three primary laws relate to children with limb conditions. The laws relate to education, rehabilitation, and accessibility. The Individuals With Disabilities Education Act (IDEA, 1990) was reauthorized in 1997 and entitles all children with disabilities to a free and appropriate education with related services in the least restrictive environment. A child may also be eligible for early intervention services starting at birth. Occupational therapy services are provided in school settings under IDEA. The Americans With Disabilities Act (ADA) extends civil rights protections to individuals with disabilities, supporting equal opportunities for employment, accessibility, transportation, and government services. The Technology Act (Technology Related Assistance for Individuals With Disabilities Act, 1988) supports the acquisition of adaptive equipment and assistive technology for people who require it.

## Lifestyle/Lifespan

It is important to help the individual and his or her family become aware of issues that will be faced throughout the lifetime of the individual with upper extremity limb conditions. Table 9.3 highlights major areas of concern.

Accessibility in the home for a child with an upper limb condition often includes using assistive devices to maximize one-handed completion of tasks. For example, a rocker knife, a cutting board, or hair dryer holder may facilitate independence. Modifications and/or careful selection of where to place objects

**Table 9.3** Lifestyle/Lifespan Factors

| Accessibility | Financial | Medical | Family | Social |
|---|---|---|---|---|
| May need adaptations for specialized sports equipment | Reimbursement for prosthetics and splints may be limited | Surgery to enhance function may be offered | Increased time for daily care | Interaction with peers |
| May need adaptations for driving a car | | Require periodic follow-up for issues of growth and new equipment, and equipment repair | Coping | Loss of upper extremity for body language/social communicator |
| Minor home modifications may be needed | | | Sibling relationships | Cosmesis versus function |

frequently used need to be considered if arm length and reaching ability are compromised. Extensive home modifications may be necessary for the child with multiple limb deformities. Adaptations, such as a knob on the steering wheel, are typically needed for driving.

Financial issues will vary depending on the family's economic resources and insurance coverage. Insurance reimbursement often has limitations, and medical equipment expenses for prosthetics, adaptive equipment, and orthoses may be encountered. It is important to recognize that the use of equipment may vary over time, depending on the needs and interests of the child and family. The occupational therapist needs to be aware of resources for the family and about equipment that can "grow" with the child to promote maximum length of use during the child's growing years.

The child with an upper extremity limb condition is often able to participate in typical community recreation programs with minimal adaptations. Many interchangeable terminal devices that are recreational-task specific are available for the unilateral below-elbow amputee. Specialized prostheses, such as a swim prosthesis, may also be an option. The therapist should encourage the child to participate in sports for the benefit of his or her physical fitness and peer relationships.

## Clinical Decision-Making Process

### Defining Focus for Intervention

In school, the foci for intervention are skills that will enable the child to benefit from the educational setting, such as handwriting, fine motor skills, the bilateral hand coordination necessary for schoolwork, and self-care skills. Hospital clinic outcomes are concerned with changes in range of motion, muscle function, and functional movement. Presurgical evaluation, splinting, prostheses, and adaptive equipment are often provided in this setting. Outpatient prosthetic training, splinting, scar management, muscle reeducation, and functional skills training may be necessary in the postoperative phase.

If the child is a candidate for a prosthesis, a passive prosthesis, along with parent education and home programming, is usually prescribed at 4 to 6 months of age. At about 18 months of age, the child should begin occupational therapy in the form of prosthetic training with a functional prosthesis. As the child matures, more technologically sophisticated equipment, such as a myoelectric prosthesis, may be employed. Also, personal goals related to school performance; prevocational skills; social acceptability; and extracurricular activities, such as sports or the arts, will govern the thrust of treatment.

### Establishing Goals for Intervention

The setting; the developmental level of the child; the family's values, interests, and expectations; and reimbursement issues often dictate the length or frequency of treatment and influence the prioritization of goals for intervention. For example, the expected proficiency with a prosthetic device for a 9-month-old differs from that for a 2-year-old or a 6-year-old. If tendon transfer surgery is anticipated, then range of motion and muscle and joint strength become treatment priorities.

## Designing Theory-Based Intervention

Although many frames of reference would be appropriately applied to this population, the biomechanical frame of reference is most frequently employed. The biomechanical frame of reference is used with individuals with neuromuscular or musculoskeletal problems. This frame of reference is based on principles of physics, physiology, neuroscience, and kinesiology (Cole & Tufano, 2008). This frame of reference is often used when adaptive equipment, orthotic devices, adapted techniques, or prosthetic intervention is required. The therapist must understand the biomechanical and physiological forces that are acting on the child, as well as the mechanical advantages and disadvantages of the specific device. Joint position, fixed deformities, sensory function, functional needs, and dynamic movement patterns may be a few of the major factors that need to be considered in determining the final orthotic or prosthetic design.

The developmental frame of reference is certainly relevant to any pediatric population. Children with upper limb deficiencies are faced with many challenges to the normal progression or acquisition of skills. Understanding normal development will assist the therapist in designing treatment plans that mitigate or compensate for these challenges and facilitate the child's ability to engage in age-appropriate life tasks that are associated with school, self-care, and play.

Many frames of reference consider the evaluation of ADL skills. The principles inherent in motor learning theory are used to teach the child specific ADL tasks. This framework might be used when teaching a child who has significant upper extremity paralysis to don a shirt. The activity would be broken down into several steps and gradually introduced into the therapy sessions. Techniques may be modified, and adaptive equipment may be introduced at various steps. Trial-and-error problem solving is then used to refine the process. Home programs might be used to provide the repeated practice that is required to reinforce the skill.

The model of human occupation is also very useful. This frame of reference focuses on the life roles that the individual needs to assume in order to develop and maintain a personally meaningful and productive lifestyle and then establishes which behaviors facilitate the performance of the life tasks and daily routines associated with those roles. This approach is driven by the values, needs, and aspirations of the child and family (Cole & Tufano, 2008).

## Evaluating Progress

Traditionally, progress is based on meeting established goals. Measurable goals typically focus on independence with ADL skills and the use and care of assistive technology. In the clinic setting, repeated measures, such as the *Functional*

*Independence Measure*, the PUFI and the UNB, and/or use of a specific checklist will help monitor the changes that occur over time. Video recording can be a powerful tool to evaluate subtle progress that is not measurable on standardized tests. Another measure of progress that is less objective is how the child and family adapt to and cope with the disability.

## Determining Change in or Termination of Treatment

Change in or termination of treatment is warranted when the child does not meet the goals established or has met all the goals established. In either event, the therapist needs to reevaluate goals for relevance. New goals could indicate a change of focus or higher levels of independence. Discharge from therapy may occur when the child has reached a maximum level of independence for his or her age and has acquired a sufficient level of foundational skills to promote independent problem solving and future skill acquisition.

### Case Study 1

*Description*

JB is an 18-month-old male with a short, left, congenital, below-elbow amputation. JB was referred to occupational therapy for his initial active prosthetic training. He has been wearing a prosthesis since he was 7 months old. He started with a passive mitt prosthesis. He was recently fitted with his first conventional body-powered prosthesis. He was provided a terminal device that is a voluntary closing system. This choice allows JB to have more feedback and control over closing force, and it works more like a natural hand in that the user closes down on an object, like a natural hand does when grasp is initiated. His harness is a figure-9 harness, and his socket is a tight self-suspending socket. He currently wears a prosthesis for about 3 to 4 hours per day, keeping the prosthesis on for about 1 hour at a time.

Developmentally, JB has been meeting all of his gross motor milestones. He is also able to perform age-appropriate fine motor skills, with the exception of bilateral tasks. Since this is his first activated prosthesis on his initial evaluation, he was not administered a formal prosthetic skill evaluation. His harness was overtightened initially to exaggerate the operation of the terminal device. He was able to activate the terminal device with encouragement to reach both his arms forward. He attends outpatient therapy for two 45-minute sessions per week at a pediatric rehabilitation facility that has experience in prosthetic care. Mom is very involved in the sessions, and home program suggestions are provided at each session.

*Long- and Short-Term Goals*

The long-term goal of intervention is for JB to develop reasonable skill with, and improve his spontaneous use of, his new prosthesis. These goals will be reached in part through successfully achieving the following short-term goals:

1. JB will be able to acquire an object 1 inch in diameter from the therapist's hand, hold it for at least 10 seconds, and release it into a large container at least 10 times in a row.

2. JB will begin to understand the need to pre-position his terminal device for differently shaped and oriented objects by rotating the terminal device with physical assistance and verbal prompting from the therapist.

3. JB will be able to maintain grasp of a small cup full of Cheerios and be able to eat 5 to 10 Cheerios with his right hand without dropping the cup.

### Therapist Goals and Strategies

The therapist's goals include the following:

1. Develop motivation to use the prosthesis and increase the level of comfort with the prosthesis to enable the child and his family to accept the prosthesis into daily life routines.

2. Ensure that the fit of the prosthesis is appropriate and that everything is functioning properly.

3. Assist with the education of the child and family in the care and use of the prosthesis.

The therapist's strategies include the following:

1. Provide opportunities to explore the adaptive equipment to facilitate skill in its use.

2. Try different techniques for positioning body or prosthesis to accomplish the task.

3. Provide opportunities for repetition and practice.

### Activity: Grasp and Release

JB will attempt to pick up 1- to 2-inch foam bath blocks from the therapist's hand. He will then carry them for a distance of less than 5 feet and drop the blocks into a large bucket or barrel. The concepts of in and out and color and shape recognition can also be incorporated into the activity.

### Treatment Objective

JB will get the blocks into the container without dropping them 75% of the time over a 5- to 10-minute period.

## Case Study 2

### Description

MP is a 15-month-old female with a right obstetric brachial plexus palsy injury involving the upper nerve roots (i.e., Erb's palsy). She had a nerve graft to the biceps 6 months ago. She receives outpatient occupational therapy services once a week at a rehabilitation facility and is followed through the clinic program at the hospital that performed the surgical procedure. MP has not had any other medical issues. She is an eldest child, born to an intact family. Her development has been mildly delayed for bilateral upper extremity weight-bearing activities, such as reciprocal creeping and pulling to stand. She is currently cruising, has learned to pull to stand using only her left upper extremity, and is able to sit independently. Social, language, cognitive, fine motor, and play skills are within normal limits, using modified techniques to compensate for her right upper extremity weakness. Table 9.4 presents the results of the initial evaluation for outpatient therapy.

**Table 9.4** Musculoskeletal Evaluation Results for MP

| Muscle/movement | Strength | Active range | Passive range |
|---|---|---|---|
| Biceps | 2+/5 | 0°–100° | WNL |
| Shoulder flexion | 2+/5 | 10°–80° | 10°–170° |
| Shoulder abduction | 2/5 | 0°–80° | WFL |
| Shoulder external rotation | 2–/5 | 0°–45° | 0°–70° |
| Wrist extension | 2/5 | 0°–45° | 0°–70° |
| Supination | 2/5 | 0°–60° | 0°–80° |

### Long- and Short-Term Goals

The long-term goal of intervention for MP is to improve bilateral coordination to develop independence in ADL skills. This goal will be reached in part through successfully achieving the following short-term goals:

1. MP will bring a two-handled cup to her mouth using both hands.
2. MP will put on and take off a hat with both hands.

### Therapist Goals and Strategies

The therapist's goals include the following:

1. Increase range of motion and strength of right elbow flexion.
2. Improve bilateral integration and spontaneous use of the right upper extremity.

The therapist's strategies include the following:

1. Improve strength by grading size and weight of objects to manipulate.
2. Engage in sensory-based activities to the right upper extremity.
3. Position activities to promote awareness of the right arm.

### Activity: Dramatic Play With Hats

Various hats used for dress-up play will be used, including items such as an army helmet, a fireman's hat, a baseball cap, a construction hat, and a space helmet. MP will place these on her head, the parent's head, and the therapist's head.

### Treatment Objective

MP will use both upper extremities to put on a hat and bend her elbow 120° against gravity.

# Resources

## Internet Resources

Association of Children's Prosthetic-Orthotic Clinics: www.ACPOC.org

Brachial Plexus Palsy Foundation: http://www.brachialplexuspalsyfoundation.org

United Brachial Plexus Network: www.ubpn.org

## Print Resources

Area Child Amputee Center. (n.d.). *Children with hand differences: A guide for families*. (Available from the Area Child Amputee Center, 235 Wealthy S.E., Grand Rapids, MI 49503)

Area Child Amputee Center. (n.d.). *Children with limb loss: A handbook for families*. (Available from the Area Child Amputee Center, 235 Wealthy S.E., Grand Rapids, MI 49503)

Area Child Amputee Center. (n.d.). *Children with limb loss: A handbook for teachers*. (Available from the Area Child Amputee Center, 235 Wealthy S.E., Grand Rapids, MI 49503)

Caseley, J. (1991). *Harry, Willy, and Carrothead*. New York, NY: Greenwillow Books.

## References

Americans With Disabilities Act of 1990, 42 U.S.C. § 12101 *et seq.* (1990) (amended 1997).

Beery, K. E., Buktenica, N. A., & Beery, N. A. (2010). *Beery–Buktenica developmental test of visual–motor integration* (6th ed.). San Antonio, TX: Pearson Assessments.

Bruininks, R. H., & Bruininks, B. D. (2005). *Bruininks–Oseretsky test of motor proficiency* (2nd ed.). San Antonio, TX: Pearson Assessments.

Cole, M. B., & Tufano, R. (2008). *Applied theories in occupational therapy*. Thorofare, NJ: Slack.

Folio, R., & Fewell, R. (2000). *Peabody developmental motor scales* (2nd ed.). Austin, TX: PRO-ED, Inc.

Furuno, S., O'Reilly, K., Inatsuka, T., Hosaka, C. M., Allman. T., & Zeiloft-Falbey, B. (1991). *The Hawaii early learning profile*. Palo Alto, CA: VORT.

Gover, A. M., & McIvor, J. (1992). Upper limb deficiencies in infants and young children. *Infants and Young Children, 5*(1), 58–72.

Haley, S., Coster, W., Ludlow, L., Haltiwanger, J., & Andrellos, P. (1992). *Pediatric evaluation of disability inventory*. San Antonio, TX: The Psychological Corporation.

Hamilton, B. B., & Granger, C. U. (1991). *Functional independence measure for children*. Buffalo: Research Foundation of the State University of New York.

Individuals With Disabilities Education Act of 1990, 20 U.S.C. § 1400 *et seq.* (1990) (amended 1997).

Jebsen, R. H., Taylor, N., Trieschmann, R. B., Trotter, M. J., & Howard, L. A. (1969). *Jebsen hand function test*. Bolingbrook, IL: Sammons Preston, Inc.

Kozin, S. H. (2007). Congenital anomalies. In T. E. Trumble (Ed.), *Hand surgery update 3* (pp. 455–468). Brooklandville, MD: Data Trace.

Krumlinde-Sundholm, L., Holmefur, M., & Eliasson, A. (2007). *Manual: The Assisting Hand Assessment* (Version 4.4). Stockholm, Sweden: Wily Blackwell.

Laub, D. R. (2002). *Congenital hand deformities*. Retrieved from www.emedicine.com/plastic/topic298.htm

Mackinnon, S. E. (2002). *Brachial plexus injuries, congenital*. Retrieved from www.emedicine.com/orthoped/topic466.htm

Martin, N. (2006). *Test of visual motor skills* (3rd ed.). Novato, CA: Academic Therapy Publications.

McDonnell, P., Scott, R., & McKay, A. (1988). Incidence of congenital upper-limb deficiencies. *Journal of the Association of Child Prosthetic–Orthotic Clinics, 23*(1), 8.

Miller, L. J. (2006). *Miller function and participation scales.* San Antonio, TX: Psychological Corporation.

Pruit, S. D., Varni, J. W., & Setogu, Y. (1996). The child amputee prosthetics projects functional status instruments. *Archives of Physical Medicine and Rehabilitation, 77*(12), 1233–1238

Sanderson, E. R., & Scott, R. N. (1985). *University of New Brunswick test of prosthetic function.* New Brunswick, Canada: Bioengineering Institute, University of New Brunswick.

Skirven, T. M., Callahan, A. D., Osterman, A. L., Schneider, L. H., & Hunter, J. M. (2002). *Hunter, Mackin & Callahan's rehabilitation of the hand and upper extremity* (5th ed.). St. Louis, MO: Elsevier Health Sciences/Mosby.

Swanson, A. B. (1976). A classification for congenital malformations. *Journal of Hand Surgery, 1*(1), 8–22.

Technology Related Assistance for Individuals With Disabilities Act of 1988, 29 U.S.C. § 2201 *et seq.*

Uniform Data System for Medical Rehabilitation. (1993). *Functional independence measure.* Buffalo: The State University of New York at Buffalo.

# Social Skills Deficits

*Nancy Allen Kauffman*

## 🌿 Synopsis of Clinical Condition

Social skills are observable actions or units of behavior, either learned or automatic, that enable a person to develop and maintain relationships. Fisher and Griswold (2008) pointed out that these skills occur within the context of engagement in an occupation that involves interaction with other people, and they label diminished skills as "performance errors" (p. 5). Horowitz (2007) defined *social skills* as the specific reactions, responses, techniques, and strategies people use in social situations. Social skills must occur appropriately within a societal and cultural system and in a variety of environments, and they require a coping style that is both effective and adaptive. *Social cognition* incorporates awareness of interpersonal skills and judgment in using them. The ability to apply positive behaviors in anticipation of social obstacles is termed *prosocial skills*. *Social competence* is a qualitative measure describing a person's general performance level in interpersonal situations.

Social interactions that allow a person to give or receive an object, instruction, or help (e.g., "Please pass the salt") or exchange factual information (e.g., "It is going to rain today") are sometimes called *instrumental interactions*, as in an implement, or tool, for accomplishing a task. On the other hand, social interactions that help to establish, sustain, or deepen a relationship (e.g., "How was your weekend?") require a more complex thought process and include the perspective of the listener. They include expressions of feelings, mutually shared humor, and reciprocal conversations about dreams and values.

Social ability requires a series of social initiative and response steps in each encounter to achieve fluidity. One must identify the social situation, select the skills needed, carry out those skills, perceive the other person's response, and adjust additional social actions accordingly. Social problem solving involves predicting consequences for each potential social response and selecting the most appropriately adaptive one.

## Prevalence and Etiology

Social skills deficits occur more often in males and in people with special needs than in the general population. Examples include people diganosed with learning disabilities, attention-deficit/hyperactivity disorder, autism spectrum disorder, spina bifida, Turner syndrome, neurofibromatosis, trichotillomania, and early gestational age or low birth weight. Other disorders that are associated with social deviations include reactive attachment disorder and obsessive–compulsive disorder (American Psychiatric Association [APA], 2000). If no known neurological handicapping condition underlies a social skill delay, then environmental conditions may be a contributing factor, for example, in the case of family modeling or cultural differences. In some cases, social skills may be learned adequately by adults or children who can describe and define them yet fail to perform them because of attention issues, expressive language difficulties, processing delays, sensory overload, organizational difficulties, or defiance.

Individuals with learning disabilities have average or above-average intelligence but have difficulty receiving, storing, processing, and responding to information and may also have difficulty with interpersonal skills and recognizing social cuing. Social and interpersonal deficits may be the primary difficulty experienced by individuals with nonverbal learning disabilities (Horowitz, 2006). Individuals with expressive and receptive language disorders are also likely to struggle with social awareness (3%–7% of the school-age population; APA, 2000).

Difficulty with social interactions; communication impairments; and restricted patterns of behavior, interests, and activities are characteristic of individuals who are on the autism spectrum. Individuals with Asperger's disorder have average intelligence, or may be intellectually gifted, but are socially awkward. The condition occurs in 2 out of every 10,000 children, and boys are 3 to 4 times more likely than girls to have the disorder (Horowitz, 2008).

Gifted students have been identified as more sensitive to their environment than children of average intelligence, and they demonstrate more heightened emotional and behavioral reactions. Those in the intellectually gifted range often demonstrate important sensory modulation differences that interfere with their attempts to socialize (Gere, Capps, Mitchell, & Grubbs, 2009). Twenty to 25% of gifted children have psychosocial difficulties, which at times result in a lack of rewarding social contacts with others (Gallagher, 1990).

Attention-deficit disorder (ADD), with and without hyperactivity, is seen in 3% to 7% of the population and is frequently accompanied by difficulties with interpersonal relations. ADD is seen in males more frequently than in females, though somewhat less so in the predominantly inattentive type (APA, 2000).

Finally, social anxiety can be found in all diagnostic categories and is characterized by fear of humiliation or embarrassment in social or performance situations that may be general or may be specific to particular settings. Although the onset may be insidious, first emerging in the mid-teens, it may abruptly emerge after an embarrassing or distressing event. The resulting withdrawal from social exposure creates or exacerbates delays or deviations in developing interpersonal skills. The lifetime prevalence for the general population ranges from 3% to 15%, and the rate of social anxiety in individuals with other anxiety disorders is between 10% and 20% (APA, 2000).

## Common Characteristics and Symptoms

People with social skills difficulty often have trouble making or keeping friends or fitting in socially. Many people with social skills deficits have difficulty seeing situations from another person's point of view or recognizing that other perspectives exist. They fail to notice the needs or feelings of others and may appear insensitive in their interactions. Some may be rigid in handling interpersonal exchanges and nonresourceful in resolving differences. Comprehension of abstract nuances and reading of verbal and nonverbal cues may elude them.

Social skills deficits, if left untreated, may result in general social adjustment problems and negative relationships in adulthood, causing problems in work relationships, family interactions, and friendship building. Social difficulties and isolation may lead to depression and other psychopathologies in later years.

## Target Areas for Intervention

The occupational therapist works as a member of a team that includes the individual client and may also include the client's family, personnel from the school or work environment, psychologists, counselors, social workers, psychiatrists, speech therapists, neurologists, and other professionals. The occupational therapist helps gather information about primary and secondary social skills deficits that interfere with adjustment in the school, home, community, or workplace and helps the team prioritize social goals. The primary focus of therapy should be on the social skills deficits, which in many cases may be directly or indirectly related to a diagnosis (see Table 10.1).

Occupational therapy for individuals with social skills deficits is usually conducted in group settings. Because of the wide range of possible treatment goals and levels of need (ranging from the seriously impaired person with autism to the mildly socially anxious person with no other diagnosis), selection of group membership will be carefully constructed. Table 10.2 lists potential target areas for intervention (Fisher & Griswold, 2008; Gresham & Elliott, 2008a; Kauffman & Kinnealey, 2006).

# 🕮 Contextual Considerations

## Clinical

The occupational therapist may interview the potential client, family members, and/or teachers in order to establish the client's level of competency in structured and unstructured social situations. Psychological, neuropsychological, or

**Table 10.1** Examples of Primary and Secondary Social Skills Deficits

| Primary deficit | Secondary social skills deficits | Treatment options to precede or run concurrently with social skills treatment |
|---|---|---|
| Sensory defensiveness | Person may withdraw from personal contact or avoid slightly crowded or mildly noisy social environments that could have been the site of friend-making opportunities. | Ameliorate interfering sensory defensiveness issues.* |
| Inadequate body scheme with resulting faulty spatial perception | Person may invade others' personal space or keep too much distance for comfortable interactions. | Use sensory integration and other techniques to improve body awareness, motor planning, and overall space perception.* |
| Coordination disorders | Young child's embarrassment about handwriting, drawing, play, or athletic competence may result in unrealistic oversensitivity and defensiveness in the presence of more competent children or actual rejection or ignoring by them. | Treat the coordination disorder.* |
| Attentional and impulsiveness issues, difficulty with self-regulation | Lack of focus during social interactions or interfering hyperactivity may spoil social opportunities. | Alert Program techniques from *How Does Your Engine Run?* (Williams & Shellenberger, 1996). Possibly refer for neurological or other medical evaluation.* |
| Learned family interaction styles that put off others | Argumentativeness, disrespectful speaking, put downs, whining, and griping may be verbal exchanges learned at home that interfere with ability to make friends elsewhere. | Possibly address this in an occupational therapist–run activity group focusing on attitude and manner of communicating, or refer to a family therapist.* |
| Language processing disorders | Failure to comprehend stated or implied social or game rules, or delays in processing information (thereby delaying social response time), may result in impatience or ignoring by others. | Refer to speech–language clinician, particularly one with a thorough understanding of pragmatics. |
| Defiance | Defiant individuals may acquire the friendship of other defiant people, but attempts to socialize them with more compliant individuals may sabotage therapeutic efforts for the whole group. | Refer deep-seated defiance to other mental health professionals if the defiance repeatedly interferes with the group process. |

*Note.* Asterisk (*) indicates a sampling of potential primary deficits suitable for occupational therapy intervention. Adapted and reprinted with permission by Occupational Therapy Programs (© 2002).

biopsychosocial reports are particularly helpful for giving an overview of the cognitive strengths and weaknesses as well as information about medications and potential side effects.

The occupational therapist uses formal and informal measures to identify primary and secondary social skills issues and establishes measurable goals for intervention. The *Social Skills Improvement System Rating Scale* (Gresham & Elliott, 2008b) assesses the social skills, problem behaviors, and academic competence of

**Table 10.2** Assessments for Areas of Intervention in Social Skills Deficits

| | Areas of Intervention | |
|---|---|---|
| *Social Skills Improvement System Intervention Guide*[a] | *Evaluation of Social Interaction*[b] | **COLLAGE Social Skills**[c] |
| Communication | Acquiring goods and services | Verbal presentation |
| Assertion | Conversing socially, small talk | Nonverbal presentation |
| Empathy | Problem solving, decision making | Emotional responses |
| Self-control | Sharing information | Play/work with others |
| Cooperation | Gathering information | Awareness and valuing of self and others |
| Responsibility | Collaborating–producing | Initiate and maintain relations |
| Engagement | 27 specific social interaction skills | Feelings about self |

*Note.* Adapted and reprinted with permission by COLLAGE/Occupational Therapy Programs (© 2010).
[a]Gresham and Elliott (2008). [b]Fisher and Griswold (2008). [c]Kauffman and Kinnealey (2006).

children ages 3 to 18 years. The accompanying *Social Skills Improvement System Intervention Guide* (Gresham & Elliott, 2008a) provides remedial strategies for the problems identified by the *Rating Scale*, allowing meaningful pre- and post-treatment assessments.

The *Evaluation of Social Interaction* (ESI; Fisher & Griswold, 2008) assesses 27 social interaction skills in a natural context with typical social partners. Developed by an occupational therapist, the ESI integrates the intended purposes of the social interactions, aspects of the environment, and characteristics of the individuals taking part in the assessment. A 2010 pilot study using the ESI outcomes identified a hierarchy of skill and quantified the quality of social interaction by age, capability level, and diagnosis (Simmons, Griswold, & Berg, 2010). Seven themes or constructs that were atypical in children with ADD who showed social skill problems were evaluated using a focused but unstructured interview of children and their parents. These domains were found to be an effective basis for social skill treatment planning for 565 socially impaired children and adults within nine diagnostic categories (Kauffman & Kinnealey, 2006). The *Canadian Occupational Performance Measure* (Law et al., 2005) is a structured interview that can be administered at the beginning of occupational therapy service and at appropriate intervals thereafter to demonstrate a baseline and subsequent changes in a client's self-perception of social skill.

The Ziggurat Model is a comprehensive intervention guide for individuals with autism that assesses social, emotional, and behavioral strengths and deficits and incorporates positive behavioral interventions and supports. The framework uses a five-level comprehensive intervention plan featuring sensory differences and biological needs, reinforcement, structure and visual–tactile supports, task demands, and skills to teach (Aspy & Grossman, 2007).

The *Early Coping Inventory* (Zeitlin, Williamson, & Szczepanski, 1988) and the social development section of the *HELP Strands* (Parks, 1992) are measures of social adaptability in the very young population (ages 4–36 months) that can serve as an informal gauge of the sequence in which early social and adaptive skills are acquired, even when assessing somewhat older children. A coping inventory is also available for assessing older children and adults (Zeitlin, 2007).

## Family

Children with social skills difficulties may appear different from other members of their families or may reflect questionable familial social behaviors. In either case, the family may benefit from specific child management suggestions from the therapist or referral to parenting classes to help expand behavioral strategies to promote social development. Parents may need reassurance to help alleviate any guilt they feel about their child's social inadequacies.

Siblings of socially impaired children may bear the brunt of ineffective or disruptive social interactions. Constant accommodation to an inflexible and disruptive child may interfere with other healthy family interactions or outings. The therapist may help the family identify potential frustrations and create family accommodations, such as arranging to prevent the socially impaired child from repeatedly spoiling playdates at home for siblings and their friends. Some families successfully hold family meetings, with all members encouraged to bring up issues they think need resolving and recommend solutions that family members could jointly carry out.

## Practice Setting

The occupational therapist in any setting should be alert to addressing social competence delays that may currently or potentially interfere with the client's interpersonal development. In the school environment, social skills difficulties emerge most often in the unstructured periods of the day, including on the playground, in the lunchroom, at the bus stop, in the hallways, and on the school bus, rather than during classroom activities. These social hot spots require reciprocal interactions and correct interpretations of other people's feelings and intended meanings.

School interventions can take the form of (a) consultation with teachers, guidance counselors, or playground and lunchroom aides; (b) classroom intervention (e.g., during project group meetings); or (c) pullout activity groups run by the therapist for children from several classes at once. Therapists and school personnel may arrange a buddy system, or "lunch pal," for a socially inept child to be paired with a socially competent model, who brings the student along for inclusion in his or her social group of lunch friends.

Playdates arranged and sometimes managed by parents may evolve into community sports teams or formal group lessons also controlled by adults. In an adult-controlled social environment, the child/young adult may have limited opportunity to practice informal chatting, reading emotions, and interpreting the intricacies of peer body language and other social cues. Occupational therapists may run activities such as lunch groups to address social goals in school. These activities provide the opportunity to address social errors as they occur, in everyday interaction with other children. Cofacilitation by an aide can allow for timely individual social coaching without disruption of the group activity.

Social goals may also be addressed in therapy groups established to address functional goals or motor skills in a variety of settings, including schools, hospitals, clinics, or therapy centers. Some social competence groups are freestanding, community-based programs, for example, at after-school care programs for children of working parents or in camp settings.

Social skills programming is also useful for adults with social delays. The adult program may be either freestanding or affiliated with a clinic, hospital, or religious organization. It can focus on interactions with family members, employers, or coworkers. It can also emphasize the social cognition skills needed for establishing independent living arrangements, including building friendships, developing relationships with neighbors, and getting along with a roommate. For any age, the presence of the therapist, the therapeutic equipment, and the members of a social group help form the parameters of the social milieu in which change is being promoted, to develop the role of friend and colleague for the participants.

## Sociopolitical

The Individuals With Disabilities Education Act was reauthorized and renamed IDEIA in 2004, and established that behavioral issues can interfere with a child's education and goals and thus should be addressed in the child's Individualized Education Program. A school social environment that includes violence, bullying, or group discrimination interferes with learning and may lead to tragedy. Many school districts are adopting whole social competence curricula for their students, faculty, and parents. A trend toward home schooling, charter schools, and online cyberschooling has expanded considerably, in part because parents have chosen to allow their children to avoid school social environments they deem unsuitable.

The ultimate social goal is to allow a person wider choices of social responses in keeping with the context of each situation. In this spirit, the American Occupational Therapy Association's (AOTA's) Societal Statement on Autism Spectrum Disorders (AOTA, 2009) holds that individuals with autism have a right to participate in all aspects of life and society, in spite of their lifelong difficulty making sense of the world because of challenges in communication, social interaction, sensory processing, and regulation of emotions and behavior. Occupational therapists collaborate with these individuals and their families, professionals, and community members to help provide needed resources and services (AOTA, 2009). Occupational therapists in private practice will need to consider the funding stream when treating children or adults for delays in social competence.

## Lifestyle/Lifespan

Social cognition difficulties are likely to emerge at certain times in the life cycle, particularly during periods of change in the social requirements of a contextual setting. For the young child with classic autism, the social impairment is first noted before or around ages 2 to 3 years. Other children's social difficulties may be first identified as they enter kindergarten or preschool, where interactions with peers outside the family are, for the first time, a major part of the child's daily experiences. During the school year, academic difficulties occur more often in students with social disorders than in other students. Difficulty with comprehension, abstract or inferential thinking, and organization may affect both the academic areas and the social domain. Upon entry into middle school and high school, children with Asperger's disorder may be more susceptible to anxiety, depression, victimization, and feelings of isolation. Their good verbal abilities may mask the severity of their social dysfunction and magnify the social challenges of the middle and high school years. During the middle and high school years, occupational therapists should be aware of and involved in the work of local school district transition councils or other systems established to help smooth transition to life after high school. A history of social skill difficulties in childhood and adolescence has been shown to be related to difficulty in adulthood with life friendships, workplace competence, marriage and parenting, work and community relationships, and adult health.

Throughout the lifespan, the abbreviated interchanges of various social media require greater adaptability in processing social cues in the absence of facial appearances, body language, or even vocal inflections. Some professionals have expressed concern that social exchanges may now be more superficial and provide less of the face-to-face interaction that helps to build a foundation for understanding of empathy, emotional nuances, and trust.

While some children and adults may be using readily available electronic communication methods to expand their personal interaction successes, others (who have more difficulty navigating the intricacies of social awareness and connection) will be hampered by the reduction in social cues that they afford. Electronics may be widening the gap between the socially cognizant individual and the less competent. The astute clinician must carefully investigate where help is needed and then facilitate access to help with social competence.

## Clinical Decision-Making Process

### Defining Focus for Intervention

Specific supportive remediation programs that teach social skills have been shown to be effective in helping individuals with nonverbal learning disabilities and Asperger's disorder (Horowitz, 2008). The therapist prioritizes the social skill difficulties (see Table 10.1.) and identifies whether referral to another professional, consultation, individual, or group treatment is required.

The focus of therapeutic intervention is to create an environment for social interaction that allows social situations that have been ineffectively resolved elsewhere to be experienced successfully. A safe, accepting environment is required, yet social challenges that entail dealing with frustration or resolving a problem must be presented. The therapist guides clients in the development of effective methods of meeting these challenges and achieving interpersonal satisfaction. Occupational therapists engage people with social impairments in activities that require interaction with others while providing verbal and visual reinforcement, social rewards for socially correct actions, opportunities to practice prosocial behaviors, and alternatives to ineffective social patterns. Table 10.3 shows examples of important clinical considerations to keep in mind when establishing or leading group therapy programs.

The individual needs of the person with social impairments must be intrinsic to intervention. For example, gifted individuals may be able to use their good language skills to effectively verbalize their own unmet social goals and to think through new solutions. Clubs that focus on chess, books, technology, or other special interests may offer environments that can be used to promote positive social change.

On the other hand, an individual with learning disabilities may benefit from more specific instruction regarding ways to change, including repeating of the same concepts several times and training in executive functioning (Horowitz, 2007). Individuals who experience inadequate social competence, in addition to a diagnoses of anxiety (social anxiety, selective mutism, stuttering, reactive attachment, separation anxiety), may require a lengthy period of experiencing an emotionally safe group environment before they can relax and try new social approaches to interactions.

Children who lack appropriate social skills may be the brunt of ridicule in school settings. This may prompt an occupational therapist to take the lead in establishing an all-school program to deal with bullying, such as *Operation Respect: The Don't Laugh At Me Program* (Yarrow, 2000) and the *Stop Bullying Now* video toolkit (U.S. Department of Health and Human Services, 2006).

## Establishing Goals for Intervention

Long- and short-term goals are established by individual interviews with the client, the family, other caregivers, and teachers. Reports identifying social skills needs may be available from schools, evaluations by other professionals, and sometimes work proficiency reports. Standardized questionnaires, such as those developed by Gresham and Elliott (2008a) and Fisher and Griswold (2008), may be helpful in identifying needs. Goals should be reevaluated periodically and revised as needed.

**Table 10.3** Sampling of Treatment Ideas for Developing Social Skills

| Categories/ constructs to be modified | Relevant treatment concepts | Potential strategies | Precautions |
|---|---|---|---|
| Verbal presentations (content) | Via modeling and coaching, group member observes and experiences successful verbal interactions. | Whole-group conversation in a circle every session. More complex small-group chat later while concurrently sharing snacks, including tastes, passing items, spills, etc. | Many members will try to direct comments to adult leaders only, not peers. Must redirect. |
| Nonverbal presentations (psychomotor) | Motivation to use self-regulation may be enhanced by improved skill at reading others' nonverbal and verbal cues depicting annoyance or frustration at irritating behaviors. | Carpet samples to delineate space in conversation circle. Techniques from *How Does Your Engine Run?* (Williams & Shellenberger, 1996). Empower members to recognize their own limits and take action (e.g., request wheelbarrow walk if feeling over-aroused, sit out game if unable to handle losing that day). | Those with ADD often hear criticism of psychomotor behaviors. Avoid repeated censoring. Instead, encourage self-awareness, reading others' reactions, and self-initiating change. |
| Emotional responses | An emotion is usually not the social problem. Person's response/behavior is the problem. | Group members act out suitable response choices. Photograph or record group members acting out emotions. Label times they recall experiencing those emotions. Keep those pictures with confidential files with no access to any individual. | Do not necessarily avoid creating unpleasant emotions in activities; instead, help group members deal with them as they arise. |
| Play and work with others | Gifted, creative, or egocentric individuals often strongly envision end products and play methods to their liking and push hard for independence or leadership. Slower or more passive members may have rarely experienced having others accept their ideas. | Constructions or murals, with requirements for jointly created end products. (Point out that the goal is for everyone to contribute and accept each other's ideas, not to win.) | May require restarting the project several times, until all members are contributing. |

| Categories/ constructs to be modified | Relevant treatment concepts | Potential strategies | Precautions |
|---|---|---|---|
| Awareness of self/others and valuing others | Use of two therapists allows one to remove a member for individual review of current social interaction and immediate feedback. Recognizing and predicting others' viewpoints is a major treatment goal. | In a confidential setting, prompt member who has been removed to identify what just happened socially and problem solve for himself/herself how to carry out the interaction more effectively and adaptively next time. (Provide support and understanding for the frustration of the former group and encouragement and patience for latter group.) | Avoid telling or even suggesting. Encourage individuals to figure out the problem and the solution for themselves, and encourage them to think about how the new solution is advantageous to them. |
| Initiating/ maintaining interpersonal relations | Speaking respectfully to others is a major treatment goal. Expect group members to speak respectfully to each other and to their families. Use "natural" opportunities during group sessions: interview newcomers, greet and handshake visitors, and send group cards to ill members. | Encourage families to record their dinner or car conversations and score themselves on respectful language and voice. Have members make phone calls for the group's pizza order or bowling alley schedule, or have them call to therapist's cell phone for practice. Indicate with colorful labels on group's big calendar all the calls/ visits initiated or received that week. | Be wary of adding a new member to a delicately bonded group that is just starting to value each other. Let the valuing swell first. |
| Feelings about self | Research implications suggest that treatment should begin early, to prevent the negative feelings of self more likely in older children. | Empower group to carry out their ideas for activities, often generated during conversation time (rather than always having leaders impose activities on them). Seeing their ideas in action often builds esteem. | Be cautious about scheduling a person with low self-esteem as one of oldest in the group. Rather than building esteem as the leader, the person may feel further intimidated by the social antics of less competent children. His or her fragile ego may be scared away. Compliments may sound hollow to the self-critic. Instead, encourage self-evaluation, but require both negative and positive aspects of performance. |

*Note.* ADD = attention-deficit disorder. Adapted and reprinted with permission by Occupational Therapy Programs (© 2002).

## Designing Theory-Based Intervention

The developmental frame of reference (Cole & Tufano, 2008) assumes that individuals achieve mastery in all areas of development in a continuous process as they age. If physical, environmental, or psychological events interrupt the process, a gap in the developmental progression may result. Occupational therapists provide activities and experiences to promote development.

The sequence of social–emotional development, social interactions, and play and work skills is acquired throughout the lifespan. The level of cognitive development should be considered in addressing social skills. For example, a gifted individual may relate better in a group of slightly older people, while an individual with cognitively impairment may be more comfortable in a mixed-age group or one of slightly younger people.

The sensory integration frame of reference (Cole & Tufano, 2008) assumes that the central nervous system receives, organizes, and uses sensory information from the environment to plan and execute appropriate and effective responses. Physical input of touch pressure or deep proprioception can have a calming and organizing effect for some children. A therapist may use this and other sensory integration techniques to supplement social skills work.

Professionals working with individuals who demonstrate sensory processing differences must consider the positive aspects as well as the negative effects of such characteristics and must interview and observe the individuals carefully before commencing interventions that could alter their sensory configurations (Dunn, 2009).

Behavior theory (positive reinforcement) and learning theory (modeling) inform the sequence and motivation of some group activities. Occupational therapy activities should be inherently motivating. As social skills develop, social rewards replace artificial rewards and intermittent behavioral reinforcement schedules can replace the need for continuous reinforcement. Verbal coaching (responding to the client's lead) will replace prompting (telling the client what to do) as soon as possible. Modeling by pointing out another group member's excellent handling of a social situation will soon supplant demonstration by adult leaders.

The model of human occupation assumes that the focus of therapy should be on the person's roles, routines, habits, and motivation in his or her environment and stresses the importance of mastering a variety of roles (Cole & Tufano, 2008). Many people with social skills delays have never mastered the role of being a friend. The occupational therapy group can establish an environment that allows group membership skills to be explored, practiced, and mastered. Group membership skills include those of group leader, follower, initiator, collaborator, and mediator–negotiator. Pre-event rehearsal allows practice of roles in social situations.

## Evaluating Progress

Although every formal treatment session is an ongoing evaluation of social growth, the progress of the client outside the clinic is the more important measure. Progress there may not evenly parallel the changes seen within the safe environment of the accepting, professionally managed therapeutic setting. Observations or periodic progress interviews or reports can be done by the occupational therapist or by other team members, the client, or family. Written comparison of current social functioning in the clinical setting with the original goals and early progress notes helps document progress. Standardized reevaluation tools and questionnaires may be important when standardized scores are required.

## Determining Change in or Termination of Treatment

The need for small modifications in the treatment approach is evaluated informally at every session. Keeping records of use of successful strategies or motivating rewards helps the therapist know which strategies are working most effectively. Change in the total approach is warranted when there is no movement toward the established goals within 6 to 8 weeks of the start of treatment. Change can take the form of referral elsewhere, addition or substitution of other forms of occupational therapy treatment, or a new approach within an existing group therapy setting. Long-term social skills work should be expected for some children with autism spectrum disorder.

Discharge is considered when social goals established by the client and family are met to a reasonable degree and/or when the client is experiencing satisfying social interactions outside the clinic setting. Discharge planning may include (a) joining or expanding involvement with relationship-building organizations in the community (e.g., Boy or Girl Scouts, church group), (b) joining programs related to the person's recreational or business interests (chess club, sports team, or horticultural group), or (c) participating in diagnosis-related groups (wheelchair basketball, Special Olympics, or a disability-related support group).

### Case Study

*Description*

TS is a 10-year-old fourth grader in a typical classroom. He is quick and accurate in math computation and can read aloud well, even when new vocabulary is introduced. He is an excellent speller. TS has difficulty understanding the full meaning of what he reads and receives resource room help for reading comprehension. His math skills have recently faltered because he is struggling to understand the more difficult word problems. In addition, he does not complete the timed math calculation "Mad Minutes" because his handwriting is so labored, and it further lowers his math average. Some kids tease him about his poor handwriting and drawing, and he silently wishes the teacher wouldn't hang his papers on the bulletin board.

Timid and shy around other children, TS often feels that they give him disapproving looks even when he tries to get their positive attention via his math computation accuracy. He feels disliked by many of his classmates. On the playground, TS watches longingly as the other kids play and often swings by himself. He doesn't catch on to the rules of four square, the current favorite recess activity, and he has felt rebuffed when he has tried to join a group playing even less complicated games.

TS plays video games in his room after school. The many kids in his neighborhood don't invite him to join their activities, and when he sees them at the school bus stop, he doesn't know what to say to them. He likes going to meetings of his Boy Scout troop, and the members are polite to him, but he overhears them speaking of visits to each other's houses, which never include him.

TS has been referred to occupational therapy because his labored handwriting slows down his written schoolwork. The therapist notices that TS rarely looks at her and does not return the greetings of children in the hall as he approaches her. She asks him who some of his friends are, and he looks blank and thinks a long time. When he begins naming children, the therapist soon realizes he has named over half the children in his fourth-grade class (an indication that he has not yet experienced a true friend).

The therapist conducts an informal structured interview with TS and learns that two of his classmates repeatedly bully him verbally during lunch and that he wishes he could find someone pleasant with whom to share both lunchtime and after-school free time. She observes him on the playground and notices that he watches the classmates engaged in group activities but fails to look at the handful of other children who, like him, also stand on the periphery of the playground. She talks to the teacher, who assures her he is a cooperative, well-behaved student. The teacher cannot think of anyone who seems like a particular friend of his and says that she has noticed that he sometimes takes offense at innocuous remarks of classmates who try to be nice to him. She reports that the last parent–teacher interview revealed that he doesn't say much to his parents about his school day and that he is becoming increasingly withdrawn from them.

In addition to working with TS's fine motor delays, the occupational therapist talks with the school counselor about starting the social skills group they have often considered. They decide to include TS and two other students from the playground periphery, as well as three students from younger classes who are antagonizing other children by their inconsiderate behavior. The goals of the group program include the following:

1. Notice and read other people's needs and feelings with accuracy.
2. Increase conversation skills and verbal negotiating abilities.
3. Ask for and offer help to others with effective results.
4. Initiate playful and verbal interactions in a manner that results in a positive response.
5. Develop confidence based on a realistic appraisal of their skills and others' perception of them.

### Long- and Short-Term Goals

One long-term intervention goal for TS is to increase his comprehension of verbal and nonverbal social cues. Related short-term goals for TS in the social skills group include the following:

1. Notice and accurately interpret three of four facial expressions displayed, devoid of verbal cues. Later, the therapist will verify the accuracy of his interpretation of feelings/emotions being expressed.
2. Using a booklet made out of magazine pictures by the group, accurately identify the social or emotional information depicted by five of five pictures

showing gestures, body movements, or positioning of people in group or crowd photographs.

3. After group rehearsal, act out three vocal inflection and tone-of-voice cues that suggest emotional content in a manner that allows other group members to correctly interpret at least two of them.

These goals must be concretely measureable for evidence-based practice in medical and educational settings.

### Therapist Goals and Strategies

The therapist's goals for the intervention include the following:

1. Use the school environment to TS's advantage for promoting social competence while also increasing confidence.
2. In addition to the whole-group social skills goals listed above, help TS to
   (a) expand comprehension of organizational structure (rules) of commonly used school games and play activities and
   (b) interpret innocuous verbal and nonverbal social cues of classmates and neighborhood peers nonnegatively or without taking offense.

The therapist's strategies for the intervention include the following:

1. Suggest to the counselor/collaborator that their weekly social skills group meet over lunch, thereby removing TS, and probably other group members, from a currently unsuccessful social environment.
2. Schedule TS's weekly fine motor therapy sessions to include one or two slightly less competent writers (to increase social opportunities under adult guidance without risking self-comparisons that would further erode self-esteem).
3. Consult with the teacher about possible confidence-building tactics. For example, the teacher could
   (a) ask TS which of his papers to display on the bulletin board or
   (b) set up times for TS to help a first- or second-grade student with word recognition reading skills or math fact computations.
4. Consult with teacher about strategies to increase TS's comprehension of reading inferences and math word problems (for insight regarding possible carryover of such strategies to improve social comprehension).

### Activity: Coach Me

Have the social skills group members each take a turn teaching (or reviewing aloud) a familiar game or other play activity to the other group members as though they were the coach. For added fun, the "coach" could speak into a (fake) microphone as though broadcasting the lesson. Encourage the coach to take the listeners' questions or comments by noticing when they look quizzical or anxious to add a brief comment (without allowing hand raising or blurting out).

### Treatment Objectives

1. Build confidence of group members in their public-speaking ability, a specific interaction that brings recognition and respect.

2. Increase members' awareness, and accuracy of interpretation, of the social cues and feelings of others (regarding the wishes of the listeners to question or speak).

3. The listeners simultaneously practice gaining entrance into a verbal exchange by demonstrating appropriate social cues that suggest their interest in participating (without blurting out and interrupting).

4. Expand skills of group members in social play activities that can be generalized to other social encounters with peers.

## Resources

### Internet Resources

Autism Asperger Publishing Company: www.aapcpublishing.net

Children and Adults With Attention-Deficit/Hyperactivity Disorder: www.chadd.org

Jessica Kingsley Publishers: www.jkp.com

National Center for Learning Disabilities: www.NCLD.org

National Institute of Neurological Disorders and Stroke: www.ninds.nih.gov

National Institute of Mental Health: www.nimh.nih.gov

OASIS @ MAAP: www.aspergersyndrome.org

StopBullying.gov: www.stopbullyingnow.hrsa.gov

Think Social Publishing: www.socialthinking.com

### Print Resources

Bellini, S. (2008). *Building social relationships: A systematic approach to teaching social interaction skills to children and adolescents with autism spectrum disorders and other social difficulties.* Shawnee Mission, KS: Autism Asperger Publishing Company.

Goleman, D. (1995). *Emotional intelligence: Why it can matter more than IQ.* New York, NY: Bantam Books.

Lavoie, R. (2005). *It's so much work to be your friend.* New York, NY: Simon and Schuster.

Williamson, G., & Dorman, W. (2003). *Promoting social competence.* Austin, TX: PRO-ED, Inc.

Winner, M. G. (2008). *Thinking about YOU thinking about ME* (2nd ed.). San Jose, CA: Think Social Publishing.

## References

American Occupational Therapy Association. (2009). AOTA's societal statement on autism spectrum disorders. *American Journal of Occupational Therapy, 63*(6), 843–844.

American Psychiatric Association. (2000). *Diagnostic and statistical manual of mental disorders* (4th ed., text revision). Washington, DC: Author.

Aspy, R., & Grossman, B. G. (2007). *The Ziggurat Model: A framework for designing comprehensive interventions for individuals with high-functioning autism and Asperger syndrome.* Shawnee Mission, KS: Autism Asperger Publishing Company.

Cole, M. B., & Tufano, R. (2008). *Applied theories in occupational therapy.* Thorofare, NJ: Slack Inc.

Dunn, W. (2009). Invited commentary on "Sensory Sensitivities of Gifted Children." *American Journal of Occupational Therapy, 63*(3), 296–300.

Fisher, A. G., & Griswold, L. A. (2008). *Evaluation of social interaction* (Research Edition IV). Fort Collins, CO: Three Star Press.

Gallagher, J. (1990). Editorial: The public and professional perception of the emotional status of gifted children. *Journal for the Education of Gifted Children, 13,* 202–211.

Gere, D. R., Capps, S. C., Mitchell, W., & Grubbs, E. (2009). Sensory sensitivities of gifted children. *American Journal of Occupational Therapy, 63*(3), 288–295.

Gresham, F., & Elliott, S. (2008a). *Social skills improvement system intervention guide.* Minneapolis, MN: PsychCorp.

Gresham, F., & Elliott, S. (2008b). *Social skills improvement system rating scale.* Minneapolis, MN: PsychCorp.

Horowitz, S. (2006, December 6). Nonverbal learning disabilities: A primer on a puzzling population. *LD News.*

Horowitz, S. (2007, December 1). The social/emotional side of learning disabilities. *LD News.*

Horowitz, S. (2008, January 6). Learning disabilities and Asperger's syndrome. *LD News.*

Kauffman, N., & Kinnealey, M. (2006). *Social skill deficits and interventions: Cross diagnosis comparisons in school aged children.* Presentation at the Annual Conference of American Occupational Therapy Association, Newtown Square, PA.

Law, M., Baptiste, S., Carswell, H., McColl, M., Polatajko, H., & Pollack, N. (2005). *Canadian occupational performance measure* (4th ed.). Toronto, Canada: The Canadian Association of Occupational Therapy Publications.

Parks, S. (1992). *Hawaii early learning profile for preschoolers: Ages 0–3 and 3–6 years, social section.* Palo Alto, CA: VORT.

Simmons, C. D., Griswold, L. A., & Berg, B. (2010). Evaluation of social interaction during occupational engagement. *American Journal of Occupational Therapy, 64*(1), 10–17.

U.S. Department of Health and Human Services. (2006). *Stop bullying now* [Video Toolkit]. Retrieved from www.stopbullyingnow.hrsa.gov

Williams, M. S., & Shellenberger, S. (1996). *How does your engine run?* Albuquerque, NM: Therapy Works.

Yarrow, P. (2000). *Operation respect: The don't laugh at me program.* New York, NY: Operation Respect.

Zeitlin, S. (2007). *Coping inventory: A measure of adaptive behavior, available for ages 3-16 years and ages 15 to adult.* Bensenville, IL: Scholastic Testing Service.

Zeitlin, S., Williamson, G., & Szczepanski, M. (1988). *Early coping inventory: A measure of adaptive behavior.* Bensenville, IL: Scholastic Testing Service.

# Learning Disabilities

*Nancy Allen Kauffman*

## 🌿 Synopsis of Clinical Condition

*Learning disability* as defined in the IDEA is "a disorder in one or more of the basic psychological processes involved in understanding or in using language, spoken or written, that may manifest itself in an imperfect ability to listen, think, speak, read, write, spell, or do mathematical calculations, including conditions such as perceptual disabilities, brain injury, minimal brain dysfunction, dyslexia, and developmental aphasia" (IDEA, 1997).

### Prevalence and Etiology

Five to seven percent of the school-age population in the United States is identified as having dyslexia, one form of language learning disabilities (Gilger, 2010; NCLD Editorial Staff, 2009). The American Psychiatric Association (APA; 2000) suggests that 2% to 10% of the student population has one or more learning disorders, depending on the criteria used. Of these, four in five may have a reading disorder (4% of students) and at least one in five may have a mathematics disorder (1% of the school-age population). Approximately 10% to 25% of people with attention-deficit/hyperactivity disorder, depression, disorders of conduct, or oppositional defiance also have learning disabilities.

According to functional magnetic resonance imaging studies, children with dyslexia exhibit unusual brain images when performing phonetic tasks while reading. Untreated, these unusual images remain into adulthood (Gorman, 2003). Birth trauma and hereditary factors have been associated with learning disorders, but no causative relationship has been established.

# Common Characteristics and Symptoms

Learning disability may be associated with abnormalities in visual processing, auditory processing, attention, or memory. Individuals with language-based learning disabilities demonstrate poor speech and/or language skills, difficulties with vocabulary and the rate or accuracy of performing language-related tasks, and problems with reading and writing. They may have receptive and/or expressive language impairment.

Individuals with nonverbal learning disabilities have difficulties with solving problems that do not involve written or spoken language. They have difficulty with staying organized in time and visual space, including the use of abstract thinking and social cuing. Motor coordination delays occur in those with nonverbal learning disabilities with more frequency than in the typical population, although the delays may be subtle and not deviant enough to be formally diagnosed as dyspraxia (impaired motor planning and manual dexterity) or dysgraphia (impaired writing ability; Thompson, 1997). Some individuals with a learning disability in one or more areas may be sufficiently competent in other areas to qualify as gifted in their general intellectual development.

Demoralization and low self-esteem are often associated with learning disabilities, particularly as individuals begin to recognize the discrepancy between their academic performance levels and that of their peers. Left untreated, a further loss of self-esteem and an actual decrease in functional capacity may occur. The school dropout rate for this population is nearly 40%, or about 1.5 times the average, and difficulties with employment and social adjustment in adults with learning disabilities are more prevalent than in individuals without learning disabilities (APA, 2000). Early educational and therapeutic interventions that help compensate for or overcome learning disabilities and associated difficulties serve an important preventative role.

The identification of children as eligible to receive special education and/or support services depends on whether the learning disability has the potential to negatively impact educational achievement and whether it can be ameliorated by specialized programming. There are myriad reasons for a discrepancy between intellectual potential as measured by IQ scores and actual academic performance. For example, a particular cognitive processing disorder or language impairment can reduce IQ scores, as can mental illness (e.g., schizophrenia), emotional disorders (e.g., anxiety), and attention issues, resulting in a reduced discrepancy between measured potential and current level of educational functioning. Other conditions that can have a negative effect on IQ scores (thereby masking the existence of a learning disability) include medical conditions (e.g., anemia), sensory deficits (e.g., visual or hearing impairment, a sensory processing disorder), ethnic and cultural factors (including English as a second language), and educational problems (e.g., poor teaching, lack of opportunity, absenteeism). If a student's IQ measures lower than actual intellectual potential, educational and therapeutic personnel may decrease the level of expectation and fail to institute remedial and therapeutic techniques that could improve academic outcomes.

## Target Areas for Intervention

The occupational therapist treating individuals with learning disabilities works as a member of an intervention team to help solve problems that negatively impact the learning process and preparation for adult living. The therapist brings a unique approach to the areas of concern listed in Table 11.1. The goal of intervention is not to improve underlying perceptual, sensory, or coordination areas but to positively affect the learning process. The table shows examples of therapeutic approaches in areas of an occupational therapist's domain that are intended to positively affect academic learning and, ultimately, adjustment to vocational, community, and adult family living (B. Maxwell, personal communication, May 16, 2003). The overriding goal for individuals with learning disabilities is to take full advantage of the academic experience without compromising the development of self-concept and social adjustment (University of North Carolina, 2010).

## ✍ Contextual Considerations

### Clinical

The occupational therapist is in a position to recommend unique sensory, perceptual, motor, or organizational enhancements to build foundation skills that benefit the learning process. The occupational therapist collaborates with other team members in consensual decision making to identify (a) problem areas interfering with educational progress and (b) plans for carrying out needed supports and services to effect success in the learning process. To do this, the therapist uses an evidence-based approach, which includes reviewing current literature, using standardized and nonstandardized assessments, conducting client and caregiver interviews, and reviewing other professionals' reports. The occupational therapist may observe clients in natural environments, such as the classroom, playground, home, or workplace, to identify factors that hamper or facilitate learning. The focus of the intervention team is the perspective of the person with learning disabilities.

Visual perception and memory may be measured by the *Test of Visual Perceptual Skills–Non-Motor–Third Edition* (TVPS-3; Martin, 2006), which consists of seven subtests for children ages 4 to 18 years. *Raven's Progressive Matrices* (Raven, 1995) may be useful for individuals age 6 years through adulthood to further define visual perception and abstract reasoning, particularly in individuals with learning disabilities in whom spatial competencies may be a strength but who have serious language processing handicaps.

Individuals with learning disabilities may have difficulty integrating spatial and motor skills. The *Wide Range Assessment of Visual Motor Abilities* (WRAVMA; Adams & Sheslow, 1995), designed for individuals ages 3 years 0 months to 17 years 11 months, separately measures fine motor skills and visual–spatial skills and measures the integration of visual and motor skills.

**Table 11.1** Examples of Occupational Therapy Process Approaches With Students With Learning Disabilities

| Underlying deficit areas that may negatively impact learning and preparation for adulthood | Examples of treatment approaches in the occupational therapist's domain |
| --- | --- |
| **Visual processing:**<br>Nonverbal learning skills<br>Visual perception<br>Comprehension of 3D space<br>Recognition of rotation<br>Ocular tracking and convergence<br>Visual memory | Introduce a moveable reading jig to expose one line at a time during reading. Eliminate the jig as soon as possible.<br><br>Advise teachers on the use of language, touch, and kinesthesia to augment visual demonstrations. For example, give considerable verbal explanations regarding graphs and tables and adapt math number lines or history timelines with raised touch points and color markers to kinesthetically and tactilely enhance understanding.<br><br>Suggest types of lined paper and lines in copy books with perceptual, motor, and attention competence in mind. |
| **Sensory processing disorders affecting attention and focus:**<br>Self-regulation<br>Sensory seeking<br>Sensory avoidance | Suggest preferential seating, probably in the front center of classroom or near the teacher's desk to avoid visual distractions, classmates' sounds, and people brushing by accidentally.<br><br>Encourage placement of special education classrooms away from the band room and views of the playground.<br><br>To increase proprioceptive input at school or home, encourage students to carry and deliver various items (e.g., boxes of snack milk cartons from the school cafeteria, Mom's laptop to the bedroom, groceries from the car during home study breaks).<br><br>Schedule sensory integration treatment, if stipulated, shortly before the class that requires the most concentration.<br><br>Store some of a child's books and materials across the room, so that the child must walk around periodically to retrieve necessary materials.<br><br>Propose heavy marching to classes, jumping or hopping during study breaks, or "pushing" walls out. |
| **Motor coordination:**<br>Written communication skills<br>Dexterity<br>Sitting balance (at desk, without leaning)<br>Back pack/book bag use<br>Architectural barriers<br>Assistive technology | Introduce dexterity tasks for classroom and home use that are interesting and self-motivating to the students (e.g. "apply 10 paper clips to this ribbon in 30 seconds"). Score progress in accuracy and speed to further motivate independent use elsewhere.<br><br>Introduce to teachers or administrators one or more suitable handwriting curricula for student, classroom, school, or district use, with ongoing consultation or individual treatment only for start-up or for particular problems that emerge. Report current research on effects of book bags on posture/motor development.<br><br>Suggest that teachers use a sideways clipboard to fasten heavy cardboard above and below the writing line to help new writers keep on lines and become accustomed to their own neat, tidy end result. |

| Underlying deficit areas that may negatively impact learning and preparation for adulthood | Examples of treatment approaches in the occupational therapist's domain |
|---|---|
| | Consider assistive technology keyboarding for children with impaired handwriting if legibility is the primary concern. Laptop computers, such as those made by NEO Direct, travel to classes and homes. Write:OutLoud software provides auditory feedback. However, if speed (not accuracy) is the primary concern, first evaluate performance skills required (especially dexterity) as deficits may prevent computer efficiency also, and computer practice is long and effortful (Weintraub, Gilmour-Grill, & [Tamar] Weiss, 2010). |
| **Organization:** <br> Processing speed <br> Abstract thinking <br> Hypothesis testing <br> Organization in time and space <br> Planning and sequencing <br> Completing responsibilities | Sort similar, but not matching, keys or buttons into groups defined by the student, requiring identification of common characteristics. <br><br> Cut comic strips into individual squares and then sort by sequence. <br><br> Make up headlines for paragraphs of information, sorting out the topic from the details. <br><br> Experiment with a variety of assignment books and calendars to individualize more effective planning methods. Emphasize this as a lifetime work habit. <br><br> Monitor book bags, desks, and notebooks for tidiness, sequencing, and completeness. Install a desk side pouch if needed for overflow. Use graphic organizer software or a personal digital assistant. <br><br> In the classroom, store a child's schoolbooks and folders in a sectioned magazine rack or file folder, separated by subject. Promote the organizing characteristics of vestibular activities. <br><br> In purchased textbooks, highlight information with different colors for section or paragraph headings versus details, to help perception of the relationship between chunks of information. |
| **Interpersonal relations:** <br> Social competence <br> Social cuing <br> Social language | Create social competence activity groups to work on projects and interact together to help <br><br> (1) individuals with language learning disabilities learn to use and recognize social language that fosters interactions (using visual cues and signals from across the room to promote learning and possibly co-leading the group with a speech therapist) <br><br> (2) individuals with nonverbal learning disabilities learn to notice and interpret visual social cues (using words and lists to call attention to those cues they themselves are exhibiting [often used accidentally] and those used by others) <br><br> (3) nonreaders to promote self-esteem and confidence in those who experience repeated failure in the single most highly valued skill in a school environment <br><br> Watch for and report to administration those students with learning disabilities who are subjected to bullying. Help establish preventive schoolwide anti-bullying programs. |

The *Beery–Buktenica Developmental Test of Visual–Motor Integration* (Beery, Buktenica, & Beery, 2010) is designed for individuals ages 2 years to 100 years. It has two supplemental standardized tests—Visual Perception and Motor Coordination—to help identify the areas of dysfunction. If impairment of optical competencies (other than acuity) appears to be contributing to learning difficulties, the therapist should screen for ocular control and for visual acuity and refer to the appropriate personnel for an in-depth assessment. The *Bruininks–Oseretsky Test of Motor Proficiency–Second Edition* (Bruininks & Bruininks, 2005), for individuals ages 4 years 0 months to 21 years 11 months, evaluates eye–hand coordination and balance, both of which are required for proper positioning and controls for handwriting skills.

Organizational difficulties often interfere with the ability of a person with a learning disability to function optimally in the work, home, or school environment. The occupational therapist may observe the manner in which a client approaches a task and identify his or her learning and memory styles. One measure of organization is the *Porteus Maze Test* (Porteus, 1933), which measures "planning capacity" and gives the participant an opportunity to realize errors, benefit from the experience, and readapt the method used. This test is not recommended as an intelligence measure, but it affords an opportunity for clients to try increasingly difficult spatial challenges and can be used for later retest for comparison scores to measure retention of nonverbal skills.

A leading measure of skills needed for everyday living is the *Vineland Adaptive Behavioral Scales–Second Edition* (Vineland-II; Sparrow, Cicchetti, & Balla, 2005). This is a semistructured interview for individuals birth through 90 years old. It consists of surveys designed to measure three main domains associated with adaptive functioning: communication, daily living, and socialization, which often pose challenges for individuals with learning disabilities. In addition, Vineland-II offers a Motor Skills Domain and an optional Maladaptive Behavior Index.

Behavioral difficulties that are reported or observed should be examined carefully to determine whether they are caused by sensory disorders. If sensory processing appears to be an obstacle to academic learning, the *Sensory Profile* (Dunn, 1999) and the *Adolescent/Adult Sensory Profile* (Dunn, 2002) with the *Sensory Profile Supplement* (Dunn, 2006a) may help pinpoint the most likely contributing factors. In addition, the *Sensory Profile School Companion* (Dunn, 2006b) uses teachers' observations and classroom behaviors to assess sensory processing skills in children with autism or other diagnoses who exhibit severe sensory processing difficulties. The *Learning Through the Senses Resource Manual: The Impact of Sensory Processing in the Classroom* (School Therapy Services, 2006) provides practical and effective strategic interventions to curtail the impact of sensory processing in the classroom.

The *Sensory Integration and Praxis Test* (SIPT; Ayres, 1989) may provide valuable information for treating the student with nonverbal learning disabilities whose academic performance may be adversely affected by difficulties with sensory processing. For example, the Space Visualization and Constructional Praxis portion of the SIPT can provide quantifiable measures of comprehension of three-dimensional space and spatial rotation, skills often associated with poor math performance.

Evidence of being bullied, rejected, or ignored by peers may indicate the necessity of a social skills evaluation and intervention. The *Social Skills Improvement System Rating Scales* enables a targeted assessment of individuals and small groups, specifically focusing on social skills, competing problem behaviors, and academic competence in school, home, and community settings (Gresham & Elliot, 2008). *Operation Respect: The Don't Laugh At Me Program* (Yarrow, 2000) and the *Stop Bullying Now* video toolkit (U.S. Department of Health and Human Services, 2006) provide valuable strategies that can help therapists, teachers, and parents to create safe, respectful environments.

## Family

Learning disabilities often follow a familial pattern, and one or more other members of the individual's family may share similar learning problems. Adults with learning disabilities in the family may feel they "made it" okay without intervention and may not favor spending the time or money associated with extra services. On the other hand, their own painful experience in school may be the basis of avid cooperation with intervention specialists on behalf of their child, or demands for increased services.

When developing treatment strategies, the impact of learning disabilities on family life must be considered. Home programs designed to supplement therapy sessions should be developed based on the needs and abilities of the family. Students with learning disabilities often take longer to carry out their required academic homework assignments because of processing, handwriting, or organizational difficulties and are easily discouraged, often becoming defensive when parental help is offered. Additional homework requirements related to therapy that require scarce after-school time and patience may only serve to increase tensions in the home.

## Practice Setting

Response to Intervention (RTI) is an educational principle grounded on the core principles of effective teaching based on ongoing professional development and adaptation of the curriculum to the needs of the student. The RTI principles also include scientific problem solving, research-based instruction and documentation, access to a standards-based curriculum, and the belief that all students can learn and achieve high standards when educated appropriately (Office of Superintendent of Public Instruction, State of Washington, 2010).

RTI provides a model for addressing students' needs in academic and behavioral/social areas by modifying the instructional quality of the curriculum and carefully monitoring progress in an attempt to rule out curriculum flaws as an explanation for learning delays. At least three tiers of increasing degrees of intervention are used to assess and remediate needs, beginning with a preventive level to proactively address all the students for screening, basic instruction, and emotional support. Tiers 2 and 3 work with increasingly smaller groups of students who have not advanced to grade level on the previous tier. Various members of the educational community are used at different levels to attain success. Curriculum-based measurement is systematically recorded at each level of intervention to provide individualized evidence needed to make ongoing educational decisions for each student (National Center on Response to Intervention, 2010).

The occupational therapist in an educational setting must engage in data-based decision making, in keeping with current educational standards (i.e., using an evidence-based approach to planning and documenting therapeutic intervention). Also, the occupational therapist should have access to job-embedded training, as the teachers do. If the school does not provide such training, the therapist must purposefully seek training to keep up with the latest in therapeutic options, particularly those suitable for educational programming.

Occupational therapists work with students with learning disabilities in a variety of settings. If occupational therapists are associated with a school, they may be employees of the school or the school district. On the other hand, they may be contracted to the school by an agency that hires private practitioners. Student placement in the least restrictive environment (i.e., in a school setting that is as close as possible to an ordinary, neighborhood setting) is required. However, there are a wide range of types of school settings currently in use, including the following:

- Mainstream general education programs, including extra supports for children with learning or other handicapping conditions or with giftedness.
- Public or private schools specifically for children with learning or other handicapping conditions or with giftedness.
- Charter schools, which receive government funding but are run by private organizations. Some charter schools have specialty course work for students with learning disabilities or special interests.
- Virtual public, private, or partial programs, which are computer-based, online programs that operate from a state or school district office. These are sometimes called "cyber" schools. Some of these private, online, virtual school programs have a few openings available that public school students can fill. Also, some charter schools are virtual programs.
- Home schooling, taught by the family, teachers from the local school, or private teachers.
- Extended school year programs, based on regression and recoupment considerations. These are summer educational experiences that are mandated for children who are expected to (a) lose ground, or regress, in their academic progress when they are not in school for the summer and (b) need prolonged help to relearn, or recoup, the information when they return to school in the fall.

The therapist's plan for defining the focus of intervention is influenced by the type of academic setting. Preferably, the therapist who works in a school setting would have access to communication with the school principal and the director of special education, to provide an accurate picture of the scope of services that the occupational therapist can provide. In some school districts, a monthly 15-minute follow-up meeting with these important administrators is sufficient to review the current effectiveness of strategies agreed on in previous discussions. School therapists who are employed by therapy contract services, not by the school district, may have more difficulty accessing the principal and other administrative personnel to make suggestions or gain information.

At least one of a school district's therapists should serve on the district-wide transition planning committee to identify and promote programming for the special education students who are 16 to 21 years old and preparing for post–high school placement. Regardless of whether students are planning to be in a vocational or college setting, supports may be needed for preparing for challenging academic or vocational competence, offering behavioral guidance, and help with friend making in the new social setting.

The occupational therapist is expected to follow an inclusion model (i.e., work with the students in their classroom setting with their peer group). The therapist also works in the playground and the lunchroom and promotes activity-focused therapy that is directly applicable to promoting success in the school setting and, eventually, in long-term employment and community living. At times, the therapist spends time educating others who have contact with the child throughout the day—teachers, bus drivers, school nurses, other support staff members, and, when possible, the parents. They pass on information designed to help the student reach his or her measureable, objective goals, giving treatment strategies that will be quantifiable, and they convey enough clinical reasoning information to help the recommended therapeutic steps make sense to the listener (Bassett, 2009). In some schools, parents are invited to attend all or some therapy sessions in order to exchange information related to the home environment.

In classrooms, the therapist may observe for sensory or organizational problems as they occur or interview teachers and aides about academic difficulties. Therapists may observe the teachers while teaching and then collaborate with them on methods or materials that might help the student with learning disabilities focus or learn more effectively (e.g., use of colored chalk, visual aids, location of materials in the classroom, sensory tips). Therapists should review classroom treatment strategies that were effective in previous years and encourage their continuation with the next year's teachers.

Therapists should exchange information through attending Individualized Education Program (IEP) meetings, instructional support team meetings, or "back to school" nights with parents and other education professionals. Therapists who contribute to the writing of goal plans should indicate methods of facilitating how academic goals are reached. The IEP should contain not "occupational therapy" goals but, rather, educational goals with suggestions from the occupational therapist about how to achieve them.

Therapists may treat individuals with learning disabilities in nonschool settings, in which there is more latitude concerning whom they treat and the areas addressed. For example, a gifted student in a private school or a charter school may be quite handicapped by a low-average ability in handwriting and may seek private therapy to address this issue. A 2010 *New York Times* article found it newsworthy and surprising that occupational therapists sometimes work with "able-bodied children," for example, those "just" needing therapy for handwriting, rather than working with only children with severe physical impairments (Gordon & McCreedy, 2010). Therapists need to make known to others the full spectrum of services they are qualified to provide.

## Sociopolitical

The Individuals With Disabilities Education Act (IDEA) of 1997 directed occupational therapists in schools to provide support services and recommendations for helping children benefit from the school environment. The act promoted a rigorous concept of objective procedures and systematic, evidence-based practice in educational settings. In 2001, the No Child Left Behind Act outlined guidelines for promoting academic improvement by screening at age 4 years and using accommodations, modifications, and alternate ways of teaching.

In 2004, the Individuals With Disabilities Education Improvement Act (IDEIA) required that all school textbooks must be available in alternate electronic format so they could be transformed into digital talking books, audiobooks, large or regular print books, and other formats. These materials must be readily available for students with disabilities, thereby rendering the curriculum adaptable to the various needs of the students. The Higher Education Opportunity Act of 2008 was the first federal legislation to define *Universal Design for Learning*, which required modern media flexibility and diversity in programming for college and university teaching. Universal Design for Learning became embedded in subsequent legislation for Grades K–12 (Rose & Vue, 2010).

The Health Information Portability and Accountability Act created federal regulations regarding privacy and security for health care providers that may serve as a reminder for all therapists regarding protected health information. School therapists who serve several schools may take records home and transform their cars into well-organized closets and filing cabinets, but they must safeguard student files from being seen through car windows or by guests or family members in the home.

School programs are legally bound to follow the IEP for each student, requiring that careful records of relevant information be kept. If an occupational therapy appointment is missed because of a class field trip, class standardized testing, or illness of the therapist or student, it usually must be made up at a later time. The therapist may need to reschedule missed school appointments through visits to the student's home.

Some clinic and private practice settings receive medical insurance reimbursement for conditions that accompany learning problems (e.g., motor coordination disorder). However, therapists may have difficulty obtaining reimbursement for novel approaches to treatment of organizational skills and academic learning disorders if the insurer considers them educational in nature.

## Lifestyle/Lifespan

Specific learning disorders are frequently identified in the early grades of school and may continue into the adult years. Sometimes these disorders are identified in high school or college, when an increase in academic expectations results in a breakdown in previously effective coping strategies.

The high school dropout rate of students with learning disorders is high, and it is important for services that support successful learning to be continued throughout the high school years. School districts are authorized to allow students with considerable learning or vocational adjustment delay to remain in public education until age 21 years. An Individualized Transition Plan is required for students who are 16 years of age or older and who qualify for special education services. Plans include transitioning from school to work and community living, as well as to additional training or higher education. Transitioning students with learning disabilities must take responsibility for their own continuing learning process, including making and using accommodations they require to succeed and advocating for themselves in requesting accommodations and assistance.

Adults with learning disabilities often experience difficulty in employment or social situations. They may encounter feelings of anxiety, discouragement, and lack of confidence because of the variability of their strengths and weaknesses, especially if they have not become self-sufficient in acquiring the accommodations necessary to succeed. The occupational therapist working with the individual with learning disabilities can help identify and implement strategies and adjustments needed at each step throughout the lifespan.

## Clinical Decision-Making Process

### Defining Focus for Intervention

The reason for the referral should be the starting point of intervention, and the data collected from reports, interviews, observations, and assessments should be prioritized and an intervention plan formulated. The impact of underlying neurological information and sensory processing considerations may be addressed by the occupational therapist. The therapist may choose to initiate direct, hands-on treatment. However, the school therapist is expected to collaborate with other professionals on the team and may have input into the curriculum by suggesting new ways for the student to work with classroom teachers, aides, individual therapeutic support staff, or parents. Occupational therapists in school settings should make themselves available to serve the students at various levels of a tiered RTI instructional program.

For example, the therapist supporting the academic learning process at a private school may, after meeting with a math teacher, design a chart of number facts that will help a spatially competent learner see a visual relationship between number facts that he or she has otherwise had difficulty memorizing. The therapist will maintain a brief, ongoing monitoring appointment with the teacher over the coming weeks and months to be certain that progress continues. The goal here is not to teach perception but to use activity and the therapist's awareness of an underlying neurological strength to build academic competence.

As another example, an occupational therapist hired by the parents of a private school student will need to focus intervention on the family's concern. This therapist may be working on organizational skills as requested by the family and may begin by suggesting that the student try several new types of books for recording homework. Together, the therapist and the family might discuss and agree on a new place to put homework to remind the student to turn it in on time.

The therapist working with students with learning disabilities in virtual, computer-based schools or in home schools may encourage families to seek opportunities for the student to interact with other peers in the community or may create a group social program for them if it seems warranted. Many children who gravitate toward a virtual or home-based school program do so because they felt that they did not fit in in their previous classroom setting, often because of their own social inadequacies. The therapist could suggest activities that promote more cooperative, collaborative teamwork with child-shared leadership and partnering opportunities.

The occupational therapist should think creatively about how to help the student with learning disabilities take advantage of nonclassroom school opportunities. Public schools have long offered extracurricular activities (such as sports, music, and theater), which can enable students with learning differences to shine socially by exhibiting skills that are strengths for them, although they may have academic problems. School talent shows and school-published newspapers can allow different kinds of students with learning disabilities to shine.

School district–wide opportunities may be a source of inspiration to the occupational therapist working with students with learning disabilities. Big school districts can offer wider selections of types of schools to attend and types of classes offered. New York City, the largest school district in the country, has its well-known High School of Performing Arts, as well as several high schools for visual arts and a high school specializing in aerospace. In New York City middle schools, students can take high-interest elective courses to help sustain their motivation and interest. Using creative thinking, the occupational therapist can find ways for some students with learning disabilities to take advantage of extracurricular activities or programs in other schools, or the therapist could even recommend a school transfer if the learning disability supports could be made available in the new setting.

## Establishing Goals for Intervention

The referral complaint, formal evaluations, other professional reports, and informal interviews inform the development of goals. Relevant academic and problem-solving goals are measureable and related to the individual's life context and learning needs.

## Designing Theory-Based Intervention

The developmental frame of reference is helpful when working with individuals with learning disabilities and assumes that an individual achieves mastery in most areas of development in a progressive, continuous fashion. If the developmental process is interrupted, there may be a gap in the process of development that undermines further development (Cole & Tufano, 2008). Not all learning problems are the result of developmental delays, and some emerge from neurological and physiological changes that never occur in the normally developing person. However, knowledge of the developmental frame of reference outlines those predictable sequences that usually occur as people learn new information and can be extremely helpful in planning effective intervention. For example, during handwriting instruction, children benefit from first watching someone write an alphabet letter before trying to copy the letter. Only later does the child write the letter from memory. A second example involves children's ability to visually perceive and motorically copy or draw a design comprising oblique lines after they are aware of verticality, horizontalness, and circularity. The second example also influences the sequence of instruction for skills such as handwriting. Knowledge of this type of sequencing aids the therapist in setting realistic learning expectations.

The sensory integration frame of reference (Cole & Tufano, 2008) assumes that the central nervous system receives, organizes, and uses information from the environment to plan and execute appropriate and effective responses. Some children have sensory modulation difficulty and cannot respond appropriately or consistently to sensory stimuli. As a result, they have difficulty attending and learning. Knowledge and insight in this area enable a therapist to provide sensory input, environmental adaptation, and learning strategies for children trying to learn in noisy and visually overstimulating learning environments. Other principles of sensory integration can influence effective learning. When a student is learning to organize a written response, using eye movements to watch another person's motor plan for writing an alphabet letter gives the new writer an internalized model of the letter-formation motor plan. Multisensory experiences, including touch and proprioception, can enhance learning. Writing letters from memory requires the further sensory challenge of visualizing the letter (ideation) while internally creating the motor plan for responding.

The model of human occupation (Cole & Tufano, 2008) assumes that effective intervention addresses a person's roles, routines, habits, and motivation within his or her environment and the importance of mastering a variety of roles and participation. Its emphasis on life roles is useful, as the child with learning disabilities is experiencing difficulty in a primary childhood role—that of student. The therapist should be as supportive and positive as possible in bringing about change for the student and in providing information to the parent. The therapist should use familiar roles in which the child excels to build confidence and new skills. For example, the therapist could introduce perceptual concepts through using aerial-view diagramming of football plays to help the child interested in football. Ineffective study and learning habits and routines should be replaced with strategies that are effective for the student.

Service delivery in schools may take the form of consultation to the administration or to teachers, classroom aides, or a child's individual therapeutic support staff. Direct therapy should be accompanied by communication with educational and family personnel (perhaps with a communication notebook that accompanies the child to school and home). The service delivery method may be to monitor progress from a distance, checking back at regular intervals to be sure progress is steady in areas that were previously the focus of direct therapy or consultation. The collaborative model of service delivery that is urged in IDEA encourages teamwork between therapists, families, and school personnel for consensual decision making regarding education.

Any classroom intervention recommendations planned by the occupational therapist must be reasonable and considerate of busy teachers, who have the responsibility for maintaining order, providing an educational environment, and keeping track of scheduling for a whole class of students. Recommendations for home activities should be incorporated into the busy family routine. For example, the therapist may suggest that the child carry heavy bags of groceries in from the car, toss the family salad with clean hands, or play penny passing or other fine motor activities during car rides. The therapist may also suggest using summers as a time to encourage extra emphasis on areas such as handwriting (including keeping a vacation journal) and to initiate time-consuming sensory protocols, which involve frequent application of tactile and proprioceptive stimulation and which may be too time-consuming to be practical during the busy school year.

## Evaluating Progress

The occupational therapist working with individuals with learning disabilities requires clear documentation of the student's progress. Evidence-based assessment records identify improvements and continuing needs, regardless of whether the therapist is working in a public school setting or is seeing a home-schooled child with learning disabilities.

To evaluate progress, the therapist must identify whether functional skills in learning and retrieving information and in applying the information to effective problem solving are increasing. Current performance levels must be compared to previous goals and objectives, standardized test results, or observation of new problem-solving abilities.

Measures of progress in learning must also evaluate independence in using strategies to compensate for the student's learning disabilities, without dependence on adult assistance. The student's rate of problem solving and processing speed must also be explored to analyze whether the learning methods adopted can be efficiently and effectively applied when carrying out daily academic tasks at home and in the classroom. The student's ability to generalize problem-solving skills to new situations and experiences must be evaluated by exposure to novel applications. Middle and high school students who are in the school's transition program are monitored for post–high school considerations as well as for high school educational criteria. Some students in this age range will have vocational placements as part of their schooling, and the monitoring of their success in the school-sponsored workplace may be in the occupational therapist's realm. Documentation of the ongoing progress levels must be clearly recorded so that results are understandable to future therapists, educators, and parents who might have cause to review them in order to benefit the student.

## Determining Change in or Termination of Treatment

The therapist regularly monitors the goals of the individual with learning disabilities to identify goal areas achieved—or, if goals are consistently not achieved, then they must be revised and refined. Plateauing may warrant discontinuation of treatment, although temporary plateauing sometimes occurs followed either by growth spurts in skill levels or further setbacks. Just because a child achieves academic grade level in a subject, or an adult achieves a desired organizational goal, does not mean therapeutic support should be removed right away. Therapeutic support may be required to reinforce newfound independent achievements and avoid regression. It is also important to avoid discontinuation of therapeutic input around the time of a major transition, such as a new educational placement, a new teacher, or changes in family structure.

In the school environment, treatment by a therapist may be terminated because a student is moved to another school, classroom, or even school district. Final termination of treatment occurs when the individual with learning disabilities is no longer impeded in his or her educational programming by deficits in the occupational therapy domain and has consistently demonstrated the ability to adapt, compensate, and succeed in the academic environment. For transitioning students (e.g., those moving out of high school), public school–sponsored occupational therapy treatment is discontinued. Individuals and/or families seeking ongoing treatment may seek private occupational therapy services.

# Case Study

## Description

DS is a fourth-grade student who reads several months below his grade level but comprehends far above his grade. His spelling is good for words that are phonetically simple (e.g., *banana, watermelon*) but poor for irregularly spelled words (e.g., *light, could*). He can cut intricately, snap his fingers, dress and undress small action figures quickly, and trace simple pictures excellently on onionskin paper. He excels in oral reports.

DS's highly informative handwritten reports that hang on the bulletin board look messy and fail to reflect his dexterity in other activities. He hates reading aloud. He can recite number facts well and can explain to other students what the word problems mean, yet he often makes errors on his math tests and homework papers. He is lax about turning in his homework, though he always claims he has done it, and he frequently has trouble finding his pencil and the book he is looking for in his untidy desk. DS's good grades are beginning to slip with the increased challenges of fourth grade. The teacher suspects underlying perceptual deficits but also wonders if he is really trying his best.

The occupational therapist administers the TVPS-3, the *Beery–Buktenica Developmental Test of Visual–Motor Integration*, and the Pegboard (Fine Motor) section of the WRAVMA. The therapist finds that DS excels in the Pegboard task but scores in the 22nd percentile on the *Beery–Buktenica Developmental Test of Visual–Motor Integration*. The TVPS-3 identifies considerable difficulty with memory for visual sequences and individual stimuli, visual–spatial relations, and visual figure–ground. The therapist notices no evidence of inattention, noncompliance, casualness, or slipshod effort during the testing. However, she notices that when DS looks at the test answers, his scanning is erratic and inefficient, and by the end of the long TVPS-3, he is rubbing his eyes. She asks him to read two paragraphs aloud and notes that on two occasions he skipped a line in the reading. He shows no evidence of using strategies to help him with the memory tasks and begins guessing wildly as the tasks become harder.

## Long- and Short-Term Goals

In the long term, DS will do the following:

1. Increase memory for irregularly spelled words.
2. Improve ocular motor control.
3. Increase awareness of part versus whole of visual stimuli.
4. Improve spacing and figure–ground aspects of written math and handwriting.
5. Organize desk, homework, and personal belongings according to a consistent plan he has established for himself.

In the short term, DS will do the following:

1. Correctly solve familiar math problems independently on full printed pages containing no more than six problems, with 95% accuracy in each of four sessions (using enlarged photocopies). Increase to 8, 10, and then 12 problems per page.

2. Independently place a frame around each math problem and solve it correctly with 95% accuracy in each of four sessions.
3. Copy math problems from book or chalkboard with correct spacing in ½-inch graph paper squares with 90% accuracy and then decrease the size of the squares.
4. Copy math problems from book or chalkboard with correct spacing on lined paper, independently using highlighter to emphasize correct spacing, with 90% accuracy.

### Therapist Goals and Strategies

1. Establish and maintain initial collaborative relationship with the classroom teacher and aide.
2. Meet individually with DS several times to help him improve memory by (a) training visualization ability; (b) applying sensory strategies, like use of color highlighting or sandpaper tracing, to stress letter groupings (such as -*ight*, -*ould*, -*eight*); and (c) using kinesthetic tracing above the word or subvocalization. Then consult with educational personnel and demonstrate memory method(s) found to be most effective. Monitor their progress together.
3. Refer DS for a developmental vision specialist screening. (This occupational therapist works in a school, so it is necessary to verify the district policy before making such a referral outside the school.) The therapist also initiates a variety of marble-rolling activities, throwing to moving targets, and throwing to stationary targets while the child is swinging on suspended equipment.
4. Use a favored activity of his—tracing—to clarify awareness of the whole versus the parts of increasingly complex pictures while still keeping outlined items separate.
5. Meet individually with DS several times to help him create a plan for organizing his belongings and demonstrate his effectiveness in using it. Then, consult with educational personnel to demonstrate the child's own plan, and follow up by monitoring for success.
6. Arrange for DS to write a letter to a teacher or relative on lined paper, having a red margin line drawn ¾ an inch in from the beginning and end of all lines. Grade up to lighter lines, and then absent lines, encouraging DS to visualize their presence. Similarly, facilitate matching verticality of letters, accuracy of touching horizontal lines, and space between words.

### Activity

Encourage DS to create a poster by (a) tracing only the mountain portion of a busy landscape picture and then (b) tracing only appropriate mountain/forest animals from another complex picture of overlapping and touching animals. DS should complete this figure–ground activity with a hand-lettered descriptive label written within the margins.

### Treatment Objectives

1. Visually discriminate foreground from background characteristics.
2. Begin and end writing within ½ an inch of left and right margins.

# Resources

## Internet Resources

AOTA backpack awareness information: www.aota.org/backpack

HEATH Resource Center at the National Youth Transitions Center: www.heath.gwu.edu

Houghton Mifflin Harcourt Education Place (resource for graphic organizer software): www.eduplace.com

International Dyslexia Association: www.interdys.org

Learning Disabilities Association of America: www.ldanatl.org

National Center for Learning Disabilities: www.ncld.org

U.S. Department of Education: www.ed.gov

## Print Resources

Bazyk, S., Michaud, P., Goodman, G., Papp, P., Hawkins, E., & Welch, M. (2009). Integrating occupational therapy services in a kindergarten curriculum: A look at the outcomes. *American Journal of Occupational Therapy, 63*(2), 160–171.

Brown, T., Unsworth, C., & Lyons, C. (2009). Factor structure of four visual-motor instruments commonly used to evaluate school-age children. *American Journal of Occupational Therapy, 63*(6), 710–723.

Cole, M. B., & Tufano, R. (2008). *Applied theories in occupational therapy.* Philadelphia, PA: Slack Inc.

Coté, C. A. (2009). Influence of a misleading context on a design copying task with children with and without learning disabilities. *American Journal of Occupational Therapy, 63*(4), 481–489.

Duff, S., & Goyen, T. A. (2010). Reliability and validity of the evaluation tool of children's handwriting—Cursive (ETCH-C) using the general scoring criteria. *American Journal of Occupational Therapy, 64*(1), 37–46.

Engel-Yeger, B., Nagauker-Yanuv, L., & Rosenblum, S. (2009). Handwriting performance, self reports, and perceived self-efficacy among children with dysgraphia. *American Journal of Occupational Therapy, 63*(2), 182–192.

Hanft, B., & Marsh, D. (1993). *Getting a grip on handwriting: A self-guided video and manual.* Bethesda, MD: AOTA.

Hwang, J.-L., & Davies, P. (2009). Rasch analysis of the school function assessment provides additional evidence for the internal validity of the activity performance scales. *American Journal of Occupational Therapy, 63*(3), 369–373.

Mackay, N., McClusky, A., & Mayes, R. (2010). The Log Handwriting Program improved children's writing legibility: A pretest–posttest study. *American Journal of Occupational Therapy, 64*(1), 30–36.

Rechetnikov, R., & Maitra, K. (2009). Motor impairments in children associated with impairments of speech or language: A meta-analytic review of research literature. *American Journal of Occupational Therapy, 63*(3), 255–263.

Thompson, S. (1997). *The source for nonverbal learning disorders*. East Moline, IL: LinguiSystems.

# References

Adams, W., & Sheslow, D. (1995). *Wide range assessment of visual motor abilities*. Lutz, FL: PAR, Inc.

American Psychiatric Association. (2000). *Diagnostic and statistical manual of mental disorders* (4th ed., text revision). Washington, DC: Author.

Ayres, A. J. (1989). *Sensory integration and praxis test*. Los Angeles, CA: Western Psychological Services.

Bassett, J. (2009). Back to school. *Advance for Directors in Rehabilitation, 18*(9), 19–21, 46.

Beery, E., Buktenica, N. A., & Beery N. A. (2010). *Beery–Buktenica Developmental test of visual–motor integration* (6th ed.). San Antonio, TX: Pearson Assessments.

Bruininks, R., & Bruininks, B. (2005). *Bruininks–Oseretsky test of motor proficiency* (2nd ed.). Upper Saddle River, NJ: Pearson Education, Inc.

Cole, M. B., & Tufano. R. (2008). *Applied theories in occupational therapy*. Philadelphia, PA: Slack Inc.

Dunn, W. (1999). *Sensory profile*. San Antonio, TX: Psychcorp/Pearson Assessments.

Dunn, W. (2002). *Adolescent/adult sensory profile*. San Antonio, TX: Psychcorp/ Pearson Assessments.

Dunn, W. (2006a). *Sensory profile supplement*. San Antonio, TX: Psychcorp/Pearson Assessments.

Dunn, W. (2006b). *Sensory profile school companion*. San Antonio, TX: Psychcorp/ Pearson Assessments.

Gilger, J. W. (2010). Dyslexics are more than people with reading problems: Genes, brains and treatment predictions for the future. *Perspectives on Language and Literacy, 36*(1), 29.

Gordon, P., & McCreedy, P. (2010, February 25). Watch how you hold that crayon. *New York Times*, E1.

Gorman, C. (2003, July 28). The new science of dyslexia. *Time, 162*(4), 52–59.

Gresham, F., & Elliot, S. (2008). *The social skills improvement system rating scales*. San Antonio, TX: Psychcorp/Pearson Assessments.

Health Insurance Portability and Privacy Act of 1996. 42 U.S.C. § 201 *et seq* (1996).

Higher Education Opportunity Act of 2008, 20 U.S.C. § 1001 *et seq.* (2008).

Individuals With Disabilities Education Act of 1997, 20 U.S.C § 1400 *et seq.* (1997).

Martin, N. (2006). *Test of visual perceptual skills–Non-motor* (3rd ed.). Los Angeles, CA: Western Psychological Services.

No Child Left Behind Act of 2001, 20 U.S.C. 70 § 6301 *et seq.* (2002).

Porteus, S. (1933). *Porteus maze test*. Wood Dale, IL: Stoelting Co.

Raven, J. C. (1995). *Raven's progressive matrices*. Los Angeles, CA: Western Psychological Services.

Rose, D., & Vue, G. (2010). 2020's learning landscape: A retrospective on dyslexia. *Perspectives on Language and Literacy*, 36(1), 33–37.

School Therapy Services. (2006). *Learning through the senses resource manual: The impact of sensory processing in the classroom.* San Antonio, TX: Pearson Education, Inc.

Sparrow, S. S., Cicchetti, D., & Balla, D. (2005). *Vineland adaptive behavior scales* (2nd ed.). Upper Saddle River, NJ: Pearson Education, Inc.

Thompson, S. (1997). *The source for nonverbal learning disorders.* East Moline, IL: LinguiSystems.

University of North Carolina. (2010, March 30). *Promoting role release on transdisciplinary teams.* Retrieved from www.cdl.unc.edu

U.S. Department of Health and Human Services. (2006). *Stop bullying now* [Video Toolkit]. Retrieved from www.stopbullyingnow.hrsa.gov

Yarrow, P. (2000). *Operation respect: The don't laugh at me program.* New York City, NY: Operation Respect.

# Neurological Disorders

*Arley Johnson*
*Scott Rushanan*

Occupational therapists frequently treat clients who have neurological disorders, such as multiple sclerosis, amyotrophic lateral sclerosis, and Guillain–Barrè syndrome. This chapter will focus on multiple sclerosis and amyotrophic lateral sclerosis. A brief discussion of Guillain–Barrè syndrome will also be provided.

## Multiple Sclerosis

### ⟨❦⟩ Synopsis of Clinical Condition

Multiple sclerosis (MS) is a neurological disease characterized by progressive demyelination of the nerve fibers of both the brain and spinal cord (Novak, 2002). Because myelin conducts impulses along nerves, demyelination of nerve fibers results in blocked or delayed nerve impulses.

### Prevalence and Etiology

Approximately 400,000 Americans have MS, and every week about 200 people are diagnosed. Worldwide, MS affects about 2.5 million people. Since the Centers for Disease Control and Prevention does not require U.S. physicians to report new cases, and because symptoms can be completely invisible, the number of MS cases can only be estimated (National Multiple Sclerosis Society, 2010). MS most often strikes people in their 20s or 30s, and women develop it twice as often as men (National Multiple Sclerosis Society, 2010). The sequence of the progression of MS is difficult to predict. After presentation of the early signs, symptoms continue to present and subside throughout life, with periods of exacerbations and remissions. MS is difficult to diagnose because other neurological conditions, such as cerebral vascular accidents and brain tumors, present with similar symptoms. It may take months or years to establish a definitive diagnosis. A diagnosis of MS is made when multiple patches of scar tissue within the central nervous system are detected via magnetic resonance imaging (MRI) and there is evidence of two separate exacerbations of the disease (Franklin, Heaton, Nelson, Filley, & Seibert, 1988).

The cause of MS is unknown, though it is generally believed to be a combination of genetic, immunological, and environmental factors. However, because it often takes many years for someone to be diagnosed, and because there are so many variables, it has been difficult to determine a specific cause or trigger (Multiple Sclerosis International Federation, 2010). There are, however, several working theories. One theory is that MS is a virus that lies dormant in the body and may be triggered by another virus, such as measles or herpes. Another theory suggests that MS is an autoimmune disease in which the body attacks its own myelin (Multiple Sclerosis International Federation, 2010).

## Common Characteristics and Symptoms

One of the first reported signs of MS is paresthesia, or tingling, in the extremities or on one side of the face. Additional early signs include muscle weakness, vertigo, and visual disturbances such as nystagmus, diplopia, and partial blindness. As the disease progresses, there may be extreme emotional lability, ataxia, abnormal reflexes, cognitive disabilities, intention tremors, swallowing deficits, and urinating difficulty (Multiple Sclerosis International Federation, 2010).

Once the disease is diagnosed, it can be classified into one of four major categories: relapsing–remitting, benign, secondary progressive, and primary progressive (Multiple Sclerosis International Federation, 2010). Relapsing–remitting MS occurs in 25% of patients and presents with unpredictable exacerbations, during which new symptoms appear or existing symptoms become more severe. This lasts for days or months and is followed by a partial or total remission. Benign MS exists in approximately 20% of patients and presents with one or two exacerbations with complete recovery. Secondary progressive MS exists in approximately 40% of patients and presents in individuals who initially have relapsing–remitting MS with subsequent progressive disability later in the course of the disease. Primary progressive MS is present in approximately 15% of individuals and is characterized by slow onset and steadily worsening symptoms, with an accumulation of deficits and disability. However, these classifications are also difficult to assign, as there tends to be some residual disability after exacerbations and a cumulative effect over time (Bhasin, 1989). Consequently, patients who are assigned to one classification at the beginning of their disease often are reclassified into other categories as it progresses. There are several precautions for those diagnosed with MS. For those who are affected with cognitive deficits, constant supervision may be required since short-term memory, attention span, problem solving, and reaction time can be impaired. There are also precautions in terms of avoiding extreme heat, cold, humidity, and stress, as these can bring on or worsen exacerbations.

## Target Areas for Intervention

Occupational therapy for individuals with MS focuses on maintaining a productive and satisfying lifestyle by enabling participation in self-care, homemaking and child care, work, and leisure pursuits. Occupational therapists use activity analysis, compensatory techniques, environmental accommodations, and energy conservation to help individuals compensate for lost or diminished skills. For example, the occupational therapist may provide driving evaluations; recommend adaptive equipment for dressing; provide consultation for home, vehicle, or computer modification; or provide instruction in manual or electric wheelchair use. In addition, the occupational therapist plays an important role during family training in educating the caregiver regarding the strengths and deficits associated with the individual with MS.

## 🌿 Contextual Considerations

### Clinical

The occupational therapist should evaluate the patient with MS in the following areas: extremity strength; range of motion and coordination; visual acuity and tracking; cognitive abilities, such as memory, problem solving, and insight into his or her own deficits; social disposition; level of self-care independence; balance during functional mobility activities; and, most important, previous functional status. The previous functional status and an occupational profile will assist in goal setting (American Occupational Therapy Association [AOTA], 2008).

In terms of treatment goals, the occupational therapist should concentrate on maintaining passive and active joint range of motion, preventing spasticity or joint contractures, improving coordination and standing balance during functional activities, and reaching maximal independence in self-care activities, using assistive devices as needed (Crepeau, Cohn, & Schell, 2008). The ability to achieve these goals is highly dependent on the previous functional level of the person and the MS category in which he or she has been diagnosed.

### Family

MS has implications for the client's spouse, children, friends, parents, and colleagues (Multiple Sclerosis International Federation, 2010). Physical assistance may be necessary to aid the individual with MS with self-care and functional mobility, and emotional support may be necessary to cope with the degenerative nature of the disease. Financial assistance may be required, as MS affects individuals in the prime of life. If cognitive deficits are present, 24-hour supervision may be required, as safety awareness and memory may be impaired and the individual may be at risk for falls. Patient and family education must also be involved to promote understanding and acceptance of the progressive course of the disease.

## Practice Setting

Rehabilitation services are frequently advocated as a means of intervention for MS patients during times of inpatient hospitalization. Inpatient rehabilitation has been linked to reduced disability in patients with progressive MS (Freeman, Langdon, Hobart, & Thompson, 1997). In addition, cognitive status can affect the type of treatment a patient will receive, as well as the amount of training the patient's family will require. Home care services are also warranted to personalize treatment within the individual's home environment.

## Sociopolitical

MS is a costly disease. It attacks individuals during their period of greatest potential and productivity. The mean age of onset for MS is between 29 and 33 years, with actual diagnosis several years after the first appearance of symptoms (Kobelt, Berg, Atherly, Hadjimichael, & Jönsson, 2005). The unpredictable nature of the disease process may limit the client's ability to maintain consistent employee roles. Treatment of MS has changed substantially during the past decade, as new biological disease-modifying treatments have been introduced in a field where only symptomatic pharmacological treatment had been available. The new treatments come at a high cost: between $8,000 and $12,000 per patient per year. Consequently, it must be expected that the percentage of total costs represented by drugs has increased, from a minor component in the 1990s (2%–5%) to a much larger proportion today (Kobelt et al., 2005).

Organizations such as the National Multiple Sclerosis Society lobby for health care legislation, disability rights, access to affordable insurance and long-term care options and public funding for MS-related research (National Multiple Sclerosis Society, 2010).

## Lifestyle/Lifespan

The lifespan for individuals with MS varies with the diagnosis and classification. It is difficult to accurately predict the course of MS for any individual. The first 5 years give some indication of how the disease will progress for that person (Multiple Sclerosis International Federation, 2010). Approximately 45% of individuals with MS are not severely affected and can live normal and productive lives, and life expectancy of individuals with MS is near normal (Multiple Sclerosis International Federation, 2010). The longer a person lives with MS, the more likely it is that interruptions in familiar activities will have psychological ramifications. It is important for individuals with MS and their family, friends, and caregivers to develop strategies to cope with stress and depression (Shadday, 2007).

## 🖾 Clinical Decision-Making Process

### Defining Focus for Intervention

The focus for occupational therapy intervention and treatment planning is based on three factors:

1. *Baseline functional level prior to the occupational therapy evaluation.* Since MS is a progressive disease, it is important to identify baseline function. An individual with MS who has required moderate assistance for self-care and has used a wheelchair for 5 years will not likely reach independence in self-care and functional mobility.

2. *Cognitive status.* The rate and extent of progress is often dependent on cognitive status. Deficits in memory and attention span will diminish the ability to comprehend and follow instructions. If there are deficits in solving problems using new information, the ability to adjust to unfamiliar situations will be impaired.

3. *Medical history and disease classification of MS.* Medical history can provide insight regarding expectations for progress. A combination of the MS classification and answers to the following questions will impact the goal-setting and treatment-planning process: How long has it been since MS was diagnosed? What were previous exacerbations like? How frequent have they been? How severe have the exacerbations been? Has the individual recovered to preadmission functional level, or are exacerbations followed by progressive deterioration? For example, someone who was diagnosed with MS 10 years ago and has had five exacerbations, all requiring hospitalization and resulting in declining functional level, would probably be classified within the primary progressive classification. Continued maintenance and family training should be initiated. However, if the individual was diagnosed 5 years ago and this is the first exacerbation, with mild weakness of the lower extremities, it would be realistic to set goals for attaining the functional level that existed prior to admission.

### Establishing Goals for Intervention

Within the acute inpatient setting, intervention goals usually address activities of daily living (ADL) and functional mobility. These goals are set, with the patient's involvement, based on a thorough evaluation of the occupational profile. The occupational profile delineates the individual's needs, problems, concerns about occupations, and daily life activity performance (AOTA, 2008). The second step of the evaluation process focuses on occupational performance. What are the functional performance levels in work tasks, ADL, homemaking, leisure activities, and functional mobility? Considerations should be made for fatigue, temperature, mood, stress level, and time of day, as all of these factors can influence functional performance on a daily basis.

Within the outpatient or home care setting, goals are often set with the maintenance of current functioning in mind. In addition, the home care setting allows the occupational therapist to more specifically design goals within the person's own environment. For example, the goal of independently performing a tub transfer with a tub bench is more realistic when actually performing the task in the person's own bathroom.

## Designing Theory-Based Intervention

The rehabilitation frame of reference emphasizes compensation for disabilities that cannot be remediated. Compensation frequently takes the form of adaptations that address self-care tasks and environmental control and mobility (Crepeau, Cohn, & Schell, 2008). Specifically, intervention strategies that are characteristic of the rehabilitation frame of reference and cogent to treatment planning for individuals with MS include adaptive devices, upper extremity orthotics, environmental modifications, wheelchair modifications, ambulatory devices, adaptive procedures, and safety education (Crepeau, Cohn, & Schell, 2008). The notion that motivation for independence cannot be separated from the individual's cognitive ability, emotional disposition, financial status, and family support is central to the rehabilitation frame of reference (Kemp, 1990). The biomechanical frame of reference maintains that purposeful activities can be used to foster range of motion, strength, and endurance.

The rehabilitative frame of reference assists with goal setting for the person with MS by using assistive devices to accomplish goals. For instance, independence in lower extremity dressing, hindered by poor trunk mobility, is fostered by the use of a dressing stick. Independence in functional mobility from a wheelchair to a commode, hindered by decreased lower extremity strength, can be accomplished with use of swing-away wheelchair arms and a transfer board. Independence in feeding, hindered by poor gross motor coordination of the upper extremities, can be accomplished by utilizing a built-up handle.

The biomechanical frame of reference assists with goal setting by addressing the performance of motor skills, such as posture, coordination, and strength. Therefore, the goal of being independent in meal preparation while standing will be accomplished through increased lower extremity strength. The goal of independence in feeding can be accomplished through increased fine motor coordination in the upper extremities. A variety of sensory and positional techniques may be used to facilitate functional movement through neurodevelopmental approaches, such as neurodevelopmental treatment and proprioceptive neuromuscular facilitation (Crepeau, Cohn, & Schell, 2008).

## Evaluating Progress

Progress can be evaluated by assessing the goals that are reached and the time period within which they are reached. Within the acute inpatient rehabilitation setting, individuals with MS are generally given 2 to 4 weeks to reach their goals.

If treatment has slowed to the point where progression toward goals is no longer occurring, the rehabilitation team must begin to investigate discharge planning. This is a process that is accomplished by the rehabilitation team, made up of the occupational therapist, the physician, the physical therapist, the nurse, the psychologist, the social worker, family members, and the individual with MS. Areas of discussion include family resources for care at the current functional level within the home environment. If the individual's family cannot provide a safe and supportive environment, long-term placement options must be explored.

## Determining Change in or Termination of Treatment

When the rate of goal accomplishment slows or plateaus in outpatient or home care settings, therapies are usually changed or terminated.

---

### Case Study

*Description*

TK is a 31-year-old female who was diagnosed with MS 2 years ago and has had five exacerbations, all requiring hospitalization and two requiring inpatient rehabilitation. Currently, she is hospitalized with the onset of dizziness, double vision, numbness on the left side of her body, and poor coordination of her left upper extremity. TK lives with her very supportive parents in a two-story home. She ambulates short distances (approximately 50 feet) with a rolling walker and is independent with all ADL. Durable medical equipment that TK owns includes a rolling walker, standard wheelchair, tub transfer bench, and 3-in-1 commode. She also owns various assistive devices, such as a reacher, a dressing stick, a long-handled shoehorn, a long-handled sponge, and a sock donner.

TK was hospitalized on the acute care floor of the hospital, administered 3 days of intravenous steroids, and transferred to the inpatient rehabilitation unit. Upon admission, TK was evaluated and found to be oriented to person, place, time, and reason for hospitalization. TK's left upper and lower extremity strength was 4/5. Her gait was determined to be ataxic. A mild intention tremor was also noted in TK's left dominant upper extremity. Sensation in all extremities was grossly intact. Speech and swallowing were noted to be grossly intact. Her sitting balance was good in both static and dynamic situations; however, her standing balance was fair both statically and dynamically. A summary of her self-care and transfer status with related goal projections can be found in Table 12.1.

*Long- and Short-Term Goals*

TK's long-term goal is to complete lower extremity dressing using a rollator walker to retrieve clothing from a closet and selected adaptive equipment (reacher, dressing stick, long-handled shoehorn, and sock donner) to dress. In the short term, TK will retrieve clothing from the closet using a rollator walker for support.

---

**Table 12.1** Multiple Sclerosis Self-Care Summary

| Performance area | Admission | Short-term goal (7 to 10 days) | Long-term goal (10 days to 3 weeks) |
|---|---|---|---|
| Feeding | Minimal assistance | Supervision | Independent |
| Grooming | Minimal assistance | Supervision | Independent |
| Bathing | Minimal assistance | Supervision | Independent |
| Upper extremity dressing | Minimal assistance | Supervision | Independent |
| Lower extremity dressing | Moderate assistance | Minimal assistance | Independent |
| Toileting | Moderate assistance | Minimal assistance | Independent |
| Bed transfer | Minimal assistance | Supervision | Independent |
| Toilet transfer | Minimal assistance | Supervision | Independent |
| Tub transfer | Minimal assistance | Supervision | Independent |

## Therapist Goals and Strategies

The therapist's goals include the following:

1. Decrease intention tremors in left (dominant) upper extremity.
2. Increase strength on left side (upper and lower extremities).
3. Increase standing balance and tolerance.

The therapist's strategies include the following:

1. Provide therapeutic exercise activities using graded wrist weights to increase upper extremity strength.
2. Apply light resistance to left upper extremity during activity to attempt to reduce intention tremor and improve control.
3. Integrate proprioceptive neuromuscular facilitation (PNF) patterns into activity to promote strength and control of movement in the left upper extremity.
4. Provide and retrain in the use of assistive devices for ADL.
5. Design activities that will challenge TK's balance while supported by a rollator walker.

## Activities

### Morning Routine

During her self-care morning routine, TK will practice using the assistive devices that she requires for lower extremity dressing (sock donner, dressing stick, long-handled shoehorn, and reacher). She will dress while sitting at the edge of her bed. It is anticipated that learning to reintegrate these pieces of equipment into her routine should be fairly easy for TK. She is familiar with the equipment and had been using it prior to admission. A challenge to TK's independence is remastering the use of the rollator walker to help her retrieve clothing from her closet in preparation for dressing. This task is complicated by her fair standing balance (static and dynamic) and the weakness and intention tremor present in her left upper extremity. An activity that challenges TK's standing balance and requires her to use the rollator walker for support is indicated. Additionally, an activity that requires her to place objects will challenge and develop the strength and control in TK's left upper extremity.

### Decorating a Holiday Tree

In preparing for TK to decorate a holiday tree, the therapist assembles the following: a small (3- or 4-foot) artificial tree, an assortment of holiday decorations that have been fitted with wire loops (2 inches in diameter) to replace traditional ornament hooks, and a 1-pound wrist weight.

To begin the activity, TK will be seated in a chair, with the tree placed on the table to her right and the box of ornaments placed on a surface (12 inches high) on her left. Placement of the tree and ornaments in these positions facilitates the use of a PNF pattern. The 1-pound wrist weight, applied to TK's left wrist, provides stability and helps to reduce intention tremors. TK is encouraged to reach for the ornaments and decorate the tree covering the front and sides. For this phase of the activity, TK will be moving in the PNF pattern using the wrist weight for stability. The nature of the activity requires that she reach and place objects using upper extremity control. This will prepare her to place and retrieve objects from a closet for dressing.

To decorate the remainder of the tree, TK will stand supported by her rollator walker. This time, the tree will be placed on the table to her left and the ornaments to her right at chair level. She will use the 1-pound wrist weights on her left hand. Placement of the tree and ornaments in this position requires TK to use another PNF pattern. Again, the 1-pound weight may help to reduce intention tremors by providing distal stability. Use of the rollator walker in the completion of this tree-trimming activity will support TK's use of this device to retrieve clothing from a closet for dressing.

### Treatment Objectives

TK will incorporate proper positioning, adaptive equipment, and energy conservation techniques into her morning routine (eating, dressing, and grooming).

## Resources

Archives of Neurology: http://archneur.ama-assn.org

Centers for Medicare and Medicaid Services: www.cms.hhs.gov

MS Watch: www.mswatch.ca

Multiple Sclerosis International Federation: www.msif.org

National Multiple Sclerosis Society: www.nationalmssociety.org

# Amyotrophic Lateral Sclerosis

## 🖑 Synopsis of Clinical Condition

Amyotrophic lateral sclerosis (ALS), or Lou Gehrig's disease, is a progressive, fatal neuromuscular disorder that can cause paralysis of all voluntary muscles.

The disease affects motor neurons in the spinal cord, brainstem, and motor cortex (Adams & Victor, 1993). ALS usually does not affect bowel and bladder function, eye musculature, sexual functioning, internal organs, or sensation.

ALS can cause both upper and lower motor neuron symptoms. Upper motor neuron symptoms include spasticity, clonus, and pseudobulbar affect (emotional lability, inappropriate laughter, inappropriate crying). Lower motor neuron symptoms include muscle weakness, fasciculations (small, localized, involuntary muscle contractions), cramping, and hyporeflexia (Rowland & Shneider, 2001).

There are three clinical subtypes of ALS: primary motor atrophy, characterized by lower motor neuron onset; progressive lateral sclerosis, characterized by upper motor neuron onset; and progressive bulbar palsy, characterized by bulbar onset. Each of these clinical subtypes leads to the onset of classic ALS. Classic ALS presents as symptoms for upper motor neuron involvement, lower motor neuron involvement, and bulbar involvement.

There are two forms of ALS: sporadic and familial. Sporadic ALS is the most common and demonstrates a random pattern of incidence throughout the world. Familial ALS accounts for 5% of those diagnosed with ALS, the victims having inherited an autosomal dominant trait (Adams & Victor, 1993). Twenty percent of patients with the familial form of the disease have genetic changes on the SOD1 gene located on chromosome 21 (Kabashi et al., 2009).

## Prevalence and Etiology

ALS affects approximately 1 to 2 in 100,000 people annually. Males are affected twice as often as females (until the age of 65 years), with the onset age of symptoms at between 50 and 70 years (Adams & Victor, 1993). Average life expectancy from onset of symptoms is 2 to 5 years, with respiratory failure being the primary cause of death (Rowland & Shneider, 2001).

The etiology of ALS had been widely unknown. Theories have posited that metal poisoning, metabolic disturbances, trauma, viruses, and autoimmune disorders play a role in the development of the disease. More recently, a problem protein, TDP43, has been discovered inside motor neurons. In healthy individuals, TDP43 is a normally occurring protein confined to the nucleus of nerve cells. The protein is used in normal cell function. In affected nerve cells, TDP43 is present in the cytoplasm of the cell and is misfolded. The accumulation of TDP43 in this area is thought to interfere with normal cell activity, affecting the viability of the cell and causing it to die (Kabashi et al., 2009). TDP43 is also present in other diseases, such as frontotemporal dementia (FTD). FTD, which can be a symptom of ALS, is a type of dementia that affects the frontal lobe, causing progressive deterioration in cognition, changes in behavior, and language dysfunction. There is much hope that the discovery of this protein will eventually lead to better treatments and, possibly, a cure for ALS.

The pathophysiology of ALS is characterized by the destruction of the motor neurons of the anterior horn and the degeneration of the white matter of the anterior and lateral columns, which mostly affect the corticospinal tract. Degeneration of the ganglion cells of the motor nuclei and pyramids of the medulla is seen in microscopic examination. The primary area of motor neuron destruction varies according to the type of ALS. For example, the primary area of destruction in progressive bulbar palsy occurs in the corticobulbar tracts and motor nuclei of the medulla, whereas in progressive lateral sclerosis, the destruction affects the cortical motor neurons of the anterior horn. There is no cure for ALS; however, one pharmaceutical drug, Rilutek, is approved for the treatment of the disease. Rilutek works on the theory that excessive glutamate (a neurotransmitter) causes neuron destruction with ALS. Rilutek lowers the release of glutamate in the nervous system. The effectiveness of Rilutek is minimal. The drug has been shown to increase survival time by 2 to 3 months in patients with ALS (Miller et al., 2007). There have been several other drugs that have showed mixed results in the treatment of ALS. Most of the medical care for those with ALS focuses on treating the side effects, such as pneumonia, respiratory failure, and dysphagia.

## Common Characteristics and Symptoms

The signs and symptoms upon presentation vary based on the type of ALS and progression. Generally, individuals may present with tongue and facial weakness, limb weakness, fasciculations (muscle twitching at rest), spasticity, muscle atrophy, slurred speech, and weight loss. In most cases, the symptoms of ALS appear as arm or leg weakness. Generally, one third of patients with ALS start off with arm weakness, one third start off with leg weakness, one fourth start off with bulbar (facial) weakness, and the remaining patients have generalized simultaneous symptoms (Mitsumoto, 2009). Although neuron degeneration predominantly affects the motor system, cognitive and behavioral symptoms have been described for over a century, and there is evidence that ALS and FTD overlap clinically, radiologically, pathologically, and genetically (Phukan, Pender, & Hardiman, 2007). Cognitive deficits can be detected in 30% to 50% of ALS patients (Lomen-Hoerth, Langmore, Kramer, Olney, & Miller, 2003; Massman et al., 1996). Functionally, the individual may complain of frequent tripping or falls, impaired fine motor dexterity, and difficulty with swallowing and breathing.

The progressive nature of ALS causes continuous changes in physical status, and medical precautions should be taken. Some of the main issues to monitor are frequent falls; swallowing and breathing difficulties (which can lead to aspiration of liquids and foods); and psychological issues regarding anxiety, denial, hopelessness, depression, and dying.

## Target Areas for Intervention

The role of the occupational therapist when treating an individual afflicted with ALS is to develop strategies to allow the patient to maintain maximum independence in the face of progressive functional decline.

# ❧ Contextual Considerations

## Clinical

The individual with ALS can present with muscle weakness, fatigue, difficulty speaking, and difficulty swallowing. As the disease progresses, the patient can show decreased functional performance in instrumental activities of daily living (IADL), self-care, leisure activities, and work-related activities. Ultimately, the patient will have to make a decision regarding whether to be ventilated as breathing becomes more difficult. Many of the medical complications related to ALS will continue to challenge the individual and family. Psychosocially, the individual may present with a multitude of issues, including anxiety, anger, and hopelessness, as well as fears of isolation, pain, dependence, and death (Umphred, Burton, Lazaro, & Roller, 2006).

## Family

The family will need to understand the prognosis of the disease, cope with the changing roles and tasks of family members throughout the process, and acknowledge the change in their own roles and tasks. Shifts of responsibilities and expectations among family members are common, and the need for high-intensity assistance can tax family resources. Referral to support groups or counseling may alleviate the effects of these abrupt changes and allow the family to develop effective coping strategies.

## Practice Setting

Occupational therapists may encounter individuals affected with ALS in the rehabilitation setting, in home care, in outpatient facilities, or at ALS clinics. Difficulty with ADL skills, IADL skills, and functional mobility resulting from muscle weakness indicate the need for a referral to occupational therapy. Inpatient acute rehabilitation may follow the acute medical intervention, but not all patients are appropriate for the traditional rehabilitation setting. Treatment will expand into the home setting because of the need for follow-up care, family training, and environmental adaptations. During the late stages of ALS, hospice care may be indicated for palliative care of the individual and family.

## Sociopolitical

The ever-increasing need for equipment, medication, and care can cause severe financial strain. Social security, Medicare, and other government programs are frequently changed and updated. The implementation of federally funded programs varies from state to state. The services of an elder law attorney or benefits counselor may facilitate clients' and caregivers' ability to access these resources.

---

## Lifestyle/Lifespan

Respite care, assisted living facilities, skilled nursing facilities, and hospice are care options that may need to be employed during the lifetime of a client with ALS. The client and his or her caregivers may need assistance in planning for and managing the transition from family-supervised home care to institutionally based care (MDA/ALS Division, 2010).

# Clinical Decision-Making Process

## Defining Focus for Intervention

Occupational therapy intervention for patients with ALS can be very beneficial. It is important for the clinician to understand that ALS is progressive. This means that traditional forms of occupational therapy used to improve function, such as therapeutic activity, therapeutic exercise, and increasing activity tolerance, are not indicated (this concept is discussed further at the end of this section). All occupational therapy interventions should be functionally based and focus on improving the safety, efficiency, and performance of appropriate ADL and IADL skills. This should be done through teaching techniques and compensatory strategies to decrease energy expenditure and efficiently use available muscle strength and energy. Strategies will include work simplification and energy conservation, self-care adaptations to promote safety, and compensation for limb weakness and balance deficits caused by weakness.

Lewis and Rushanan's (2007) article outlined best practice for physical and occupational therapy clinicians to use for the treatment of patients with ALS. This article justified the use of adaptive equipment and compensatory techniques to improve functional performance with ADL and mobility. The article also cautioned that, as with any adaptive device or technique, the use of such equipment must not decrease efficiency or increase energy expenditure. There comes a point during the course of the disease where no amount of adaptive equipment or technique is appropriate to be used. At this point, it is best that the focus of treatment switch to family training and that the patient accept help with his or her self-care and mobility needs. Family training should include handling and transfer techniques for completing all self-cares and transfers from ADL surfaces.

It is also important to note the controversy over the use of therapeutic exercise as a treatment for patients with ALS. There are studies that show exercise is beneficial for patients with ALS and that it increases or maintains muscle strength; however, many of these studies focus on patients who have a slow progression of the disease, high vital capacities, and very few lower motor neuron symptoms. For example, Dal Bello-Haas et al. (2007) showed that patients who participated in a home exercise program had a decreased rate of lower extremity weakness, compared with patients who only engaged in a passive stretching. However, study participants all had a functional vital capacity of 90%, and no one in the trial had even moderately advanced ALS. Other studies have shown that exercise has either no effect or adverse affects on the strength of patients with ALS. Drory, Goltsman, Reznik, Mosek, and Korczyn (2001) showed that after 6 months, there was no statistical difference between an exercise group and a control group of patients with ALS in strength, fatigue level, pain, and quality of life.

It is easy to think that muscle atrophy as a symptom for ALS is partially due to lack of muscle use, but no study has linked disuse atrophy with disability in individuals with neuromuscular disease (Hallum, 2001; Kilmer & Aitkens, 2006). In fact, participating in normal, everyday activities, including ADL and IADL, is enough for patients to prevent atrophy from lack of muscle use. It is not necessary for patients with ALS to engage in extra activity, exercise, or strength training in an effort to increase or maintain muscle strength.

Kilmer (2002) demonstrated that high-resistance strength training in patients with neuromuscular disease can have adverse affects and induce overwork weakness. Patients who have ALS and engage in too much exercise or physical activity may become overly fatigued and be unable to safely participate in ADL, decreasing function and increasing the chance of injury due to falling. It is advised that patients with ALS engage in no exercise other than that inherent in everyday activities (Dal Bello-Haas, Kloos, & Mitsumoto, 1998).

## Establishing Goals for Intervention

Occupational therapy goals are established based on an understanding of the disease process and the physical and psychological presentation during the evaluation of task performance and the patient interview.

## Designing Theory-Based Intervention

Because of the progressive nature of the disease, occupational therapy intervention is focused on adaptation and optimization of residual abilities, rather than the remediation of the disability. The rehabilitation frame of reference will be used to develop interventions that include the use adaptive equipment and compensatory techniques to maintain independence. In addition, the biomechanical frame of reference will serve as a guide in the design of activities that maintain joint and muscle integrity and range of motion.

## Evaluating Progress

Progress is difficult to achieve in ALS because of its rapid progression and consequential deterioration of function. Occupational therapy intervention should be continued with the patient until the later stages of the disease, when dependence in ADL and functional mobility is identified. At that point, family training becomes the focus of intervention. Caretaker independence in carrying out passive range of motion and handling techniques becomes the desired outcome, as well as psychological support for the individual.

## Determining Change in or Termination of Treatment

Goals continue to be downgraded as functional ability deteriorates. Caretaker education continues to be an important component of the plan. Treatment is terminated when the caretaker is able to demonstrate competence in strategies required to meet patient needs or a comprehensive support system is in place.

### Case Study

*Description*

LL is a 52-year-old woman who lives in a two-story house with a strongly supportive husband. She has been living with ALS for 2 years. She is presently unemployed but was working as a bank teller a year ago. Her major life roles are those of wife, mother, grandmother, friend, and confidant. Her leisure interests include reading, writing, singing, talking on the phone to her friends, and spending time with her granddaughter. LL is a very charismatic and insightful person and loves to talk with everyone. LL has made it a point to educate herself about ALS but does not discuss the prognosis of the disease with her therapists or other health care team members. During this admission, she has noticed a change in her lower extremity strength and her writing abilities and occasional slurred speech. Her shoulder and interphalangeal joints bilaterally are somewhat painful with passive range of motion, and she is unable to achieve full passive range of motion in shoulder flexion and abduction and interphalangeal flexion. LL reports that the active and passive range of motion of both upper extremities has been decreasing over the last 3 months.

LL reports that she can still dress, bathe, and groom independently and that she has developed slight difficulty with feeding utensils because of hand weakness. She ambulates with a rolling walker and uses a tub chair for bathing and a raised toilet seat. Her husband performs all household cleaning and maintenance and prepares and cooks all of her dinners. A home health aide assists with breakfast and lunch preparation. A summary of her self-care status and goal projections are found in Table 12.2. Note the inconsistencies of self-care level of assistance during initial evaluation.

*Long- and Short-Term Goals*

As a long-term goal, LL will complete feeding with supervision and adaptive equipment in 15 minutes while using a compensatory strategy for upper extremity support. The short-term goal is for LL to complete feeding with minimum assistance and adaptive equipment in 30 minutes while using a compensatory strategy for upper extremity support.

*Therapist Goals and Strategies*

The therapist's goals include the following:

1. Improve passive range of motion and reduce joint pain.
2. Educate family in passive range of motion.

**Table 12.2** Amyotrophic Lateral Sclerosis Self-Care Summary

| Performance area | Admission | Short-term goal (5 days) | Long-term goal (10 days) |
|---|---|---|---|
| Feeding | Moderate assistance | Minimal assistance with adaptive devices and compensatory strategy for upper extremity support in 30 minutes | Supervision with adaptive devices and compensatory strategy for upper extremity support in 15 minutes |
| Grooming | Moderate assistance | Minimal assistance with adaptive device to brush hair in 3 minutes | Minimal assistance with adaptive device to brush hair in 1 minute |
| Upper extremity dressing | Maximal assistance | Moderate assistance to thread shirt over both arms in 2 minutes | Moderate assistance to thread shirt on both arms and over head in 2 minutes with assistive device |
| Lower extremity dressing | Maximal assistance | Moderate assistance to put legs into sweatpants with assistive device while seated | Minimal assistance to don sweatpants with assistive device |

3. Provide compensatory strategies for upper extremity weakness during self-care tasks.
4. Prevent shoulder subluxation.
5. Prevent upper extremity contractures through splinting and passive range of motion.
6. Educate patients on energy-conservation techniques.
7. Provide appropriate assistive equipment to improve functional performance with ADL and IADL. The assistive equipment prescribed should not increase the difficulty of the task or increase energy expenditure.
8. Teach proper positioning and support to prevent discomfort and pain.

The therapist's strategies include the following:

1. Provide built-up utensils.
2. Teach use of proximal upper extremity support on an elevated surface to compensate for shoulder weakness during tasks.
3. Illustrate use of adapting environment for activity.

### Activities

#### Morning Routine

During her morning self-care routine, LL completes feeding using a large lightweight mug with handles and utensils with built-up handles. She sits at a bedside table that is raised to the height of her chest. While eating, LL supports her elbows on the table. The support of the table allows LL to compensate for the lack of strength and endurance in her shoulders. LL is also practicing the use of adaptive equipment and techniques for dressing and grooming. Any activity that is designed for LL should incorporate lightweight materials, use equipment that has large handles or could be adapted to have large handles, and be able to be positioned on a raised bedside table. It should be short in duration and provide LL with the opportunity to engage in her leisure interests. Focusing an activity in the leisure domain will allow LL to see how the compensatory strategies and adaptive equipment utilized in self-care can be translated to support her leisure skills.

### Book With Grandchild

To prepare to engage LL and her granddaughter in the activity, the therapist will assemble a bedside table, an activity book, a set of colored markers, and foam to build up handles. LL and her granddaughter will be on the same side of the bedside table. LL should be seated, with the bedside table raised to chest height. The granddaughter may sit or stand. A set of markers and the activity book are placed between them. LL places her elbows on the table to provide proximal support. LL's granddaughter is instructed to insert markers into foam grips. LL and her granddaughter take turns completing selected puzzles and pictures in the activity book. As LL completes this activity, she is reinforcing the skills and adaptive strategies that she will need to attain her long-term feeding goal while spending quality time with her family.

## Resources

ALS Association: www.alsa.org

MDA/ALS Caregiver's Guide: www.als-mda.org/publications/alscare/default.htm

# Guillain–Barrè Syndrome

## ⬔ Synopsis of Clinical Condition

Guillain–Barrè syndrome (GBS) is also known as acute inflammatory polyneuropathy, idiopathic polyneuritis, acute inflammatory polyneuritis, Landry's paralysis, Landry–Guillain–Barrè syndrome, and autoimmune neuropathy. It involves acute weakness of the extremities, in which the body's immune system attacks part of the peripheral nervous system (Umphred et al., 2006).

### Prevalence and Etiology

This disease affects people worldwide, regardless of age, ethnicity, race, or gender. It has no seasonal or epidemic incidence, and it affects approximately 2 of every 100,000 people. It has been documented in both children and adults (Umphred et al., 2006).

The etiology of GBS is unknown; however, viral infections, respiratory infections, and gastrointestinal bacterial infections usually precede symptoms by 1 to 3 weeks. Approximately 50% of GBS patients have had a viral infection within the 2 to 4 weeks before symptoms appear. In rare instances, surgery, vaccinations, pregnancy, cancer, or lymphoma will initiate the disease process. These listed conditions trigger an immune response against the myelin sheath of the peripheral nerves. One theory of causation implies that the viral infection changes the nature of the cells in the peripheral nervous system, and these cells are then treated as foreign bodies. Another theory suggests that the immune system becomes less discriminatory, allowing for lymphocytes and macrophages to attack the axonal myelin sheath. Also, it is believed that the invading antigen has antigenic similarity to the myelin antigens (Umphred et al., 2006).

## Common Characteristics and Symptoms

The initial clinical presentation of this syndrome will be somewhat symmetrical muscle weakness and paraesthesias of the lower extremities, with ascending weakness to the upper extremities and trunk musculature within 4 weeks. Decreased or absent reflexes, increased presence of protein in the cerebral spinal fluid, slow nerve conduction velocity, and accompaniment of the rapid onset of symmetrical weakness are good indicators of GBS. Cranial nerve impairment can lead to dysarthria, dysphagia, and ptosis. Complaints of generalized pain, especially at the joints, and tenderness at the muscle bellies are common. The intensity of weakness can increase to the point of leaving those severely affected with total paralysis. Within 2 weeks of the onset of symptoms, most people will have reached the most severe level of weakness they will encounter during this course. Complications and precautions of GBS may include abnormal heart rate and blood pressure, deep vein thromboses, infections, and insufficient respiration, indicating the need for possible mechanical ventilation. Skin decubiti, hemodynamic instability, increased risk of falling, and range of motion limitations, such as adhesive capsulitis, are other precautions for the occupational therapist to recognize during treatment. The medical treatment for GBS lessens the severity of the illness and facilitates recovery. Plasmaphoresis and high-dose immunoglobulin therapy are the current choice for treatment. These two interventions are generally successful, although the reason for their success is unknown.

Recovery time varies based on the amount of axonal damage that has occurred. Axonal damage is usually mild after GBS, often leading to complete recovery. Sixty-seven percent of those with GBS will present with no residual weakness 3 years after onset. However, if axonal degradation has occurred, complete recovery will be limited (Goodman, Boissonnault, & Fuller, 2003).

## Target Areas for Intervention

The role of the occupational therapist when treating those afflicted with GBS is to facilitate the patient's ability to achieve maximal independence in all areas of occupation performed prior to onset of disability.

## ⚘ Contextual Considerations

### Clinical

The biomechanical and rehabilitative frames of reference are most commonly employed in the treatment of individuals with GBS. These two approaches are used together because while the patient is learning ADL strategies to compensate for temporary muscle weakness, he or she must continue to perform activities to improve motor skills. During the initial phase of intervention, the occupational therapist will identify problem areas of occupation and performance skills. Body position, ADL, and communication are pertinent skills to evaluate in this population. Treatment intervention focuses on proper instruction in the use of compensatory strategies for ADL, splinting, and activities to improve motor skills.

## Family

Ongoing assessment of the psychosocial impact of the disease process on the patient and family should be addressed. The abruptness of this disease can adversely affect the patient's ability to engage in life roles and tasks and can cause family disruption.

## Practice Setting

Occupational therapy professionals may encounter clients with GBS in inpatient and outpatient settings, as well as in community-based wellness programs.

## Sociopolitical

Organizations such as GBS/CIDP (chronic inflammatory demyelinating polyneuropathy) Foundation International provide support, education, resource guides, research updates, and legislative advocacy.

## Lifestyle/Lifespan

The impact of GBS on clients' participation in meaningful activities is considerably altered even after the acute phase of the disease has passed. The continuing support of family, friends, organizations, and professionals may be required (Bersano et al., 2006; Rudolph, Larsen, & Farbu, 2008).

## Resource

GBS/CIBP Foundation International: http://www.gbs-cidp.org

## References

Adams, R., & Victor, M. (1993). *Principles of neurology*. New York, NY: McGraw-Hill.

American Occupational Therapy Association. (2008). *Occupational therapy practice framework: Domain and process* (2nd ed.). Bethesda, MD: Author.

Bersano, A., Carpo, M., Allaria, S., Franciotta, D., Citterio, A., & Nobile-Orazio, E. (2006). Long term disability and social status change after Guillain-Barre syndrome. *Journal of Neurology, 253*(2), 214–218.

Bhasin, C. (1989). Occupational therapy in the management of multiple sclerosis. *AOTA Physical Disabilities Special Interest Section Newsletter, 12*(4), 1–4.

Crepeau, E., Cohn, E., & Schell, B. (2008). *Willard and Spackman's occupational therapy* (11th ed.). Philadelphia, PA: Lippincott, Williams & Wilkins.

Dal Bello-Haas, V., Florence, J., Kloos, A., Scheirbecker, J., Lopate, G., Hayes, S., Pioro, E. P., & Mitsumoto, H. (2007). A randomized controlled trial of resistance exercise in individuals with ALS. *Neurology, 68*, 2003–2007.

Dal Bello-Haas, V., Kloos, A., & Mitsumoto, H. (1998). Physical therapy for a patient through six stages of amyotrophic lateral sclerosis. *Physical Therapy, 78*, 1312–1324.

Drory, V., Goltsman, J., Reznik, J., Mosek, A., & Korczyn, A. (2001). The value of muscle exercise in patients with amyotrophic lateral sclerosis. *Journal of Neurological Science, 191*, 133–137.

Franklin, G., Heaton, R., Nelson, L., Filley, C., & Seibert, C. (1988). Correlation of neuropsychological and MRI findings in chronic/progressive multiple sclerosis. *Neurology, 38*(12), 1826–1829.

Freeman, J., Langdon, D., Hobart, J., & Thompson, A. (1997). The impact of inpatient rehabilitation on progressive multiple sclerosis. *Annals of Neurology, 42*, 236–244.

Goodman, C., Boissonnault, W., & Fuller, K. (2003). *Pathology: Implications for the physical therapist* (2nd ed.). Philadelphia, PA: Saunders.

Hallum, A. (2001). *Neurological rehabilitation* (4th ed.). St. Louis, MO: Mosby.

Kabashi, E., Li Lin, L., Tradewell, M., Dion, P., Bercier, V., Bourgouin, P., Rochefort, D., . . . Drapeau, P. (2009). Gain and loss of function of ALS-related mutations of TARDBP (TDP-43) cause motor deficits in vivo. *Human Molecular Genetics, 19*(4), 671–683.

Kemp, B. (1990). *The psychosocial context of geriatric rehabilitation*. Boston, MA: Little, Brown & Co.

Kilmer, D. (2002). Response to resistive strengthening exercise training in humans with neuromuscular disease. *American Journal of Physical Medicine & Rehabilitation, 81*, S121–S126.

Kilmer, D. D., & Aitkens, S. (2006). Neuromuscular diseases. In W. R. Frontera, D. M. Slovik, & D. M. Dawson (Eds.), *Exercise in rehabilitation medicine* (2nd ed., pp. 180–191). Champaign, IL: Human Kinetics.

Kobelt, G., Berg, J., Atherley, D., Hadjimichael, O., & Jönsson, B. (2005). *Costs and quality of life in multiple sclerosis: A cross-sectional study in the USA*. Retrieved from http://ideas.repec.org/p/hhs/hastef/0594.html

Lewis, M., & Rushanan, S. (2007). The role of physical therapy and occupational therapy in the treatment of amyotrophic lateral sclerosis. *NeuroRehabilitation, 22*, 451–461.

Lomen-Hoerth, C., Langmore, M., Kramer, J., Olney, R., & Miller, B. (2003). Are amyotrophic lateral sclerosis patients cognitively normal? *Neurology, 60*, 1094–1097.

Massman, P., Sims, J., Cooke, N., Haverkamp, L., Appel, V., & Appel, S. (1996). Prevalence and correlates of neuropsychological deficits in amyotrophic lateral sclerosis. *Journal of Neurology, Neurosurgery & Psychiatry, 61*, 450–455.

MDA ALS Division. (2010). *MDS/ALS caregiver's guide*. Tucson, AZ: Author.

Miller, R., Bradley, W., Cudkowicz, M., Hubble, J., Meininger, V., Mitsumoto, H., Moore, D., . . . The TCH346 Study Group. (2007). Phase II/III randomized trial of TCH346 in patients with ALS. *Neurology, 69,* 776–784.

Mitsumoto, H. (2009). *Amyotrophic lateral sclerosis: A guide for patients and families* (3rd ed.). New York, NY: Demos Medical Publishing.

Multiple Sclerosis International Federation. (2010). *About MS research.* Retrieved from. http://www.msif.org/en/research/index.html

National Multiple Sclerosis Society. (2010). *What is multiple sclerosis?* Retrieved from http://www.nationalmssociety.org/about-multiple-sclerosis/what-we-know-about-ms/faqs-about-ms/index.aspx#whatis

Novak, P. (2002). *Mosby's medical, nursing, and allied health dictionary* (5th ed.). St. Louis, MO: Mosby.

Phukan, J., Pender, N., & Hardiman, O. (2007). Cognitive impairment in amyotrophic lateral sclerosis. *The Lancet Neurology, 6,* 994–1003.

Rowland, L., & Shneider, N. (2001). Amyotrophic lateral sclerosis. *The New England Journal of Medicine, 344*(22), 1688–1700.

Rudolph, T., Larsen, J., & Farbu, E. (2008). The long-term functional status in patients with Guillain-Barre syndrome. *European Journal of Neurology, 15*(12), 1332–1337.

Shadday, A. (2007). *Understanding and treating depression in MS: Recognizing the symptoms and learning the solutions.* Cherry Hill, NJ: The Multiple Sclerosis Association of America.

Umphred, D., Burton, G., Lazaro, R., & Roller, M. (Eds.). (2006). *Neurological rehabilitation* (5th ed.). St. Louis, MO: Mosby.

# Amputations | *James Foster*

## 🎗 Synopsis of Clinical Condition

### Prevalence and Etiology

Dysvascular limb loss is an increasing problem within the diabetic community and throughout the country. There are approximately 1.7 million people in the United States living with limb loss (Ziegler-Graham, MacKenzie, Ephraim, Travision, & Brookmeyer, 2008). Leg amputations make up 90% of all cases, and at 77%, males make up the overwhelming majority of cases. Approximately 50% of individuals with limb loss are between the ages of 21 and 65 years. If unchecked, there are estimates that the number of dysvascular amputees may double by 2050 (Ziegler-Graham et al., 2008). Between 1988 and 1996, there were an average of 133,735 people discharged from hospitals after amputation (Dillingham, Pezzin, & MacKenzie, 2002a). Of individuals discharged, 82% of their amputations were caused by dysvascular disease (Dillingham et al., 2002a). The incidence of vascular leg amputation is 8 times higher in diabetic than in nondiabetic individuals (Johannesson et al., 2009). Dillingham et al. (2002b) also noted significant racial differences, finding that African Americans were 2 to 4 times more likely to lose a lower limb than were European Americans of similar age and gender.

Other causes of amputation include bone cancer, trauma, and congenital deformities (Carroll & Edelstein, 2006). Improvements in the early detection and treatment of bone cancer will be accompanied by an increase in amputations, with surgeons attempting to remove the shortest amount of limb while still maintaining vascular integrity to the residual limb.

Rate of reamputation of the ipsilateral lower extremity has been shown to be as high as 60.7 % within 5 years of the original surgery (Izumi, Satterfield, Lee, & Harkless, 2006). In addition, amputation of the contralateral lower extremity is as high as 33% (Izumi et al., 2006).

## Common Characteristics and Symptoms

Each type of amputation is characterized by an array of traits, symptoms, and challenges. From distal to proximal, lower extremity amputations can be classified into the following categories: toe amputations, transmetatarsal amputations, partial foot amputations (Chopart or Symes amputations), below-the-knee amputations (BKAs), knee disarticulations, above-the-knee amputations (AKAs), and hip disarticulations. At 55% of all amputations, BKAs are the most common amputation (Muilenburg & Wilson, 1996a, 1996b). Upper extremity amputations can be digit amputations, wrist disarticulations, below-the-elbow amputations, elbow disarticulations, above-the-elbow amputations, and shoulder disarticulations.

The closer to the body that the amputation occurs, the more stability that will be provided by a prosthesis. Longer limb length, compared with shorter limb length, has been proven to result in less atrophy and more strength in amputees (Isakov, Burger, Gregoric, & Marincek, 1996). This is because less muscle is attached to bone, so the remaining musculature needs to work harder to stabilize the remaining joint.

## Target Areas for Intervention

Upper and lower extremity rehabilitation can be broken down into three stages: preprosthetic, prosthetic, and postprosthetic. The occupational therapist has an important role in the preprosthetic and prosthetic stages. In the preprosthetic stage for lower and upper extremity amputation, the occupational therapist concentrates on limb desensitization, edema control, limb shaping, limb positioning, and safe functional mobility training. Self-image issues need to be addressed during this stage as well. For the occupational therapist, the prosthetic stage includes teaching the patient to put on and take off the prosthetic and the understockings and to perform functional activities with the new limb. The postprosthetic stage includes fitting for a final prosthetic and helping the amputee reach higher functioning prosthetic use.

## 🌿 Contextual Considerations
### Clinical

During the preprosthetic stage, the focus for treatment is limb and incision inspection, limb wrapping, limb desensitization, limb positioning, and functional mobility training. The preprosthetic stage lasts approximately 2 to 4 months. According to Dillingham, Pezzin, and MacKenzie (2003), 40.6% of dysvascular lower limb amputees in the state of Maryland were discharged from acute care hospital directly to home, 37.4% to a nursing home, 9.2% to home care, and

9.6% to an inpatient rehabilitation unit. The location of discharge often speaks to the patient's level of function. Higher functioning people can often be discharged directly to their home or to an acute rehabilitation setting, whereas lower functioning individuals are discharged to skilled rehabilitation at a nursing home setting.

The patient should inspect the incision and residual limb 2 to 3 times daily. This process can be assisted using an inspection mirror to view distal and posterior aspects of the limb. The patient should look for areas around the incision that blacken, redden, or become pale, all of which could suggest vascular changes or necrosis of the distal aspect of the limb. Incisions that are not healing should also be noted, as should amounts and color of any drainage. Sutures or staples will be removed when the incision is fully healed, usually within 2 to 4 weeks. Sutures/staples may be partially removed at individual aspects of the incision, as the wound may not uniformly heal throughout the entire incision.

There is much debate over the use of rigid versus soft postoperative residual limb dressings (Smith, McFarland, Sangeorzan, Reiber, & Czerniechi, 2003). Examples of rigid and semi-rigid dressings include plaster casting material, Unna's paste dressing, and bivalved splints. The benefits of these dressings include good contracture prevention, total contact to the incision, and good shaping. The disadvantages include poor ability to monitor the incision and increased probability of pressure sores if applied incorrectly.

Examples of soft dressings include Ace wrap and Tubigrip bandages. Advantages of soft dressings include good limb shaping, allowance of daily incision inspection, and ease of application. Disadvantages include difficulty for some patients to apply and variance in pressure with application. Rigid dressings have been shown to increase wound healing (Deutsch, English, Vermeer, Murray, & Condous, 2005), decrease time to first prosthetic casting, and decrease acute hospital length of stay (Taylor, Cavenett, Stepien, & Crotty, 2008).

Limb wrapping, or covering the limb with elastic dressing, can occur while the patient is inspecting the limb. Limb wrapping is necessary to control edema, to shape the limb, and to provide sensory input and pressure to the limb. During the acute stage, the residual limb should be covered with both an inner and an outer wrap. The inner wrap should consist of absorbent gauze, such as sterile 4 × 4 Kling wrap or Kerlix bandage rolls, to collect any drainage and keep it from soaking the outer wrap. The outer wrap should initially be Ace wrap and should be applied in a figure-8 method, utilizing a diagonal pattern. For the patient with a BKA, the Ace wrap should extend up to the knee for more uniform edema control and to prevent knee contractures.

The wrap should be tighter at the distal aspect of the limb and looser at the proximal aspect to allow for circulation proximally. Special attention must be paid to the medial and lateral distal edges of the limb and incision. Fleshy folds (referred to as "dog ears"), which can occur at these areas, need to be flattened via the wrapping process for the proper shaping to occur.

Generally, the wider and shorter the residual limb, the more difficult it is to wrap and for the wrap to remain in place. This is especially true for AKAs, which can leave wide and short residual limbs. In these cases, an Elastinet covering over the Ace wrap will help keep the wrap in place. The Elastinet covering can also incorporate a belt to wrap around the waist and then tie off at the distal end of the limb.

The wrap should be secured to itself using medical tape and not the metal clips that usually accompany the wrap. Many amputees have decreased sensation in the residual limb and may not feel the metal clip against their skin. The patient should also be instructed to wear the wrapping 24 hours a day unless performing self-care.

The patient should be instructed via a physical demonstration in addition to illustrated handouts. An "artificial limb" can also be fabricated from sheets that have been rounded at the edges, to provide the patient another medium to practice wrapping. The residual limb should be unwrapped and wrapped 2 to 3 times a day, as the wrap's elasticity decreases after several hours. If drainage is present on the inner wrap, it should be replaced every time the limb is wrapped. Circumferential measurements should be made to track the effectiveness of the wrapping in terms of edema management. These measurements should be shared with the patient to demonstrate the importance of limb wrapping.

Limb wrapping also provides constant pressure to the limb. This is beneficial for several reasons. First, consistent and equal pressure on a wound or incision promotes healing and prevents scar formation. Second, it provides sensory and tactile input to the limb. This is necessary because initially the limb will be painful and sensitive to touch, but it must be desensitized in order for the patient to tolerate the use of a prosthetic.

As noted previously, the bandage of choice should initially be Ace wrap. Many patients, however, have difficulty utilizing the figure-8 method because of issues related to their vascular disease. Poor vascular flow to the peripheral extremities can result in poor sensation in the upper extremities and consequently affect fine motor coordination during limb wrapping. Many individuals with compromised vascular systems also have poor visual acuity and cannot see the end of the limb or fully appreciate the figure-8 technique required for proper wrapping.

For these reasons, it may be easier to apply a Tubigrip stocking to the limb. This can be done by measuring the limb for the correct width of stocking and applying it with a Tubigrip applicator, proximally to distally, to avoid shearing of the incision. A double layer should be used, and there should be a twist between layers at the distal end of the limb. The second layer should also be shorter, to provide increased pressure at the distal aspect of the limb.

The increased inspection and touching of the limb will help the patient become more self-aware of the new image that their amputation displays. There are people who will avoid touching and looking at their residual limb. Wegener, MacKenzie, Ephraim, Ehde, and Williams (2009) demonstrated that increased self-management interventions lead to positive mood, increased self-efficacy, and decreased depression in persons with limb loss after 6 months.

When the physician and rehabilitation team decide that the incision can sustain minimal sheering force, a limb shrinker, or gel limb sock, can be used. The limb shrinker, a tightly sized elastic sock that can be donned and doffed over the residual limb, will be explained further during discussion of the prosthetic and postprosthetic stages.

Limb desensitization is important in order to allow prosthetic usage in the future. Desensitization begins by having the patient envision placement of the prosthetic over the limb. The patient should be instructed to physically feel and palpate the residual limb. This is important for both sensory and self-image purposes. Some patients may have emotional difficulty accomplishing self-palpation of the limb. The patient can tap the limb using a "limb tapper," a foam-handled instrument that the patient should carry with him or her at all times. Alcohol-free and fragrance-free lotions can also be used to provide tactile input to the limb. During this process, deep massage and pressure should be applied to accomplish skin mobilization. This will prevent any skin-to-muscle adhesions, which can occur after surgery. These sensory input and skin mobilization processes should last 10 to 15 minutes and should take place 2 to 3 times daily.

Amputee patients may also experience phantom sensation and phantom pain. Phantom sensation is a painless sensation or awareness that gives form to a body part with specific dimensions, weight, or range of motion (Gailey, 1994). Examples of phantom sensations include feelings of touch, pressure, cold, wetness, or movement. Kern, Busch, Rockland, Kohl, and Birklein (2009) reported that 73.4% of amputees experience phantom sensations. Amputees frequently report phantom sensations when they move from supine to sitting while getting out of bed.

Phantom pain is a painful feeling experienced below the residual limb. Examples of phantom pain are dull aching, burning, and knife-like stabbing. Approximately 74.5% of amputees report having phantom pain experiences (Kern et al., 2009). The etiology of both phantom sensation and phantom pain has been debated, with some researchers offering the explanation that the homunculus for the leg remains in the brain and produces abnormal neurological signature patterns (Melzack, 1992). Treatment methods such as use of heat, proprioceptive input, use of prosthesis, and stretching have not consistently been shown to be effective (Sherman, 1989). Other approaches include pharmaceuticals, spinal cord stimulation, deep brain stimulation, hypnosis, biofeedback, and other holistic methods.

Positioning issues must also be addressed within the preprosthetic stage. These issues are especially evident for BKAs and below-elbow amputations, as range of motion of the knee and elbow will be critical during the prosthetic and postprosthetic stages.

The patient should be educated to maintain full extension of the knee and elbow joints when not ambulating or using residual limbs. When extension is not maintained, a flexion contracture can occur. Range of motion exercises, in addition to heat combined with a sustained passive stretching of the contracted joint, can be used.

For a lower extremity, full extension can be assisted through several means. If the patient will be immobile or supine during a lengthy hospitalization, a dorsal knee extension splint can be fabricated from thermoplastic splinting material and applied to the limb while in bed or in a chair. Surgeons often apply a knee extension splint after surgery. Serial casting of the knee joint in extension can be utilized in more extreme cases; however, this makes it difficult to address sensory and shaping issues. While supine in bed, the patient should be instructed not to place a pillow under the knee, as this will only encourage a flexion contracture. When the patient is in a wheelchair, an amputee leg rest should be used to maintain knee extension.

For elbow contractures, an anterior extension splint can be fabricated from thermoplastic splinting material and applied to provide force and encourage elbow extension. The splint may need to be modified as more extension is gained. Goniometer measurements should be recorded on a daily basis and shared with the patient to encourage proper positioning of the residual limb.

Goals of independence in functional mobility and self-care are also addressed within the preprosthetic stage. Independence in functional mobility and lower extremity dressing may prove to be especially challenging to the lower extremity amputee because of decreased standing balance. Generally, the higher the amputation, the greater the standing balance deficit will be. This is true because longer limbs allow for increased righting reactions. Individuals with AKAs will have less limb to assist in righting reactions. Independence in these areas may require the use of assistive devices, such as rolling walkers, auxiliary crutches, tub seats, or tub transfer benches.

Safety in functional mobility is important so as to limit harm from falling. Approximately one in five amputee patients will fall during inpatient rehabilitation, with 18% experiencing a subsequent injury from the fall (Pauley, Devlin, & Heslin, 2006). Dyer, Bouman, Davey, and Ismond (2008) noted that 71% of all falls involving amputees occur while transferring to and from a wheelchair.

During the preprosthetic stage, patients should be encouraged to interview and meet several certified prosthetists. The selection of a prosthetist should not be left solely to a physician or therapist, as it will be the patient who will have a lifetime relationship with the person creating and fitting his or her prosthesis. A good way to begin is to verify the prosthetist's certification with the American Board for Certification in Orthotics, Prosthetics and Pedorthics (www.abcop.org). Prosthetists should offer references for the patient to contact as well.

A prosthetist creates a mold of the residual limb once the incision is fully healed and the limb is completely shaped with little or no edema present. This generally occurs 2 to 4 months after the amputation surgery. A positive plaster mold is created from a negative cast of the limb and then hardened. Thermoplastic material is heated and draped over the plaster mold and shaped to the form of the mold to create a socket. Prior to delivery of the temporary prosthesis, the prosthetist will often perform a home visit to check the fit of the socket and gauge the amount and thickness of limb socks that will be required.

For a lower extremity prosthesis, a lightweight metal pole (also know as a *pylon*) is connected to the socket with a foam or plastic foot attached to the end. This is known as the *initial prosthesis*, or *temporary pylon*. For an upper extremity prosthesis, the socket is attached to a hook-like terminal device with a pull cable looped around the opposite shoulder that serves to open and close the hook for grasping.

Upper extremity amputees will require instruction in one-handed techniques for a variety of self-care tasks, such as manipulating clothing fasteners, cooking, and eating. If the dominant extremity has been amputated, the challenge presented by this aspect of treatment is increased.

There are emotional issues that will need to be addressed within the preprosthetic stage as well. Approximately two thirds of all amputees will experience symptoms of depression (Schulz, 2009). A certified peer visitor from the National Peer Network of the Amputee Coalition can provide the new amputee the opportunity to discuss his or her feelings and experiences with someone who has already been through the process. Nationwide, there are nearly 300 amputee support groups (Amputee Coalition, n.d.).

The prosthetic stage consists of application of a temporary prosthetic and, ultimately, a permanent prosthetic. The entire rehabilitation team will determine the type of prosthesis that will best suit the needs of the patient. The team may recommend to begin use of a gel liner over the residual limb, which will also aid in maintaining good shape and controlling edema. This gel liner may be used to assist in suspension of the prosthesis to the residual limb.

The occupational therapist, along with the prosthetist, the physical therapist, and the physician, instructs the patient on how to put on and take off the temporary prosthetic. For upper extremity amputees, this is generally accomplished in an outpatient therapy setting, but for lower extremity amputees, this may involve inpatient hospitalization. The patient must also become accustomed to wearing the prosthetic. There are many types of suspension methods for a prosthesis. For BKAs, the most common are a silicone gel liner with pin, plain elastic sleeve, and supracondylar brim with belt. These are all mainly patellar-tendon-bearing systems. For AKAs, the most common types of suspension include total elastic suspension, suction suspension, or suspension using a silesian bandage or a pelvic belt. A wearing schedule should be set, with the patient wearing the prosthetic no longer than 30 minutes to 3 hours per day by the end of the first week. After the first week, the schedule should consist of two 2- to 3-hour wearing sessions each day. Prosthetic limbs should not be worn overnight, as prolonged wear can compromise skin integrity. After the second week, the prosthetic can be worn as tolerated, with multiple inspections for areas of redness. It is not uncommon for the prosthetist to make changes in the foam insert or thermoplastic socket. This usually includes "blowing out" certain areas to relieve pressure points. It also must be stressed to the patient that the limb shrinker or gel liner must continue to be worn when the prosthetic is not. Without use of these devices, there will be great variability in edema and shape of the limb, affecting prosthetic use and fit.

Generally, a cotton limb sock, or socks, is placed on the limb in the socket for several purposes. First, it absorbs the sweat or moisture within the area. Second, the number and thickness (also known as *ply*) of the socks can be changed to improve the fit of the limb within the socket. The size of the residual limb is dynamic during the first several months of prosthetic use because of changing edema levels within the limb. The prosthetic user and the rehabilitation team must constantly evaluate the fit of the limb within the socket and change the ply of the socks as warranted. For individuals with BKAs, a light foam custom-molded insert is often used either in addition to or instead of the cotton sock.

To avoid constant changing of the limb socks or irritation from the cotton socks, some prosthetists suggest using an inner Alpha Gel sock, which is a sock that is made of gel and will change with the shape of the limb. These socks do have drawbacks, including the trapping of moisture within the liner. Also, they are much more expensive than a cotton limb sock. If a gel sock is used, it must be washed with alcohol on a weekly basis to avoid mold or bacterial buildup, which could cause an infection on the residual limb.

Function with the lower limb prosthetic is accomplished through high-level standing balance activities, such as cooking at the stove or putting on and removing the prosthetic for bathtub transfers. The new prosthetic user must also achieve independence in self-care and functional mobility with the prosthetic. For some, this mobility can be accomplished through outpatient therapy, but others accomplish these goals, in addition to independence in ambulation and stairs, within an acute or skilled inpatient rehabilitation setting. One must consider that some patients might require supervision while others might be independent at home for 1 to 2 months while their incision heals. Thus, the goal is not to achieve independence in self-care and functional mobility but to achieve independence in self-care and independence with the prosthetic.

Upper extremity amputees often develop prosthetic functionality in an outpatient setting. The decision to use a hook or a cosmetic hand is made during the prosthetic stage of rehabilitation. Prosthetic hands can be used for fine motor tasks, although they are mainly used for cosmetic purposes.

Satisfaction with the prosthesis will vary and is dependent on a multitude of factors. Pezzin, Dillingham, MacKenzie, Ephraim, and Rossbach (2004) found that most people (94.5%) who wore their prosthesis extensively (71 hours per week) were satisfied with its overall performance. However, nearly one third of these individuals expressed dissatisfaction with the comfort of their prosthesis. In addition, frequency of prosthesis usage and satisfaction were shown to be significantly higher for those with a shorter time to prosthesis fitting.

The postprosthetic stage involves fitting for a permanent prosthetic and is generally accomplished on an outpatient basis with the assistance of a physical therapist and a prosthetist. The main issues that concern prosthetic wearers during these latter stages are comfort and function (Nielsen, Psonak, & Kalter, 1989). The patient should have his or her permanent upper extremity prosthetic within 1 year of the original surgery.

## Family

There are several considerations concerning the family of an amputee through-out all of the prosthetic stages. Family members should be enlisted in education programs during the preprosthetic stage so they feel involved from the very beginning. Tasks such as limb wrapping and limb desensitization may fall upon a primary caretaker if the patient is not able to complete these tasks independently. The patient requires emotional support and encouragement from the family. Roles and hobbies that were performed prior to amputation may need to be adjusted or altered to fit the patient's new functional status. The use of a local support group can involve both the amputee and his or her spouse or family members.

## Practice Setting

The practice setting for occupational therapy treatment of the amputee varies for upper and lower extremity amputations. The preprosthetic stage for both types of amputee will include some inpatient hospitalization. The lower extremity amputee's hospitalization length will likely be longer and may include inpatient rehabilitation at either the acute or the subacute setting during the prosthetic stage. The upper extremity amputee will likely achieve most goals in an outpatient setting during the prosthetic and postprosthetic stages.

## Sociopolitical

Medicare will reimburse a patient for a prosthesis when it is medically necessary and when the person is classified as K1 through K4, with K4 being the highest in function, in the Medicare Functional Classification Levels, which describe the functional levels of individuals with a lower extremity prosthesis. This is covered under Medicare Part B and will apply to 80% of costs, including those for related prosthesis equipment (Medicare.gov, 2011). Private insurance companies differ in their coverage for a prosthetic. The worst-case scenario is that private companies will only cover one prosthetic per lifetime. If a patient is of working age, his or her state Office for Vocational Rehabilitation (which assists individuals with disabilities in returning to work) can help provide funding for a prosthetic.

The frequency of prosthetic replacement depends on several factors, such as the activity level of the patient, the way the prosthetic is used, and the complexity of the actual prosthetic. The moving parts of a prosthetic (such as knee and elbow joints) will eventually break down. Also, the insert within a lower extremity requires replacement on a yearly basis. The timely processing of all reimbursement claims is essential because delays in receipt of the prosthetic will interfere with the therapeutic process. The prosthesis should be delivered to the patient's home, as Medicare and most private insurances will not reimburse for medical equipment delivered during an inpatient hospitalization.

It is important for the occupational therapist to collaborate with the prosthetist, and it is important that the prosthetist understands the patient's functional goals because he or she is usually responsible for submitting reimbursement claims to Medicare and private insurance companies.

## Lifestyle/Lifespan

The needs of an amputee will vary throughout his or her lifespan. Prosthetics for both the upper and lower extremities can be created or adjusted for almost any need imaginable. Advancements in lightweight graphite and metals continue to advance athletic and active prosthetic technology. C-Legs, by Otto Bock, have become popular with younger amputees. A C-Leg has a microprocessor-controlled knee that speeds up and slows down gait and is able to manage uneven surfaces, such as hills and steps. These high-technology prosthetics, however, are much costlier than the prosthetics required for basic ambulation needs. In addition, prosthetics for the active user need to be replaced more often because of their increased usage.

# Clinical Decision-Making Process

## Defining Focus for Intervention

Occupational therapy intervention is based on the prosthetic stage and the patient's premorbid disposition, cognitive ability, and social support systems, as well as the physical arrangement of the individual's living quarters. For persons with upper extremity amputations, limb dominance is an issue. In addition, the patient's expectations with regard to postamputation activity resumption must be taken into consideration when establishing goals for treatment.

During the postprosthetic stage for upper extremity amputations, a definitive, or permanent, prosthetic will be applied. This may include delivery of both a cosmetic hand and a terminal hook device. Most upper extremity prosthetics include interchangeable terminal devices. Focus will be on using the prosthetic for fine motor tasks and instruction for when to use each device.

## Establishing Goals for Intervention

Occupational therapy goals are set by the therapist and the patient. During the preprosthetic stage for lower extremity amputation, goals concerning limb care, functional mobility, and self-care are generally made. The level at which the patient will be able to perform these tasks depends on many factors, including the patient's cognition, standing balance, fine motor coordination, and visual acuity.

The availability of assistance, the home environment, and premorbid functioning will determine goals with regard to ambulation and mobility. If a wheelchair is necessary, a goal of independence in wheelchair mobility will be set. If the patient is cognitively impaired and has the social support to return home, family training in safe transfer methods will also be an important goal. For patients who are anxious to return to previous roles, such as head of household, goals include practicing these roles within the rehabilitation setting. The patient should be encouraged to participate in these roles soon after discharge from the hospital.

The upper extremity amputee will also need to achieve goals in limb care during the preprosthetic stage, with a focus on many of the same factors as the lower extremity amputee. The main difference is whether the dominant hand has been amputated. This will dictate whether dominance transferal training will occur. One-handed techniques will not be as challenging if the dominant hand can be used for fine motor tasks.

During the prosthetic stage, patient education about the appropriate thickness, or ply, of limb sock and how and when to change the sock is necessary. A goal will also be set for increased wearing tolerance. This goal will greatly depend on the patient's skin integrity and his or her compliance with limb wrapping or use of the limb shrinker since the surgery.

For lower extremity amputees, a goal will also be set to reach independence in functional mobility and self-care with the prosthetic. This may or may not occur in an inpatient setting, and the patient may already be independent in functional mobility and self-care without the prosthetic. If the latter is true, the goals will likely be achieved quickly.

For upper extremity amputees, the goals during the prosthetic stage will likely be achieved in an outpatient setting. It is important to note that the longer the patient is without a prosthetic, the more he or she will get accustomed to not needing it. It is important that clear and precise goals be set with the patient long before delivery of the upper extremity prosthetic.

## Designing Theory-Based Intervention

There are several frames of reference utilized with the amputee patient, including the biomechanical and rehabilitation frames of reference and the model of human occupation. The biomechanical frame of reference states that purposeful activities can be used to treat loss of range of motion, strength, and endurance (Crepeau, Cohn, & Schell, 2011). Within the function–dysfunction continuum, the domains of concern include edema control, passive range of motion, strength, and high-level endurance. These are all areas addressed with amputees via independence in certain areas of occupation.

The rehabilitation frame of reference addresses underlying deficits that cannot be remediated or compensated. Domains of concern included within this frame of reference are activities of daily living, work, and leisure tasks, which are all areas affected by a limb amputation. This frame of reference stipulates rehabilitation methods such as adaptive devices, ambulatory devices, wheelchair modification, environmental modification, adaptive procedures, and safety education (Crepeau, Cohn, & Schell, 2011).

The model of human occupation is appropriate for amputees using the volition, habituation, and performance subsystems. Values and interests are assessed during the preprosthetic stage for amputees. Roles and habits are kept in mind when designing and selecting the proper prosthetic or prosthetics for the patient.

## Evaluating Progress

Progress can be evaluated by assessing the goals that are accomplished and appreciating the time periods involved. The most important goal to be accomplished within the preprosthetic stage is independence in limb care and functional mobility. Often, the ability to reach independence in these areas is a predictor of future success in the prosthetic and postprosthetic stages. Another important goal within the preprosthetic stage is for the patient to return home being able to perform functional mobility and independent self-care. The level at which the patient returns home will not be the permanent level of function. Once the prosthetic training occurs, the level will likely change and possibly improve.

## Determining Change in or Termination of Treatment

Once goals are achieved within the preprosthetic stage, the patient can be discharged until the prosthetic is available for use. During the prosthetic stage, patients with lower extremity amputations will be discharged from all therapies when they are independent in applying the prosthesis and in ambulation, and upper extremity amputees will be discharged when they are independent with high-level fine motor tasks.

Between the preprosthetic and prosthetic stages, the rehabilitation team and prosthetist will decide if the patient is a good prosthetic candidate. Factors that assist in this decision include the patient's level of performance in functional mobility, compliance with limb care, safety, and family support. A combination of patient self-report tools and professional reporting tools can be used, although there is much debate over the validity and reliability of these tools (Gailey, 2006). One tool with high validity to predict ambulation outcome is the *Amputee Mobility Predictor* (Gailey et al., 2002). If the team believes that the functional level will not be improved or may worsen with the prosthetic, the team may decide not to proceed into the prosthetic stage. As stated above, the person must score between K1 and K4 in the Medicare Functional Classification Levels. If a score of K0 is given, it has been determined that the patient does not have the ability or potential to ambulate or transfer safely with or without assistance and that a prosthesis does not enhance the quality of life or mobility (Medicare.gov, 2011).

# Case Study

## Description

KR is a 30-year-old female with a history of intravenous drug use, endocarditis, hepatitis B and C, chronic liver disease, and sepsis. She was admitted to the hospital with complaints of bilateral leg pain. Upon examination, KR demonstrated gangrenous bilateral calf and foot areas. It was later determined that she had developed multiple septic emboli to her lower extremities. She had also been noncompliant with past drug rehabilitation and antibiotic therapy for her endocarditis. Approximately 2 weeks after admission, KR underwent amputation of the right and left legs below the knee. Originally, all wounds were left open. The lower extremity amputations underwent a skin graft closure approximately 2 weeks after the original surgery.

Occupational therapy and all rehabilitation services initiated therapy 3 days after surgery. The patient was in a considerable amount of pain and was only able to demonstrate bed mobility and bilateral upper extremity active range of motion. Both of her lower extremity amputations had flexion contractures and were covered in soft dressings. The remainder of her self-care and functional mobility activities were not tested because of complaints of pain and fatigue. These areas were ultimately assessed within the first week, and goals were set. KR's sitting balance in bed was fair. In addition, there was a considerable amount of patient education in terms of her long-term rehabilitation needs and the settings within which they would be accomplished.

KR's social situation was an obstacle to achieving her rehabilitation goals. KR was homeless and estranged from her family. She also had a 6-year-old son who was living with his father. The months leading up to her hospitalization had been spent in shelters or on the streets, and she had no medical insurance coverage. Her admission status and goals projections for activities of daily living and functional transfers are summarized in Table 13.1.

As part of her comprehensive occupational therapy program, KR will be educated in limb wrapping, skin inspection, and limb desensitization. These requisite components of her program will remain in place and integrated into her day as the healing process progresses. Fabricated knee extension splints will be checked on an ongoing basis and adjusted to reduce her contractures and facilitate full knee extension bilaterally. In choosing and designing an activity for KR, the therapist notes that she will be completing all activities from a wheelchair or in unsupported sitting throughout the preprosthetic stage. Using a wheelchair, in combination with sitting unsupported at the edge of the bed, is the way she will approach her morning self-care routine. Specifically, the night before, KR will use her wheelchair to secure her clothing for the next day and place it within easy reach of her bed. She will then be able to dress in the morning before transferring to the wheelchair. In the early stages of rehabilitation, the transfer will be a challenge for KR, and grooming, hygiene, and toileting will require the assistance of the staff.

A key component of KR's ability to be successful at developing independence in the wheelchair and sitting at the edge of the bed will be sitting balance. As a new bilateral lower extremity amputee, KR has experienced a change in her center of gravity and an alteration of her sense of balance. She adapts by using her upper extremities to support sitting. Using her arms to maintain balance will severely impact her efforts to be independent. A new sense of her center of gravity and balance will be important to her independence.

**Table 13.1** KR's Admission Status and Goal Projections

| Performance area | Admission | Short-term goal | Long-term goal |
|---|---|---|---|
| Feeding | Independent | Independent | Independent |
| Grooming | Maximal assistance | Minimal assistance | Independent |
| Bathing | Moderate assistance | Minimal assistance | Independent |
| Upper extremity dressing | Minimal assistance | Independent | Independent |
| Lower extremity dressing (including limb care) | Maximal assistance | Minimal assistance | Independent |
| Toileting | Moderate assistance | Minimal assistance | Independent |
| Bed transfer | Moderate assistance | Minimal assistance | Independent |
| Toilet transfer | Moderate assistance | Minimal assistance | Independent |
| Tub transfer | Dependent | Moderate assistance | Independent |

Because the primary focus is to assist KR in developing sitting balance, a simple activity that is easy to understand, allows KR to concentrate on keeping her balance, and can readily be graded to challenge her is best. As her sitting balance improves, KR will become more confident that she will be able to move forward with more complicated tasks.

### Long- and Short-Term Goals

KR's long-term goal is to be able to dress independently while seated unsupported in bed. In the short term, KR will be able to securely reach for a shirt from a closet without losing her seated balance.

### Therapist Goals and Strategies

The therapist's goals include the following:

1. Reduce flexion contractures in the knees bilaterally.
2. Improve sitting balance to allow both upper extremities to be free to engage in activity from wheelchair level or seated at the edge of the bed.

The therapist's strategies include the following:

1. Fabrication of knee extension splints bilaterally. Splints will be constructed from thermoplastic materials and will be designed to facilitate full knee extension.
2. Design of functional activities of daily living, independent activities of daily living, and leisure activities that can be graded to challenge KR's sitting balance.

### Activity: Ball Toss—O–U–T

KR is positioned sitting unsupported on a mat. The therapist stands in a 3-foot square outlined on the floor. A large beach ball is tossed between KR and the therapist. Each time a person misses, he or she receives a letter: O–U–T. The first person to miss three throws and spell *OUT* loses the game. The activity of catching and throwing is familiar to KR. Use of a large beach ball helps KR use both upper extremities in the game. This requires her to rely on her developing sitting balance. The therapist challenges KR's sitting balance in all directions by targeting the ball.

*Treatment Objective*

KR will achieve simultaneous bilateral upper extremity extension without loss of seated balance.

# Resources

Alberta Amputee Sports and Recreation Association: http://www.aasra.ab.ca

American Association of Retired Persons: www.aarp.org

Americans With Disabilities Act Home Page: http://www.ada.gov

Amputee Coalition: http://www.amputee-coalition.org

Centers for Medicare and Medicaid Services: www.cms.gov

National Amputee Golf Association: http://www.nagagolf.org

Orthotics and Prosthetic Information for Practitioners, Amputees, and Healthcare Professionals: www.oandp.com

# References

Amputee Coalition. (n.d.). *National Limb Loss Information Center/Amputee Coalition fact sheets.* Retrieved from http://www.amputee-coalition.org/fact_sheets/index .html

Carroll, K., & Edelstein, J. (2006). *Prosthetics and patient management: A comprehensive clinical approach.* Thorofare, NJ: Slack.

Crepeau, E., Cohn, E., & Schell, B. (2011). *Willard and Spackman's occupational therapy* (11th ed.). Philadelphia, PA: Lippincott, Williams & Wilkins.

Deutsch, A., English, R. D., Vermeer, T. C., Murray, P. S., & Condous, M. (2005). Removable rigid dressings versus soft dressings: A randomized, controlled study with dysvascular, trans tibial amputees. *Prosthetics and Orthotics International, 29*(2), 193–200.

Dillingham, T. R., Pezzin, L. E., & MacKenzie, E. J. (2002a). Limb amputation and limb deficiency: Epidemiology and recent trends in the United States. *Southern Medical Journal, 95*(8), 875–883.

Dillingham, T. R., Pezzin, L. E., & MacKenzie, E. J. (2002b). Racial differences in the incidence of limb loss secondary to peripheral vascular disease: A population based study. *Archives of Physical Medicine and Rehabilitation, 83*(9), 1252–1257.

Dillingham, T. R., Pezzin, L. E., & MacKenzie, E. J. (2003). Discharge destination after dysvascular lower limb amputations. *Archives of Physical Medicine and Rehabilitation, 84*(11), 1662–1668.

Dyer, D., Bouman, B., Davey, M., & Ismond, K. P. (2008). An intervention program to reduce falls for adult in-patients following major lower limb amputation. *Healthcare Quarterly, 11*(3), 117–121.

Gailey, R. (1994). *One step ahead: An integrated approach to lower extremity prosthetics and amputee rehabilitation*. Miami, FL: Advanced Rehabilitation Therapy, Inc.

Gailey, R. S. (2006). Predictive outcome measures versus functional outcome measures in the lower limb amputee. *Journal of Prosthetics and Orthotics, 18*(1), 51–60.

Gailey, R. S., Roach, K. E., Applegate, E. B., Cho, B., Cunniffe, B., Licht, S., Maguire, M., & Nash, M. S. (2002). The Amputee Mobility Predictor: An instrument to assess determinants of the lower-limb amputee's ability to ambulate. *Archives of Physical Medicine and Rehabilitation, 83*(5), 613–627.

Isakov, E., Burger, H., Gregoric, M., & Marincek, C. (1996). Stump length as related to atrophy and strength of the thigh muscles in trans tibial amputees. *Prosthetic and Orthotics International, 20*(2), 96–100.

Izumi, Y., Satterfield, K., Lee, S., & Harkless, L. B. (2006). Risk of reamputation in diabetic patients stratified by limb and level of amputation: A 10 year observation. *Diabetes Care, 29*(3), 566–570.

Johannesson, A., Larsson, G. U., Ramstrand, N., Turkeiwicz, A., Wirehn, A. B., & Atroshi, I. (2009). Incidence of lower-limb amputation in the diabetic and non-diabetic general population: A 10 year population based cohort study of initial unilateral and contralateral amputations and reamputations. *Diabetes Care, 32*(2), 275–280.

Kern, U., Busch, V., Rockland, M., Kohl, M., & Birklein, F. (2009). Prevalence and risk factors of phantom limb pain and phantom limb sensations in Germany: A nationwide field survey. *Schmerz, 23*(5), 479–488.

Medicare.gov. (2011). *Artificial limbs and eyes coverage*. Retrieved from http://www.medicare.gov/Coverage/Home.asp

Melzack, R. (1992, April). Phantom limbs. *Scientific American*, pp. 120–126.

Muilenburg, A., & Wilson, A. (1996a). *A manual for above-knee (trans-femoral) amputees*. Retrieved from http://www.oandp.com/resources/patientinfo/manuals/akindex.htm

Muilenburg, A., & Wilson, A. (1996b). *A manual for below-knee (trans-tibial) amputees*. Retrieved from http://www.oandp.com/resources/patientinfo/manuals/bkindex.htm

Nielsen, C., Psonak, R., & Kalter, T. (1989). Factors affecting the use of prosthetic services. *Journal of Prosthetics and Orthotics, 1*(4), 242–249.

Pauley, T., Devlin, M., & Heslin, K. (2006). Falls sustained during inpatient rehabilitation after lower limb amputation: Prevalence and predictors. *American Journal of Physical Medicine and Rehabilitation, 85*(6), 521–532.

Pezzin, L. E., Dillingham, T. R., MacKenzie E. J., Ephraim, P., & Rossbach, P. (2004). Use and satisfaction with prosthetic limb devices and related services. *Archives of Physical Medicine and Rehabilitation, 85*(5), 723–729.

Schulz, M. (2009). Coping psychologically with amputation. *Vasa, 38*(74), 72–74.

Sherman, R. A. (1989). Stump and phantom limb pain. *Neuro Clinics, 7*(2), 249–264.

Smith, D., McFarland, L., Sangeorzan, B., Reiber, G., & Czerniecki, J. (2003). Postoperative dressing and management strategies for transtibial amputations: A critical review. *Journal of Rehabilitation and Development, 40*(3), 213–224.

Taylor, L., Cavenett, S., Stepien, J. M., & Crotty, M. (2008). Removable rigid dressings: A retrospective case note audit to determine the validity of post amputation application. *Prosthetics and Orthotics International, 32*(2), 223–230.

Wegener, S. T., MacKenzie, E. J., Ephraim, P., Ehde, D., & Williams, R. (2009). Self-management improves outcomes in persons with limb loss. *Archives of Physical Medicine and Rehabilitation, 90*(2), 373–380.

Zeigler-Graham, K., MacKenzie, E. J., Ephraim, P. L., Travison, T. G., & Brookmeyer, R. (2008). Estimating the prevalence of limb loss in the United States: 2005 to 2050. *Archives of Physical Medicine and Rehabilitation, 89*(3), 422–429.

# Chapter 14

# Orthopedics
## *Fractures and Joint Replacements* | *Marlene J. Morgan*

## ⚑ Synopsis of Clinical Condition

Orthopedics is the specialty concerned with the preservation, restoration, and development of the form and function of the musculoskeletal system, extremities, spine, and associated structures by medical, surgical, and physical methods (Cyriax, 1982). Medical conditions addressed in the field of orthopedics include fractures, strains and sprains, tendon or ligament repairs, joint replacements, and numerous associated soft tissue injuries. This chapter will focus on orthopedic conditions as they affect the hip, knee, wrist and hand, elbow, and shoulder, and related occupational therapy interventions.

### Prevalence and Etiology

During the aging process, loss of bone density and calcium increases the chance that falls will result in fractures, especially in the spine, forearms or wrists, and femurs (the site for most hip fractures). Fractures affect roughly 6.8 million Americans each year, with a higher prevalence in men below age 45 years and women above age 45 years. Fractures commonly occur in the extremities. The most common fracture to the upper extremity is a distal radius fracture, or Colles fracture. The most common fracture to the lower extremity is the hip fracture, resulting in roughly 300,000 cases per year in the United States.

Hip and knee replacements are the most common joint replacement surgeries performed, frequently resulting from degenerative diseases (e.g., degenerative joint disease, arthritis, osteoporosis). Joint replacements performed in the upper extremities are most commonly performed at the wrist (the proximal row more

The editors gratefully acknowledge the contributions of Jonathan Niszczak and Abu Panackal to earlier versions of this chapter.

than the distal row) and at individual metacarpophalangeal (MCP) joints and individual proximal interphalangeal joints, usually as a result of rheumatoid arthritis. The shoulder (i.e., the glenohumeral joint) and the elbow (i.e., the humeral–ulnar joint) also can be replaced, but these replacements are less common than those of the wrist and phalanges. Although joint replacements in the shoulder and elbow can result from degenerative conditions, a history of trauma (e.g., a fall on the outstretched extremity) is usually involved. Joint replacements are not permanent, usually lasting 10 to 15 years.

## Common Characteristics and Symptoms

### Fractures

Fractures are classified as diaphyseal (a fracture in the midportion of the bone), metaphyseal (a fracture within close proximity to the flare of the bone at the articular joint surface), or articular (a fracture within the joint surface at the end of the bone). Fractures are also classified by the involved joint, the angle of fracture, the number of fragments produced in the bone, and whether they are closed or open. Fracture angles are described as *transverse*, *oblique*, *longitudinal*, or *stellate* (star-like). Simple fractures result in two major components, and comminuted fractures produce multiple fragments. Fractures that are contained within the bone or joint are considered closed, and those that protrude through the soft-tissues and skin are considered open (Hunter, Mackin, & Callahan, 2002; Rockwood, 1984).

Closed fractures are those fractures that are relatively stable and only require an orthosis (e.g., a splint or cast) to maintain good, anatomic positioning of the joint, which will allow natural healing to occur. Fractures can also be repaired using many different surgical means. Common internal fixation includes Kirschner wires (i.e., K-wires), cerclage wires, tension band wires, screws (lag and pressure), intramedullary rods and nails, and plate and screw combinations (Kauer, 1980). However, some complex fractures with multiple fracture sites and unstable fixation may require external fixation as well. External fixators (most commonly intramedullary pins) provide a stable force to oppose strong muscle compressive forces across the injured joint and allow healing to occur by pulling on ligamentous attachment points (known as *ligamentotaxis*) and maintaining good anatomic joint position for healing (Rockwood, 1984). Healing of fractured bones typically takes 4 to 6 weeks. Healing time can be protracted by complications such as diabetes, poor nutrition, more compound injuries, and vascular insufficiency (Cyriax, 1982).

Weight-bearing activity contributes to the healing process and helps the bone remodel through callous formation. Patients are assigned weight-bearing status based on the mechanism of injury and surgical repair. The health care professional promotes strict patient compliance to the weight-bearing status during mobilization. Continued communication among the patient, the therapist, and the physician regarding the progress of the healing process, compliance with weight-bearing restrictions, and effective pain management facilitates patient independence in activities of daily living (ADL) and helps to reduce the length of hospital stay.

## Wrist and Hand Injuries

The Colles fracture, one of the most common fractures of the upper extremity, is a fracture involving the distal radius with dorsal displacement. This fracture disrupts the delicate degree of normal palmar tilt between the radius and the carpal bones—proximally, the scaphoid and lunate and, distally, the capitate (Kauer, 1980). If left untreated, the mobility and dexterity of the hand may be lost as a result of immobility of the wrist joint. Depending on the type and degree of injury involved, the Colles fracture may be immobilized in a cast and/or external fixation for 3 to 6 weeks. The physician will determine the period of immobilization in a cast, splint, and/or external fixation. It is the responsibility of the occupational therapist to limit the potential for secondary complications, such as stiffness in the affected shoulder, elbow, forearm, and digits; edema; and loss of active range of motion (AROM; Hunter et al., 2002).

## Elbow Injuries

Orthopedic injuries that affect the elbow disrupt the fine motor coordination and dexterity of the hand in space and limit the flexibility and reach of the shoulder girdle. The elbow provides a solid, weight-bearing structure for the entire upper torso along with the flexion, extension, and supination patterns that allow for discreet finger, hand, and wrist movements (Smith, Weiss, & Lehmkuhl, 1996). At the elbow, ligamentous flexibility coupled with bony stability allows the mobile radial head to rotate upon the fixed and rigid ulna. Without this efficient and unique design, most simple ADLs (especially feeding, grooming, and bathing activities) become almost impossible to perform (London, 1981).

Fractures to the olecranon and radial head are the most common sites of injury to the elbow. These conditions require management to maintain AROM and passive range of motion (PROM) within the joint. Usually, the radial head will incur the majority of damage in a fracture involving the elbow.

A nondisplaced fracture (Mason Type I) will usually require no immobilization, and quick return to mobilization is encouraged. In moderate fractures (Mason Type II and III), an open reduction internal fixation (ORIF) operation is performed and protective motion is initiated as soon as possible. In all three of these fracture types, the goal is to maintain PROM and begin gentle AROM for flexion and extension motions only. By the third week, supination and pronation motions are initiated and focus is given to regaining this motion.

## Shoulder Injuries

Orthopedic injuries that affect the shoulder girdle ultimately impact the function of the hand. The shoulder girdle (i.e., the clavicle, scapula, humerus, and thoracic spine and sternum) is multifunctional. The interplay of the humerus and scapula, commonly referred to as the scapulohumeral rhythm, provides for increased range of motion (ROM) in a number of different planes. This relationship is based on the interplay between muscular and ligamentous structures, which effectively suspends the humeral head within the glenoid fossa (Hengeveld & Banks, 2005). In acute care, the occupational therapist may encounter the lack of AROM of the shoulder above 100 degrees of flexion and the lack of external rotation greater than 30 degrees. Simple explanations for this loss of motion, especially in the elderly population, can be attributed to a kyphotic position of the thoracic spine as well as common arthritic changes in the acromioclavicular joint itself, which affects the available ROM around the shoulder (France, 2004).

## Hip Fractures

Hip fractures are common diagnoses treated in an acute care hospital setting. Women sustain three quarters of all hip fractures. The incidence of fracture rates increases with age. People age 85 years and older are 10 to 15 times more likely to sustain a hip fracture than are those ages 60 to 65 years. The incidence of hip fracture increases with osteoporosis. This is important to note. The National Osteoporosis Foundation has estimated that more than 10 million people in the United States over the age of 50 years have this disease (Centers for Disease Control and Prevention, 2010). In 2006, there were more than 316,000 hospital admissions for hip fractures, a 7% increase from the previous year. However, from 1996 to 2004, after adjusting for the increasing age of the U.S. population, the hip fracture rate decreased 25% (from 1,060 to 850 per 100,000 individuals). More than 90% of hip fractures are caused by falling, most often sideways onto the hip (Centers for Disease Control and Prevention, 2010). Three common surgical interventions that an occupational therapist will encounter are total hip arthroplasty/replacement, ORIF, and hemiarthroplasty (McGann, 1991).

## Femoral Fractures

The primary site of hip fractures is at the femoral neck and intertrochanteric region of the femur. If no displacement is noted in the fracture site, the physician will opt for ORIF or hip pinning (i.e., insertion of metal screws to stabilize the fracture). If the damage results in the disunion of the bone in the femoral neck area, the physician may opt to perform a hemiarthroplasty, or replacement of one part of the hip joint. If the damage is related to degenerative disease affecting the acetabulum as well as the femoral head and neck, the physician may opt to replace the entire joint surface through a total hip replacement (Melton, 1995).

## Total Hip Replacements

When other forms of intervention to decrease pain and improve mobility have failed, total joint replacement surgery is considered. There are three types of procedures: the anterolateral approach, the posterolateral approach, and the transtrochanteric approach. The age and health of the patient are considered in deciding on the surgical procedure (Pendelton & Schultz-Krohn, 2006).

## Target Areas for Intervention

Occupational therapy goals following fracture and joint replacement surgery include (a) reduction of pain and edema in the affected joint after surgery, (b) maintenance of early AROM and PROM of the joint after surgery, (c) restoration of independence in functional ADL skills, and (d) return to premorbid occupational life roles.

## Contextual Considerations

### Clinical

The occupational therapist will usually encounter the patient 1 to 3 days after the operation and will find the patient in a hospital gown, immobile, and in mild to moderate discomfort. The occupational therapist will complete a screening assessment to determine the need for adaptive devices and techniques and the degree of services that will be required at discharge to facilitate the person's resumption of life roles.

The early postoperative contact facilitates functional recovery and is cost effective. The initial evaluation is a brief summary of the patient's medical history, social history, presentation, sensory and perceptual assessment, cognitive evaluation, and neurological and muscular assessment. The evaluation should include ROM and manual muscle testing; functional assessment, including performance in self-care and mobility; a problem list; a summary assessment of the findings; an estimated length of stay; equipment needs; long-term goals and short-term objectives (made in collaboration with the patient); and discharge recommendations.

Information gathering is a team effort. The physiatrist or physician often makes first contact and assesses the rehabilitative prognosis for the patient, including orthopedic and medical ongoing treatments, weight-bearing and ROM limitations, and the patient's pain and activity tolerance. Once the patient's readiness for physical and occupational therapy is determined, the physiatrist's orders are placed and physical and occupational therapy is initiated. Alternatively, the orthopedic service may alert the rehabilitation service of pending or completed surgical procedures that require services. Information needs to be gathered on the social and physical environments to which the patient will return.

### Family

Family involvement of individuals with orthopedic diagnoses is critical to patients who may be discharged at a supervision or assistance level. Regular contact with family, including formal family training, can secure a safe discharge for the patient into his or her environment.

## Practice Setting

The initial occupational therapy consult or referral for orthopedic diagnosis is most commonly encountered in the acute care hospital setting. The occupational therapist initiates and plans a continuum of care, initiates ROM as permitted by the surgeon, introduces and initiates self-care and functional transfers, and determines the follow-up need for inpatient rehabilitation or a discharge to home with the necessary equipment and therapies. Areas that are addressed in the evaluation in acute care include ADL, ROM, strength, functional mobility, skin integrity, cognitive–perceptual skills, and the need for orthotics. In the acute care setting, the occupational therapist often works closely with the physical therapist to initiate bed mobility and transfers. Time in acute care is limited, and self-care training may include the introduction of assistive devices and their use.

After acute care, the rehabilitation setting is typically the next step in the continuum of care for many patients with orthopedic problems. Typically, the therapist is given an hour and a half daily to work with the patient to return him or her to functional independence. In this high-intensity setting, the focus of occupational therapy is to expand on the skills initiated in the acute care setting. Daily participation in self-care, bathing, grooming, upper extremity dressing, lower extremity dressing, and hygiene becomes routine for the patient until short-term and long-term goals are achieved. Transfer training expands to bathroom and kitchen mobility with an assistive device. Therapeutic exercise expands into light meal preparation and participation in home management tasks. Simple cognitive and perceptual activities expand into instrumental ADL (IADL), including money management, shopping, driving, and so forth. The occupational therapist, through ongoing reevaluation and assessment of progress, will determine the possibility of the patient achieving functional independence and/or the necessity of family or caretaker involvement.

## Sociopolitical

The primary sociopolitical issue facing individuals with orthopedic injuries is payment for services. Older individuals who require hospitalization after a fall or fracture will typically have inpatient, outpatient, and home care costs covered by Medicare. Commercial insurance and workers' compensation may also cover hospitalization and related costs. The failure of both Medicare and commercial insurance to cover the cost of durable medical equipment and assistive devices for self-care may create a hardship for the patient who requires these tools to support ADL or IADL during the healing process.

## Lifestyle/Lifespan

The recovery from orthopedic injuries is, for most patients, a short-term process. With proper medical and therapeutic intervention, major lifestyle changes are not required.

# ![] Clinical Decision-Making Process

## Defining Focus for Intervention

The treatment focus for orthopedic patients is to improve ROM and strength, increase pain tolerance, increase activity tolerance, improve performance in ADL, and return the patient to a normal routine with the aid of durable medical equipment, assistive devices, education in energy conservation, and adaptation of the home environment to facilitate functional independence.

The focus of treatment is related specifically to the injury or body part. Treatment approaches for Colles fracture, stiff shoulder, and total hip replacement will serve as examples for how the focus of treatment changes as the healing process progresses.

### Colles Fracture

Early in treatment, the person with a Colles fracture should learn to "salute the ceiling." In order to reduce edema, lifting the affected extremity over the head and maintaining the arm on an elevated plane above the level of the heart will allow for good venous return and support the lymphatic system during the inflammatory phase of healing. Active motion is optimal, with movement at each joint (shoulder, elbow, forearm, and digits) at least twice every waking hour. If the patient has difficulty moving any of the joints, the therapist should take each joint gently through its available ROM to prevent joint stiffness and aid in edema reduction. Elevation with a pillow or foam wedge is ideal for maintaining position above, or at least level with, the heart. Use of a sling to support the affected extremity is almost always contraindicated because it tends to foster the immobility of the extremity and can increase stiffness of the entire extremity. If the extremity is in a cast, care should be taken that thumb motion is not restricted. The cast should only reach the distal palmar crease and should allow for full MCP extension and at least pinch to the third digit.

Tendon gliding exercises, which allow for full excursion of the long digital flexor and extensor tendons and prevent ligamentous shortening during the wrist immobilization phase, are also important. In addition, these exercises help stimulate circulation and reduce edema in the digits. Persistent digital edema can be reduced with the use of Coban wrapping and retrograde massage. The Coban is wrapped in a figure-8 style, beginning at the distal end of the digit and proceeding down to the level of the cast. The Coban can be left in place for up to 24 hours but should be changed daily for hygiene and skin checks. Retrograde massage is performed by milking the digit, beginning at the distal end and moving back to the MCPs proximally. The use of lotion will aid in the movement over the digits as well as provide some lubrication to the skin.

Once the cast and/or external fixation are removed, therapy becomes more intense. The therapist's goal during this phase is to mobilize the wrist joint. A fabricated thermoplastic splint can be used to support the weakened wrist extensors and provide stability to the digits as well. The splint can be made with either a dorsal or a volar design with a bar that supports the distal palmar crease. It is imperative that the splint allow for full digital flexion and extension of the joints, as well as full mobility of the thumb with opposition available to the fifth digit. Out of the splint, the patient is guided through gentle active assistive ROM and PROM for wrist flexion and extension, as well as radial and ulnar deviation. It is also important to work on full supination, which is likely to be limited initially because of the pronation positioning in the cast. Initial movement will be very weak at first, so movement begins gently in gravity-eliminated planes, to assist with good muscle recruitment throughout the wrist joint. The wrist joint will be stiff, so moist heat is often applied prior to mobilization. Gentle joint mobilization is also used, especially at the radiocarpal and midcarpal joints, to further enhance the motion.

From an occupational therapy perspective, light bimanual activities can be most rewarding to the patient and allow for increased mobility throughout the wrist joint. Weaving, knitting, kneading light dough or putty, buttoning, wringing out a rag, or threading nuts and bolts are just a few examples of exercises that require a variable amount of wrist and digital mobility that can be employed as part of a therapy regime at this stage of recovery. Another hallmark exercise is the prayer position, which puts maximal stretch on the wrist and digital flexors and extensors and provides the patient with a simple reference guide for increasing joint mobility and AROM.

In the later phase (roughly, by Week 10), the most crucial motion that needs to be relearned is independent wrist extension. Because of the weakness of the wrist extensors (i.e., the extensor carpi radialis brevis, the extensor carpi radialis longus, and the extensor carpi ulnaris), active wrist ROM can be compensated using the long axis of the digital extensors. (These are the extensor digiti communis and, to a lesser extent, the extensor indicis and extensor digiti minimi.) A fully closed, tightly packed fist during wrist extension eliminates the force arm of the digital wrist extensors and puts the load of wrist extension primarily on the extensor carpi radialis brevis, which gets assistance from the extensor carpi radialis longus and extensor carpi ulnaris. With the loss of independent wrist extension, the power grip and pinch of the hand are affected, as well as the power of the wrist joint itself. Without independent wrist stability, the mobility of the hand is significantly limited. As the stability of the wrist increases, the splint can be discontinued in favor of increasing the overall stability of the wrist joint. However, for individuals who will perform heavy and repetitive activities, the splint can provide increased stability until the muscular endurance around the joint is regained.

## Stiff Shoulder

Conservative management of the stiff shoulder that is acute in origin and for which other possible pathologies have been ruled out usually begins with a therapeutic modality such as moist heat. Placing the individual's shoulder in a lengthened position in which the joint is comfortable is usually optimal. Once the soft tissues have been heated, a gentle stretch can be applied. Placing the individual in a supine position allows the shoulder joint to become relaxed and helps facilitate relaxation of the muscles, which, in turn, allows the therapist greater control of the joint. Gentle distractive forces can be applied to loosen the connection of the humeral head within the glenoid fossa. Additionally, gentle distractive and externally derived forces can be applied to unwind the humeral head within the glenoid. Usually, this external rotation force will be the most upsetting to the patient, and care must be taken to allow the patient to relax and not recruit muscular forces to block PROM. Gently, passively guiding the joint through its available ROM and applying a gentle, sustained stretch at the available end ROM will help slowly increase shoulder joint mobility.

Overhead pulleys can further help mobilize the shoulder by allowing the individual to aid his or her own muscular system to incrementally guide the shoulder through active assistive ROM. This system also provides the individual with increased control over his or her mobility and allows participation in therapy at his or her own schedule. In addition, Codman's exercises, or pendulum exercises, will help provide stretch to the shoulder joint and allow for slow, gentle motion. Graded exercise should begin in supine to take further pressure off the joint, allow for gravity-minimized motion, and provide stability to the scapula throughout its ROM. Also, a dowel provides a visual and physiological feedback mechanism to compare motion with that of the other shoulder and allows the unaffected upper extremity to assist the weaker shoulder through its ROM. Exercise should be provided not only for the shoulder itself but also for the scapula and upper back extensors, to provide a stable base for shoulder mobilization.

## Total Hip Replacement

The occupational therapist may begin treatment for a person with a total hip replacement on the first, second, and third day after the operation. The physical therapist, often first on the case, may perform the initial assessments of bed mobility and transfer out of bed, per the physician's orders. The occupational therapist frequently arrives at the bedside to find the patient in a hip chair (an elevated chair that promotes ease of transfers), in a hospital gown, often orthostatic, in mild to moderate discomfort, and possibly requesting to return to bed. The purpose of the therapist's visit and the frequency and the role of occupational therapy in the acute setting are explained to the patient. Vital signs are taken and compared to the parameters set by physicians (usually, systolic blood pressure anywhere from 90 to 150 or 180 and diastolic blood pressure from 60 to 90, oxygen saturation between 92% and 100%, and pulse rate between 60 and 100 bpm). Pain is assessed using the 0-to-10 pain scale.

## Establishing Goals for Intervention

Physical limitations, including those involving ROM, strength, endurance, activity tolerance, balance, coordination, sensation, and overall ADL skill performance, need to be addressed. Appropriate goals are set considering the patient's physical, social, and environmental factors. When considering goal setting and treatment focus, the occupational therapist focuses on discharge planning. The question one should ask is, Where is this person going when he or she leaves the acute care environment? The options, although many, can include an acute rehabilitation setting, where the person extends his or her hospital stay with emphasis on physical rehabilitation; a skilled nursing facility, in which the person is transferred to a rehabilitative center where moderate-intensity therapies are given; a nursing home, in which the patient is given daily, low-intensity physical and occupational therapies; a boarding home with few physical or occupational therapies offered; an independent living or assisted living center, where low-intensity therapies may be provided; and, simply, the patient's home, with home-based therapies provided.

The next question to be addressed is, Who is at home with the patient? If the patient lives alone, it may be imperative that he or she be independent in ambulation and self-care upon discharge. Even though a person living alone may have neighbors, grown children, or grandchildren who can provide intermittent supervision, the patient must be independent and safe.

The person's spouse may be capable of providing assistance as needed, in which case the patient's goals can be to reach independence with supervision. If the person lives with an elderly or disabled spouse with limited ability to help, the goals of the patient will reflect independence, or discharge planning will include continued home therapies and home health services. In other cases, placement in a long-term-care facility with physical and occupational therapies may be the best option.

Another question is whether the patient's living space is conducive to his or her recovery. Beyond the issue of supervision, is the patient safe? Falls resulting in orthopedic impairments are generally accidental in nature, such as tripping over an unsecured throw rug or slipping on icy pavement. However, abuse and negligence (malnutrition, undernutrition, history of previous burns, or multiple falls where no known neurological impairments exist) are also factors to be considered. Health professionals are required by law to report any and all cases of suspected abuse to authorities.

The next question is, Does the patient plan to return to his or her prior living space? The patient's family members may offer temporary or permanent living quarters until the patient is ready to return home. The patient may have to consider moving to another location more conducive to his or her current situation.

## Designing Theory-Based Intervention

The biomechanical and rehabilitation frames of reference are extremely useful for orthopedic patients in the hospital, rehabilitation, outpatient, or home care settings. The biomechanical frame of reference assumes that activity is used for the treatment of loss of ROM, strength, and endurance due to accident, injury, or surgery. As ROM, strength, and endurance improve, function is regained. Stress and rest need to be appropriately incorporated. This frame of reference is best suited for individuals who are cognitively intact. The biomechanical approach emphasizes structural stability, edema control, ROM, strength, and low-level and high-level endurance.

The rehabilitation frame of reference focuses on having the patient compensate for underlying deficits that cannot be remediated. The underlying assumptions for this frame of reference are that independence will be achieved through compensation, that the person is motivated to be independent, that the environmental context and the emotional and cognitive skills needed for independence are present, and that adaptations and compensations are designed for the person to function in the discharge environment. The goal of rehabilitation is participation in ADL, work, and leisure tasks in spite of physical limitations. Some of the tools used in rehabilitation are (a) adaptive equipment, including adaptive devices and assistive technology, (b) upper extremity orthotics, (c) wheelchair modification, (d) ambulatory devices, (e) adaptive procedures, (f) environmental modification, and (g) safety education.

## Evaluating Progress

As long as the patient continues to progress, occupational therapy intervention is warranted. Progress is continually evaluated via daily progress notes, weekly conferences if the patient is in a rehabilitation or subacute nursing facility setting, and monthly reevaluations if the patient is in an outpatient or home care environment. Goals are patient centered, so that upon culmination of occupational therapy intervention, the patient has achieved functional independence and can return to former occupational roles.

## Determining Change in or Termination of Treatment

Ultimately, change in or termination of treatment is attained when the individual has achieved all of the goals or when the patient has reached maximal therapeutic benefit. Usually, a team familiar with the case will meet with the individual and his or her family to recommend the best place to serve the person and to recommend equipment as needed.

## Case Study

### Description

KO is a 56-year-old female who suffered a fall on the ice while returning from lunch to a local bank, where she works as a teller. She is married with three grown children and is expecting her first grandchild in 6 months. She fell onto her right upper extremity and landed on her outstretched arm. She remembers hearing an audible crack and feeling intense pain in the dorsal and volar aspects of her wrist. She returned to the bank and immediately iced her wrist and finished her shift. The next day when she awoke, her hand and wrist were severely swollen. Her husband took her to the emergency room. Her X-rays showed a distal radius fracture with an avulsion of the radial styloid. She was immediately taken to surgery. Her fracture was reduced, an external fixation system was applied, and her hand was cast in plaster.

After surgery, KO was sent to a bed in an acute care setting, and the occupational therapy department received an order to evaluate and treat her for a distal radius fracture, with stable fixation, digital mobilization, ROM exercises, and edema management. The acute care therapist assessed KO; instructed her in edema management, proper pin care, and cast management; and issued a home program for KO to complete that included ROM exercises and tendon gliding exercises. KO was discharged to home.

KO's fracture has healed, and her cast and pins have been removed. She is now being seen for more intense therapy in an outpatient setting. Her wrist, as expected, is stiff. She has been fitted with a volar wrist splint that immobilizes the wrist and supports the distal palmar crease. KO is spending more and more time in therapy without the splint. She moves her wrist in all positions. In addition, she is encouraged to supinate. Although her muscles and movement are weak, it is important for KO to move actively and recruit muscles throughout the areas of the wrist. Continuous movement and participation in activities that require graded increases in strength will assist her in achieving an optimal recovery.

### Long- and Short-Term Goals

In the long term, KO will demonstrate sufficient AROM, strength, coordination, and endurance in the right wrist and hand to support full independence in ADL and IADL. In the short term, KO will demonstrate sufficient AROM, strength, coordination, and endurance in the right wrist and hand to engage in a light, bimanual activity for 3 minutes.

### Therapist Goals and Strategies

The therapist's goals include the following:

1. Reduce joint stiffness.
2. Increase ROM.
3. Increase muscle strength.
4. Improve coordination.
5. Increase endurance.

The therapist's strategies include the following:

1. Provide heat modality prior to activity.
2. Provide gentle joint mobilization prior to activity.
3. Provide a series of graded activities that facilitate ROM, muscle strength, coordination, and endurance.

### Activity: Knitting a Small Baby Blanket

At this point in her recovery, KO will benefit from an activity that is bimanual and offers light resistance, requires movement throughout the wrist joint, and emphasizes wrist extension. Knitting is such an activity. It is easy to learn, it will offer light resistance, and it requires her to move her right wrist and fingers repetitively. Wrist flexion and extension are emphasized. KO can work on the project at home, and the baby blanket will allow her to focus her recovery on the impending happy occasion of the birth of her grandchild.

### Treatment Objectives

The patient will demonstrate the AROM, strength, coordination, and endurance in the right hand and wrist necessary to cast on 50 stitches and complete two rows of a knitting project.

## Resources

American Occupational Therapy Association: www.aota.org

Erstad, S. (2009). *Hip replacement surgery: Procedure and recovery.* Retrieved from arthritis.webmd.com/hip-replacement-surgery

Rasul, A. T., Jr. (2010). *Total joint replacement rehabilitation.* Retrieved from emedicine.medscape.com/article/320061-overview

Wedro, B. C. (n.d.). *Fracture causes, symptoms, diagnosis, and treatment.* Retrieved from www.medicinenet.com/fracture/article.htm

## References

Centers for Disease Control and Prevention. (2010). *Hip fractures among older adults.* Retrieved from http://www.cdc.gov/HomeandRecreationalSafety/Falls/adulthipfx .html

Cyriax, J. (1982). *Textbook of orthopedic medicine: Vol. I. Diagnosis of soft tissue lesions.* London, England: Bailliere Tindall.

France, M. (2004). Anatomy and biomechanics of the shoulder. In R. Donatelli (Ed.), *Physical therapy of the shoulder* (pp. 42–73). Edinburgh, Scotland: Churchill Livingstone.

Hengeveld, E., & Banks, K. (2005). *Maitland's peripheral manipulation.* Amsterdam, Netherlands: Elsevier Health Sciences.

Hunter, J., Mackin, E., & Callahan, A. (2002). *Rehabilitation of the hand: Surgery and therapy* (5th ed.). Amsterdam, Netherlands: Elsevier Health Sciences.

Kauer, J. (1980). Functional anatomy of the wrist. *Clinical Orthopedics and Related Research, 149*(9), 92–106.

London, J. (1981). Kinematics of the elbow. *Journal of Bone and Joint Surgery, 63,* 529.

McGann, W. (1991). History and physical examination. In M. Steinberg (Ed.), *The hip and its disorders.* Philadelphia, PA: Saunders.

Melton, L. (1995). How many women have osteoporosis now? *Journal of Bone Mineral Research, 10,* 175–177.

Pendelton, H., & Schultz-Krohn, W. (2006). *Pedretti's occupational therapy: Practice skills for physical dysfunction* (5th ed.). St Louis, MO: Mosby.

Rockwood, C. (1984). Subluxations and dislocations of the shoulder. In C. Rockwood & D. Green (Eds.), *Fractures in adults* (pp. 21–42). Philadelphia, PA: Lippincott, Williams & Wilkins.

Smith, L., Weiss, E., & Lehmkuhl, L. (1996). *Brunnstrom's clinical kinesiology* (5th ed.). Philadelphia, PA: FA Davis.

# Burns | *Josette Merkel*
*Jonathan Niszczak*

## 🌿 Synopsis of Clinical Condition

### Prevalence and Etiology

In the United States, 1.4 to 2 million people are burned each year, and 75,000 of the victims require hospitalization for at least 2 days. Of those hospitalized, 85% have injuries to the hand or upper extremity. Approximately 3,500 deaths each year result from a burn injury or related complications. The most common ages of injury are between 16 and 40 years. Burns are the primary cause of accidental death for children between the ages of 1 and 14 years and the second most common cause of accidental death in the elderly. Burns are the second most common form of child abuse, and men have the highest incidence of being burned (Staley & Richard, 2004).

Burn injuries are classified into three major types: thermal, chemical, or electrical. Thermal injuries may include flame, scald, and contact. There are innumerable causes of injury, such as motor vehicle accidents, house fires, work-related accidents, and kitchen accidents. Children are often burned as a result of scalding (frequently, by the child pulling down a cup or pot full of hot water or other liquid or being put in a tub of hot water), playing with matches, and contact with a hot surface, such as an iron.

### Common Characteristics and Symptoms

The four major classifications of burn injury are as follows:

🌿 First-degree burns (also called *superficial burns*) are usually characterized by red, dry, and edematous skin that is painful to touch and involve only the epidermal layer of the skin. It usually heals in 3 to 5 days, with possible slight discoloration and peeling but no scarring. The most common cause of first-degree burn is sunburn.

- Second-degree burns are divided into two categories: superficial partial thickness and deep partial thickness. Superficial partial thickness burns are characterized by red, blistering, weeping, and moist edematous skin that is very painful and sensitive to temperature. This burn involves the epidermis and some papillary dermis. It should heal in 7 to 21 days without skin grafting. Minimal scarring and pigment change result. Deep partial thickness burns are pink, cherry red, or, in the most severe cases, mottled white. There may also be small or large thick-walled blisters. This burn involves the entire epidermis, multiple layers of the dermis, and possibly the subcutaneous fat layer. It may heal in 21 to 35 days without skin grafting; however, significant pigment changes and scar contractures will develop.
- Third-degree burns (also called *full thickness burns*) are characterized by skin that is dry, leathery, and nonpliable. No blisters appear, but the skin does have a mixed white or waxy white appearance. There is typically little to no pain. This burn involves the epidermis, the majority of the dermal and fat layers, and possibly the underlying fascial and muscular layers. This burn requires grafting; however, small burns (<2% of the total body surface area) may heal without grafting after several months but with significant scarring.
- Fourth-degree burns (also called *dermal injury burns*) are characterized by skin that is dry and white to dark charred in color. It appears mummified and is anesthetic. This injury involves epidermis, dermis, and fat layers and commonly is associated with exposed bone and tendon. If the burned skin is not grafted (usually with a muscle flap or full thickness graft), it will not heal. Amputations are often required, and in the absence of surgical wound closure, these burns may result in death.

There will often be a combination of burn classifications in the same person. For example, a person involved in a house fire may suffer first- and second-degree burns to his or her face and third-degree burns to his or her hands as a result of crawling out to escape the burning house. The physician will estimate the total body surface area (TBSA) burned. The methods most commonly used to obtain this estimation are the Lund and Browder method and Berkow's percentages chart (Lund & Browder, 1955). First-degree burns are not included in the estimation. An estimate of the TSBA burned allows the physician to determine the resuscitation calculation and the severity of the injury. Generally, the higher the burn area percentage, the more critical the injury and the more involved the rehabilitation will be. Specifically, when TBSA burned is 20% or greater in adults, 10% in children and older adults, or 5% or greater for full thickness burns, the patient will require hospitalization. Other patients who require hospital admission are those with chemical and electrical burns and suspected inhalation injury (Staley & Richard, 2004).

In addition to the obvious injury to the skin, the respiratory system can be injured as a result of inhaling toxic substances. This injury is referred to as a *smoke inhalation injury.* A severe inhalation injury alone or combined with a skin injury can indicate a poor morbidity and mortality prognosis. Mortality rates with inhalation injury are reported to be greater than 50%, with little change over the last 30 years (Roth, Hughes, & DeClement, 1999). Inhalation injury is reported to be found in 3% to 21% of burn patients. The pulmonary injury is usually proportional to the depth and size of the cutaneous burn (i.e., those with severe burn injuries commonly have an inhalation injury). As a result of severe inhalation injury, patients may need to be on mechanical ventilation and/or supplemental oxygen for a long period of time.

## Target Areas for Intervention

Occupational therapy should begin as soon as the patient is medically stable. The occupational therapist focuses on maintaining range of motion (ROM), positioning, edema control and reduction, splinting, education, scar prevention and management, activities of daily living (ADL) adaptation and remediation, and return to occupation.

# 🔥 Contextual Considerations

## Clinical

The clinical evaluation must incorporate information about the depth of the burn injury, the psychological status, and level of ADL independence. Data must be gathered regarding the nature of the injury, any comorbidity, and the leisure and occupational roles of the client. A thorough evaluation must be performed that assesses the patient's active and passive ROM, strength, sensation, coordination, ADL status, and functional mobility. Any joint involved in a burn should be measured and reassessed for changes on a daily basis.

Strength testing is particularly important after an electrical injury. An electrical injury is manifested in progressive weakness of affected muscles in the first days and weeks after the injury. Sensory testing helps to determine the classification of the burn injury and to ascertain the level of risk for further injury because of diminished sensation. Self-care frequently begins with tasks at the bedside, including feeding and grooming tasks, toileting, and hygiene. Assessment regarding how the patient transfers and ambulates is also needed.

The *Functional Independence Measure* (Uniform Data Systems for Medical Rehabilitation, 1993) can provide information on many of these areas. Another widely used assessment for burns is the *Vancouver Scar Scale* (Baryza & Baryza, 1995). This instrument objectively assesses scar maturation across four distinct variables and provides a basis for the patient and therapist to chart progress. Pain is an inevitable consequence of burn injury and can be assessed in many formats. The most commonly used formats are the *FLACC Scale* (Merkel, Voepel-Lewis, Shayevitzer, & Malviya, 1997) and the *Wong-Baker FACES Pain Rating Scale* (Wong et al., 1999). The *FLACC Scale* can be used on unresponsive adults and children. The *Wong-Baker FACES Pain Rating Scale* may be used with children and with individuals who speak a foreign language. Edema is measured with a tape measure over common joint areas and bony prominences (e.g., the wrist crease at the level of the styloids or at the level of the proximal interphalangeal joint in the finger).

## Family

Family support and encouragement is a critical component throughout the recovery process. Many patients require constant encouragement and persuasion to participate in the program. This is most critical when pain limits movement. Family members need to be encouraged and educated in the burn recovery process. It is important for them to understand that movement must ensue before healing has occurred. Family education in positioning, wound healing, scar management, home exercises, and participation in ADL and instrumental ADL (IADL) is important. Family members may require emotional and psychological support to help the patient through episodes of depression, withdrawal secondary to disfigurement, and/or anxiety related to returning to school or work.

## Practice Setting

Individuals are usually treated at a formalized burn center in a trauma hospital. Once the critical and surgical phase of recovery is complete, the patient can be transferred to an inpatient rehabilitation setting for further recovery and rehabilitation, if warranted. Outpatient therapy can be performed at various settings, including a hospital, a hand center, or a work hardening center.

## Sociopolitical

Patients who are recovering from a severe burn injury will require services from an acute care hospital, rehabilitation inpatient services, and/or outpatient programming. Commercial insurance will be relied on to cover acute care, rehabilitation, and outpatient services. For patients who sustain a work-related burn, workers' compensation will provide funds for rehabilitation and the return to work. Patients who return to work will be covered under the Americans With Disabilities Act (ADA), which provides mechanism for reasonable workplace accommodations.

## Lifestyle/Lifespan

Although most burn survivors can expect to return to their roles and a level of independence close to premorbid levels, the process of complete recovery may be long and difficult. The acute care experience for inpatients is often fraught with fear of mortality, dependency, pain, stress, anxiety, and isolation. Further into the recovery process, the patient may experience depression, as well as fear of and withdrawal from social situations, work, or school because of disfigurement and the need to wear pressure garments or splints. Patients will face a long process of rehabilitation, requiring compliance with a program of exercise, pressure garment use, and scar management until the burns are completely healed. Patients may experience prolonged periods of unemployment during recovery, and some may require a change in occupation and lifestyle.

# Clinical Decision-Making Process

## Defining Focus for Intervention

The focus of occupational therapy depends on the location of the burn, the severity or depth of the burn, the TBSA burned, associated injuries (i.e., fractured leg as a result of jumping out a window), the patient's age, the presence of an inhalation injury, the patient's past medical history, and the patient's occupation prior to admission. The therapist must also consider which phase the patient is at in the recovery process. The two phases in the recovery process are the acute phase and the rehabilitative phase. In the acute phase, from Day 0 to approximately Day 21, the critical factors that the therapist must address are edema management, positioning and splints, mobilization, maintaining active and passive ROM, patient education, self-care skill and adaptation, and skin and scar management. In the rehabilitative phase, from approximately Day 22 until full recovery (which may take 6 months to several years), the critical factors that the therapist must address are the same areas as in the acute phase, in addition to cardiovascular and strength training, psychosocial adaptation, and return to participation in life roles.

Psychosocial adaptation is a constant focus for occupational therapy in the acute and rehabilitative phases and poses a lifelong challenge for the patient. Burn injuries create potential for pain, disfigurement, and the loss of independence. The challenge of therapy is to provide activity that fosters physical as well as psychosocial well-being.

## Establishing Goals for Intervention

The goals for intervention can be classified according to the phases, or stages, of recovery. In the acute phase, avoidance of deepening the burn injury and destroying the surrounding tissue is paramount. This translates into a treatment plan that will focus on reducing edema, preventing further loss of strength and endurance, preventing loss of mobility in the skin and joints, promoting independence in self-care, and providing education to the patient and family. During the rehabilitative phase of recovery, the focus for occupational therapy intervention shifts toward providing patient and family education; promoting independence in self-care; controlling edema; managing scars; teaching compensation techniques; fitting splints and pressure garments; restoring muscle strength, endurance, and hand function; and restoring activity tolerance. The development of discharge plans that facilitate the return to school or work forms the final phase of the rehabilitation process.

## Designing Theory-Based Intervention

Successful long-term rehabilitation requires the combined application of the biomechanical and rehabilitation frames of reference. The biomechanical approach is used to address remedial issues, such as edema control, scar management, strengthening and improvement of ROM, and hand and upper extremity function.

Several strategies address edema control; one of the most common is elevation of the extremities with pillows, bedside tables, or IV poles. Hand edema responds well to the muscle pumping of active ROM exercises and retrograde massage, Coban wraps, and Isotoner gloves. Patients should be encouraged to use and move their hands actively as much as possible through simple self-care tasks. Upper extremity and lower extremity edema may respond well to gradient pressure material, such as Tubigrip bandages. In the rehabilitation frame of reference, issues of patient and family education and the use of adaptive equipment and strategies are the focus of intervention.

Upon admission, the patient needs to be positioned to minimize the potential for deformity and contracture. The ideal position is to stretch the burned skin. For example, if the burn is on the anterior surface of the elbow, the person should be positioned in elbow extension. If the burn is in the axilla, the person should alternate the positions of shoulder abduction and flexion to a least 90 degrees. If the patient is actively moving and performing self-care ADL, this activity should be encouraged. But the person should resume positions of stretch during rest periods. A primary role of the occupational therapist is the fabrication of splints. Splints are used to prevent deformity, lengthen soft tissues, promote graft take, and prevent graft loss. A burn that will require grafting and crosses a joint surface must be splinted. The recommended position for upper and lower extremities is shoulder abduction 90 to 100 degrees; elbow extension, neutral forearm, and wrist extension to 30 degrees; thumb abduction and extension and metacarpal phalangeal flexion 50 to 70 degrees; and interphalangeal extension. Splints are used to immobilize joints for the first 3 days after the graft. After the graft is stable, splints can continue to be used to stretch the healed skin and increase motion in the joint and extremity.

In order to maximize pulmonary function and prevent weakness, the burn patient should begin to move around as soon as possible. Mobilization, depending on the patient's condition, may mean bed mobility, sitting upright in bed, sitting out of bed in a chair, or ambulating short or long distances. For a more involved patient, the therapist (in progressing the patient to get out of bed or at least move from supine) will need to consider many factors. The patient's medical status is imperative. Critical attention must be given to heart rate, oxygen saturation, respiration, and blood pressure initially and in response to position changes and movement. The patient may need to start slowly by having the head of the bed elevated to 30 degrees and progressed to 90 degrees. Mechanically ventilated patients may be medically stable enough to sit up in bed, at the edge of the bed, or even in a chair.

Date and location of skin grafts are very important. A skin graft less than 3 days old is at risk for shifting and loss. Generally, grafts more than 3 days old are not at great risk for loss and can withstand more aggressive movement. The patient with a burn injury will most likely experience pain with mobility. Pain can be addressed with medication. Lower extremities can be wrapped with Ace bandages to prevent blood-pooling.

A goal of occupational therapy is to maintain ROM of the involved joints. As skin heals, it will resist motion and contract. Second- and third-degree burns left in positions of comfort will develop limitations and contracture. Joints particularly at risk are the neck, axilla, shoulder girdle, elbow, wrist, thumb, and digits. ROM must be performed daily, unless contraindicated by a new graft. An optimal time to perform ROM is during dressing changes, when the occupational therapist can visualize the joint's motion and see how the joint reacts to stretch. Tightness and skin blanching indicate that the patient is at risk for scar bands and contracture. Accurate assessment of both active and passive ROM measurements must be used to determine gains and losses of joint ROM.

The injury, the skin grafting, the recovery process, and rehabilitation will be a new experience for the patient. Education is vital. The more a patient understands the reason for therapeutic intervention, the more likely it is that he or she will be an active and empowered participant in the process. For example, explaining to a patient that the purpose of a splint is to prevent contracture and showing the patient a photograph of a person with a contracture can elicit better compliance. Education should start in the hospital as soon as possible. During hospitalization, education focuses on the need for movement, the risk of contracture, ideal positioning, and splints.

In preparing the patient for discharge to home, education should include sun precautions, skin care needs, and follow-up instructions, such as doctor visits and outpatient therapy appointments. Most patients need to learn an exercise program to perform at home as an adjunct to outpatient therapy visits. The ongoing care of healing skin is very important. Open, unhealed wounds need to be dressed with an antimicrobial topical dressing (typically silver sulfadiazine) and covered with bandages. This procedure will prevent infection and promote wound healing. Nongrafted and grafted skin are dressed with bandages until the wound has fully closed. Nurses usually perform dressing changes while the patient is hospitalized.

Once skin is closed and no longer needs dressing, the patient needs to be educated about skin and sun precautions. New skin is sensitive and fragile and is at risk for scratches and cuts. Friction should be avoided, as it can cause blisters and reopening of the wound. Skin that has suffered a burn of any classification needs to be protected from the sun. The ultraviolet rays of the sun can damage the epidermis by increasing melanin production and therefore permanently darken the complexion of the burned skin. Protective clothing, such as a hat with a wide brim, long sleeves, and socks, should be worn to cover newly healed skin. Once skin has closed, the patient should apply a sunblock with an SPF of at least 45. Sunblock needs to be used even under clothes and on inclement-weather days. A patient should avoid prolonged sun exposure during the first year after a burn injury.

Scars are an unfortunate consequence of burns. Grafted skin, as well as burned skin that is not grafted and takes longer than 14 days to heal, is highly susceptible to scarring. Scars are the result of an overproduction of collagen deposited in a disorganized fashion in the healing wound bed. The immature scar begins in the acute phase of recovery. The hallmark signs of the immature scar are red, raised, rigid skin and, most often, limits to motion. *Scar management* is the employment of techniques to minimize scarring. Scars need to be managed immediately and continuously. It is never too early to begin scar management. Scars form quickly and will continue to grow until maturity.

In the acute phase, scar management includes active ROM, passive ROM, splinting, and positioning. Once the wound has closed, pressure therapy can begin. Pressure works to limit and organize the overproduction of collagen bundles. In the acute phase, pressure can be applied with Tubigrip bandages, Coban wraps, custom-sewn spandex gloves, or Isotoner gloves. The patient should wear the pressure garment 23 hours per day and remove it for bathing and skin care.

Patients can begin self-care tasks in the burn unit. Depending on the patient's level and area of involvement, adaptations may need to be made for casting, grooming, dressing, bathing, and toileting. An effort should be made to encourage the patient to participate in self-care to promote his or her independence and recovery.

In the rehabilitative phase, approximately Day 22 until full recovery, the critical factors that the therapist must address are the same areas as in the acute phase, in addition to cardiovascular and strength training, psychosocial adaptation, and return to occupational life roles. Edema may continue to be a problem in this phase. It will most likely have evolved from a pitting, soft edema to a more brawny type. The same interventions used in the acute phase can apply. More aggressive techniques, such as retrograde massage, contrast baths, or temporary fabricated garments, may be required. Since hand edema is usually most prominent, the use of resistive active ROM activities tends to be the most effective intervention. Whereas the goal in the acute phase was movement, patients in the rehabilitation phase should do more resistive exercises and self-care tasks. At this time in recovery, the therapist will identify joints at risk for loss of ROM and contracture. This is manifest in decreasing, more restricted ROM measurements; scar bands and blanched skin with movement; and lack of active movement by the patient. Positioning techniques and splints are used to maintain a low-load, prolonged stretch on the healing skin. The patient should be positioned so that the stretch occurs against the direction in which the scar is pulling. For example, an anterior chest and neck burn will pull the patient into flexion as the scar contracts. To counteract the flexion force, the patient should be in extension and, at times, exercise into hyperextension. For example, the patient might be advised to sleep without a pillow or wear a neck collar positioned in neutral.

If the patient is still in an inpatient hospital setting, every effort should be made to return the person to his or her former mode of ambulation. If no medical contraindications exist, efforts should be made to discontinue assistive devices and restore prior ambulatory status. Active and passive ROM exercises are an essential focus of therapy and recovery. The therapist and, most important, the patient need to be aggressive in this area. Active ROM is performed against the pull of the burn scar. Every joint affected by the burn must be stretched to its full available motion. This will usually be painful to the patient; however, joints not pushed to their limit will become contracted and nonfunctional. The burned hand needs to be stretched at every joint both in isolated passive ROM and active ROM as well as in total passive motion and active motion, to fully stretch the scar.

Scars form quickly and will continue to grow until maturity, usually 1 to 1½ years after a burn. Several techniques are used to decrease the chances for hypertrophic scars. Pressure modalities and silicone gel sheeting are paramount. The use of gradient pressure (i.e., Tubigrip bandages) and custom-fit pressure garments is a staple of burn treatment in this phase. For facial burns, a clear plastic mask can be custom molded to fit facial features.

At this level, patients are expected to perform (or at least participate in) every aspect of the self-care activities of their daily routine. The movement and independence will be beneficial. Adaptive devices can be used when needed, but most important, the joint motion during daily skills will serve to increase overall ROM and decrease the chance for contracture. Loss of muscle mass and girth is common. Cardiovascular and strength training are employed as further adjuncts to active ROM. Stressing the cardiovascular system will help to challenge the skin and stretch the muscle tissue. In addition, the skin's ability to respond to change in temperature, perspiration, and blood flow can be monitored.

## Evaluating Progress

Periodic reassessments evaluate progress in areas such as edema and deformity control, scar mobilization, restoration of ROM, strength, endurance, and coordination. Demonstration of facility with adaptive equipment and techniques and compliance with home programs signal a positive outcome of patient and family education strategies. Improvement in these areas will be reflected in progressively higher levels of independence in ADL and IADL.

## Determining Change in or Termination of Treatment

The wound-healing process dictates treatment for the patient recovering from a burn injury. The status of the healing skin and related physical structures will be indicative of the course for therapy throughout all phases of recovery. Termination of treatment is indicated after the skin and structures have healed, the threat of scar or deformity formation has passed, and maximum function has been restored.

# Case Study

*Description*

JJ is a 45-year-old male who has been referred to an outpatient clinic. He is employed in a warehouse, stocking shelves and filling orders. JJ lives with his wife and two small boys, ages 8 and 4 years. His wife stays at home and cares for the children. JJ is an active and involved father. He and his wife are restoring a historic home, and JJ enjoys working on the house. In his spare time, he fly-fishes and coaches his son's soccer team. He is right-hand dominant. Prior to his injury, he was employed full-time and was independent in all ADL and IADL.

JJ was involved in a chemical explosion when a coworker inadvertently combined two reactive chemicals. JJ sustained second-degree burns to the anterior chest on his right side and third-degree burns to the right upper extremity (RUE) from the dorsal proximal interphalangeals to the axillary fold. Immediately after the accident, JJ was transported to the acute care hospital and admitted to the burn unit. He underwent a split thickness skin graft to the RUE. JJ received occupational therapy in acute care for 7 days. The focus of treatment was positioning to control edema and minimize deformity. The therapist provided JJ with eating utensils that had built-up sponge handles and encouraged him to use his RUE. On the eighth day after the burn, JJ was transferred to the rehabilitation unit. His progress was steady but slow. His graft sites and skin healed well, and strength and ROM improved throughout his RUE. His skin continued to heal, and he was fitted with splints and pressure garments. Throughout his recovery, JJ's wife provided support and encouragement. JJ is now at the point of sorting out vocational options. He would like to be able to return to work in the warehouse and looks forward to resuming work on the house.

Initial evaluation reveals that JJ has resumed independence in ADL. He demonstrates some residual deficits in RUE function. Specifically, shoulder flexion is lacking 30 degrees, and elbow extension is lacking 25 degrees. Muscle strength, tested grossly throughout his RUE, is 4 (*good*). Coordination, as measured by the *Nine Hole Peg Test*, is below average. JJ exhibits decreased endurance for completing upper extremity activities that require reaching while standing. He continues to wear pressure garments on his RUE.

The interview indicates that JJ would like to return to the job that he held before his accident, and his employer is willing to have him return if he is able to complete the job safely and efficiently. JJ's job consists of two distinct parts. Restocking shelves is a task that occurs early in his shift. There are no specific time limits or requirements for this task, and JJ is confident that he will be able to do this efficiently. The second component to his job requires that he read and fill orders on a conveyor belt. JJ must read the order, obtain inventory from the shelf, and place it in a box before the conveyor moves the box out of his reach. In this job operation, timing is critical. JJ is not as confident in his ability to complete this job task.

*Long- and Short-Term Goals*

The long-term goal of intervention for JJ is to demonstrate the ability to fill orders by reading the request, securing products from a shelf behind him, and placing products in a shipping box at the rate of one order per minute (i.e., the industry standard). The short-term goal of intervention for JJ is to demonstrate the ability to fill a simulated order by reading the request, securing products from a low shelf, and placing them on a table in 2 minutes.

### Therapist Goals and Strategies

The therapist's goals include the following:

1. Increase active ROM in the right shoulder and elbow.
2. Increase strength throughout the RUE.
3. Increase endurance in the RUE.
4. Improve activity tolerance.
5. Improve skin tolerance to movement.
6. Educate JJ about his body response to temperature during work.

The therapist's strategies include the following:

1. Have patient wear compressive garments during treatment.
2. Encourage attention to skin response and temperature.
3. Provide patient with the opportunity to complete activities requiring combination movements of the shoulder, elbow, forearm, wrist, and hand.
4. Provide graded activities that challenge ROM, strength, endurance, and activity tolerance.

### Activity: Whole Body Range of Motion

The *Valpar 9–Whole Body Range of Motion* is a module (Valpar International Corporation). It requires a patient to remove and reposition a variety of shapes on a frame, using screws to remove and reattach each piece. As the name implies, the *Whole Body Range of Motion* requires the patient to demonstrate flexibility in the upper extremities, lower extremities, and trunk. It provides opportunities for the patient to produce combination movements of the shoulder, elbow, wrist, and hand. Removal and replacement of the shapes using screws requires sustained effort against gravity, which will help improve JJ's strength and endurance. Graded wrist weights could be used to increase the challenge for JJ. Performance on the *Whole Body Range of Motion* may be timed and related to industry standards. Throughout completion of the activity, JJ will be able to judge the impact of such movement on the shearing forces between his compression garments and skin.

JJ has come to this clinic with the goal of returning to work. He has been through ongoing rehabilitation since his injury and has received occupational therapy in both acute care and rehabilitation. It is important that the activities in which he engages now are clearly work related. The job to which JJ will be returning requires him to stand and use both upper extremities to place and retrieve objects of varied weights and sizes on shelves. JJ will complete all activities with his compression garments on. It may take up to 18 months for scar tissue to mature. JJ will return to work with pressure garments in place.

### Treatment Objectives

JJ will remove and reposition all shapes of the *Whole Body Range of Motion*, taking rest breaks as required.

# Resources

Baryza, M. J., & Baryza, G. A. (1995). The Vancouver Scar Scale: An administration tool and its interrater reliability. *Journal of Burn Care and Rehabilitation, 16*(5), 535–538.

Merkel, S., Voepel-Lewis, T., Shayevitz, J. R., & Malviya, S. (1997). The FLACC Scale: A behavioral scale for scoring postoperative pain in young children. *Pediatric Nursing, 23*(3), 293–297.

Uniform Data Systems for Medical Rehabilitation. (1993). *Functional independence measure*. Buffalo: The State University of New York University at Buffalo.

# References

Baryza, M. J., & Baryza, G. A. (1995). The Vancouver Scar Scale: An administration tool and its interrater reliability. *Journal of Burn Care and Rehabilitation, 16*(5), 535–538.

Lund, C. C., & Browder, N. C. (1955). The estimation of areas of burns. *Surgery, Gynecology, and Obstetrics, 79,* 352–358.

Merkel, S., Voepel-Lewis, T., Shayevitz, J. R., & Malviya, S. (1997). The FLACC Scale: A behavioral scale for scoring postoperative pain in young children. *Pediatric Nursing, 23*(3), 293–297.

Roth, J., Hughes, W., & DeClement, F. (1999) *The Philadelphia burn unit handbook.* Philadelphia, PA: Merck Pharmaceuticals.

Staley, M. J., & Richard, R. (2004). Burns. In S. B. O'Sullivan & T. J. Schmitz (Eds.), *Physical rehabilitation assessment and treatment* (pp. 845–873). Philadelphia, PA: FA Davis.

Uniform Data Systems for Medical Rehabilitation. (1993). *Functional independence measure*. Buffalo: The State University of New York University at Buffalo.

Wong, D. L., Hockenberry, M. J., Wilson, D., Winkelstein, M. L., Ahmann, E., & DiVito-Thomas, P. (1999). *Whaley and Wong's nursing care of infants and children* (6th ed.). St. Louis, MO: Mosby.

# Spinal Cord Injuries

*Kendall Daly*
*Ellen Rosenberg Pitonyak*

## 🔥 Synopsis of Clinical Condition

### Prevalence and Etiology

To understand the etiology of spinal cord injury (SCI), the occupational therapist must have a basic knowledge of the anatomy of the spinal cord, the vertebral column, the spinal nerves, and the spinal cord's vascular supply. The spinal cord, along with the brain, composes the central nervous system. It is responsible for sending messages from the brain to the muscles, to produce voluntary movement. The spinal cord also controls involuntary functions not associated with the autonomic nervous system, including skin sensation and respiration. On average, the spinal cord is half an inch wide and 18 inches long, extending from the medulla oblongata (high in the neck) to the level of the L1 or L2 vertebrae (in the lower back). The bony structure that supports and protects the spinal cord, known as the *spinal column*, consists of 33 vertebrae: 7 cervical, 12 thoracic, 5 lumbar, 5 sacral, and 4 coccygeal. A typical vertebra consists of a body, located anteriorly, and an arch. The spinal cord is encased in the spinal canal formed and protected by the vertebral bodies and arches. The cervical, thoracic, and lumbar vertebrae are separated by intervertebral discs and are connected and stabilized by ligaments. The sacral and coccygeal vertebrae are fused (Lundy-Ekman, 2007; National Spinal Cord Injury Network, n.d.; Smith, Weiss, & Lehmkuhl, 1996).

A cross section of the spinal cord reveals an H-shaped area in the center referred to as the *gray matter* and a surrounding area called the *white matter*. The dorsal horn of the gray matter contains cell bodies that are predominantly sensory, and the ventral horn contains cell bodies that innervate the skeletal muscles that control motor function. The white matter contains various motor and sensory tracts. The nerves that lie within the spinal cord are called *upper motor neurons*, and their function is to carry messages back and forth from the brain to the spinal nerves along the spinal tract. There are also spinal nerves called *lower motor neurons* that branch out from the spinal cord to specific areas of the body.

There are motor and sensory portions of the lower motor neurons. The motor portions send messages from the brain to various body parts to initiate movement. For example, the C7 spinal nerve controls the movement of the biceps. The sensory portions carry messages about sensations from the skin and other organs to the brain (Lundy-Ekman, 2007; National Spinal Cord Injury Network, n.d.; Smith, Weiss, & Lehmkuhl, 1996).

There are 8 cervical, 12 thoracic, 5 lumbar, 1 coccygeal, and 5 sacral pairs of spinal nerves. The C1 through C7 spinal nerves exit the vertebral canal above the corresponding numbered vertebrae. The C8 spinal nerve exits the canal below the C7 vertebrae, because there is no C8 vertebra. Because the spinal cord is shorter than the vertebral column, the spinal nerves need to travel caudally to exit the column, forming the cauda equina. The spinal cord receives its blood supply from a single anterior artery and from two posterior spinal arteries (Lundy-Ekman, 2007; National Spinal Cord Injury Network, n.d.; Smith, Weiss, & Lehmkuhl, 1996).

SCI is damage to the spinal cord that results in loss of motor function and sensation. SCI is catastrophic and impacts almost all aspects of the injured person's life. It is estimated that 7,500 individuals experience spinal cord trauma every year in the United States (National Spinal Cord Injury Statistical Center, 2006). The recovery is often long and frustrating for the person with the injury, as well as for his or her family and friends. It is estimated that 250,000 to 400,000 individuals in the United States are living with SCI (National Spinal Cord Injury Statistical Center, 2006). The etiology of the condition may be either traumatic or nontraumatic. There are many causes of SCI, including motor vehicle accidents (38.5%), violence (24.5%), falls (21.8%), sports (7.2%), and others (7.9%; National Spinal Cord Injury Statistical Center, 2006). Sixty percent of individuals with SCI are 30 years old or younger. Most injuries occur between 16 and 30 years of age. The majority of individuals with SCI are men, with a 4:1 male-to-female ratio (National Spinal Cord Injury Statistical Center, 2006).

Fracture dislocation is the most common injury to the cervical spine at C5 through C6. Gunshots and stab wounds may damage the cord either by direct penetration or by bone fragments causing laceration of the cord. This type of injury can occur at any level. Hemorrhage, aneurysm, thrombosis, or emboli can disrupt the blood supply to the cord, resulting in an SCI. Compression resulting from tumors may also cause permanent damage (Lundy-Ekman, 2007).

An SCI may be either complete or incomplete. The designation of the level of SCI is determined by the most caudal normally functioning segment. A complete injury involves the loss of all motor and sensory function in the dermatomal distribution below the level of the lesion. In incomplete lesions, some combination of neurologic function is retained below the level of the injury. Residual muscle function depends on which spinal fibers remain intact. With incomplete lesions, sensation may be intact, impaired, or absent below the level of the lesion. Incomplete SCIs are often described as *syndromes* (Lundy-Ekman, 2007).

Central cord syndrome and Brown-Séquard syndrome are the most common types of incomplete SCIs. In central cord syndrome, the middle of the cord is more damaged than are the outer areas, resulting in more upper extremity than lower extremity involvement. This syndrome occurs most often in older individuals who fall and experience neck hypertension. It can also occur in any age after a flexion injury. Brown-Séquard syndrome is characterized by one side of the spinal cord being damaged, causing motor and proprioceptive loss on one side of the body and loss of pain and temperature on the other side of the body. This is the most common SCI after a ruptured disc, burst fracture, or penetrating trauma. Almost all people with this syndrome ambulate and regain a large part of their independence (Altrice, Morrison, McDowell, & Shandalov, 2006; Lundy-Ekman, 2007).

Anterior cord syndrome results from trauma to the anterior cord or to the anterior spinal artery or both. This is caused by flexion injuries and/or pressure to the anterior cord from a ruptured disc or fracture. Loss of pain and temperature sensations and loss of motor function is noted, whereas proprioception remains intact (Altrice et al., 2006; Lundy-Ekman, 2007).

Posterior cord syndrome describes damage to the dorsal columns, causing loss of proprioception while other sensory and motor function remains intact. Damage to the cauda equina is usually due to massive disc herniation at the level of the lowest discs in the spinal column. It can also stem from vertebral collapse, which is caused by tumors, infections, or trauma and results in bowel and bladder dysfunction and lower limb involvement. Conus medullaris syndrome, which describes injury to the sacral cord above the cauda equina, also results in bowel, bladder, and lower limb dysfunction (Lundy-Ekman, 2007).

SCIs may be grossly divided into two categories: tetraplegia and paraplegia. Tetraplegia, which consists of injury to one of the high cervical segments, is characterized by a pattern of motor and sensory deficits in all four extremities. Paraplegia, which involves injury to the thoracic, lumbar, or sacral regions, is characterized by a pattern of sensory and motor deficit in the lower extremities. Since 1990, the most frequent distribution of SCIs has been as follows: incomplete tetraplegia, 39.5%; complete paraplegia, 22.1%; incomplete paraplegia, 21.7%; and complete tetraplegia, 16.3% (National Spinal Cord Injury Statistical Center, 2011).

## Common Characteristics and Symptoms

The most obvious symptom of SCI is the loss of voluntary muscle control in the trunk and extremities. With the loss of muscle control, impaired sitting posture and balance also become evident. This affects control over the body and the ability to manipulate the environment, resulting in loss of independence. In the months and years following, most people with SCI experience some recovery in the musculature, which is innervated by cord segments one to two levels below the lesion (Schonherr, Groothoff, Mulder, & Eisma, 2000).

Sensory impairment is evident in most SCIs. A loss of sensation can lead to incoordination of body movements, decreased body awareness, and vulnerability to trauma. Initially, after the injury, there is a period of spinal shock lasting 1 day to 8 weeks. *Spinal shock* refers to a state of decreased excitability of the spinal cord secondary to withdrawal of the excitatory influences from higher centers (Lundy-Ekman, 2007; Schonherr et al., 2000).

During spinal shock, muscles are flaccid. As spinal shock resolves, muscle reflexes below the level of the lesion return, causing spasticity. Spasticity is characterized by flexor or extensor tone, or by myoclonus. This increase in tone can be uncomfortable or painful and can limit function or lead to contractures. Contractures can also result from disuse, overuse, or poor positioning (Hill, 1986; Lundy-Ekman, 2007).

A person with a complete SCI experiences loss of body temperature regulation. Sweating is not evident below the level of the lesion, and an inability to sweat can lead to overheating. Individuals also experience frequent intolerance to either hot or cold.

Respiratory dysfunction is another symptom of SCI. Because the muscles involved in respiration are not functioning, individuals with high tetraplegia may require a ventilator. Some individuals, but most likely not those with injuries at C1, C2, or even C3, can be weaned off the ventilator eventually. Respiratory problems, including difficulty coughing and clearing the lungs of secretions, can lead to pneumonia and other respiratory complications, which are the most common causes of death resulting from SCI. Decreased endurance can also result from respiratory insufficiency (Somers, 2010).

Cardiovascular function can also be altered after SCI. Common problems are slowed heart rate, hypotension (low blood pressure), and orthostatic hypotension, which is a decrease in blood pressure that occurs with movement into an upright position. An abdominal binder and compression stockings are indicated in order to reduce orthostatic hypotension (Hill, 1986; Somers, 2010).

Most SCIs result in an inability to voluntarily control bowel and bladder function. Voluntary control requires an intact sacral cord, and most injuries occur above this level. Bowel and bladder dysfunction varies with incomplete injuries. Incontinence must be managed carefully, as it can cause a variety of physical and psychological problems (Consortium for Spinal Cord Medicine, 1998b; Kirshblum, Gulati, O'Connor, & Voorman, 1998).

SCI can also result in a loss of sexual functioning. The genitals receive their innervations from the thoracolumbar and sacral regions of the spinal cord. With an SCI, messages from the genitals to the brain are disrupted, and men may experience difficulty with erection. Female fertility remains unchanged. Many people also have problems related to body image and feelings of unattractiveness (Ducharme & Gill, 1997).

Feelings of loss, depression, anger, and anxiety are common psychological symptoms of SCI. Changes in an individual's roles, social functioning, and interests can be very challenging. Adjusting to disability requires patience, education, and communication (Consortium for Spinal Cord Medicine 1998a).

The medical complications that can occur as a result of SCI include autonomic dysreflexia, deep vein thrombosis, osteoporosis, heterotopic ossification, and gastrointestinal tract and urinary tract dysfunction. Autonomic dysreflexia can occur in people who sustain an SCI at T6 level or above. Complete and incomplete injuries are vulnerable to this condition. Autonomic dysreflexia is a hyperreflexia caused by an irritation or other noxious stimulus, such as a full bladder or bowel, a blocked catheter, a skin ulcer, a muscle spasm, and sexual activity. Signals from the affected area cannot reach the brain, so the body continues to send the message, and the reflex becomes "hyper." Symptoms of autonomic dysreflexia include a sudden increase in blood pressure, a pounding headache, a flushed face, goose bumps, sweating above the level of lesion, a slowed pulse, and anxiety. Treatment requires sitting the person up and looking for the stimulus to relieve the irritation. An untreated autonomic dysreflexia can result in a serious medical condition with risk of stroke or seizure (Consortium for Spinal Cord Medicine, 1997; Hill, 1986; Somers, 2010).

Individuals with SCI are also at risk for deep vein thrombosis. A deep vein thrombosis is a blood clot that can occur in the lower extremities as a result of decreased circulation and inactivity. Pulmonary embolism is one of the leading causes of death in individuals with SCI, and it usually occurs within 3 months after injury. Anticoagulants and compression stockings are indicated (Consortium for Spinal Cord Medicine, 1997; Somers, 2010).

After SCI, bones lose both calcium and collagen. Osteoporosis progresses gradually and increases the likelihood of fractures. Heterotopic ossification is the formation of new bone, which occurs below the level of injury. This usually occurs in the first 4 months after the injury, and treatment includes aggressive range of motion and radiation. Surgery is indicated if changes in function and positioning problems arise (Garland, 1991; Somers, 2010).

Pressure sores are caused by loss of blood supply to an area, secondary to prolonged pressure over a bony prominence. In patients with SCI, muscle atrophy and sensory loss complicate the process. Skin abrasion during movement is also a problem. Symptoms of pressure sores include a red or discolored area, blistering, or an opening in the skin (Hill, 1986).

Gastrointestinal complications of SCI include stomach ulcers, gastrointestinal bleeds, paralytic ileus, gastric dilation, fecal impaction, and bowel obstruction. Proper medical management can prevent these complications. Bladder dysfunction resulting from SCI can lead to multiple medical issues, including urinary retention, bladder infection, reflux of urine into the ureters, kidney stones, and kidney failure (Somers, 2010).

Life after SCI can be enjoyable and productive. In 1999, the average length of stay in the hospital was 16 days in acute care and 44 days of rehabilitation (National Spinal Cord Injury Statistical Center, 2006). Eighty-eight percent of individuals with SCIs return to their homes; the remainder find residence in group homes or other lodging. Approximately 40% of individuals with paraplegia and 30% with tetraplegia eventually return to work.

## Target Areas for Intervention

Occupational therapy intervention provides unique opportunities for people with SCI to return to their prior life roles. Through purposeful functional activity, education, and support, occupational therapists facilitate increased independence. A thorough initial interview is conducted with the patient and family in order to determine the patient's prior level of function, as well as his or her interests and hobbies. It is also important to understand the roles, such as those of parent, spouse, worker, or homemaker, that the patient engaged in prior to the injury.

Areas that the occupational therapist should initially address are feeding, self-care, skin care, bed mobility, and transfers. Instruction in the appropriate weight shift is an immediate concern because of the high risk of pressure ulcers. Often, self-care skills need to be performed at the bedside until the patient can progress to a seated level. Once the patient progresses, more complex skills, such as bowel and bladder management, home management, and meal preparation, are addressed. Further progression leads to participation in community activities, such as shopping, driving, using public transportation, and working. Occupational therapists provide the necessary resources in order to help people achieve future goals and to plan for future needs.

Accessibility is a major concern for people with SCI. Occupational therapy plays a major role in evaluating the home environment and in making the appropriate recommendations for home setup, equipment, and strategies to increase independence, safety, and accessibility. Since not all people with SCI ambulate, wheelchair skills and accessibility are a major focus of intervention. Occupational therapists also involve the family to a great extent in the form of education and training in order to prepare everyone for discharge (Hill, 1986; Somers, 2010).

## 🖉 Contextual Considerations

### Clinical

The clinical evaluation incorporates biographical information, sensorimotor components, cognitive components, psychological components, activities of daily living performance, and functional mobility performance (American Occupational Therapy Association, 2008). Biographical information, which is obtained through an interview with the patient, includes information about prior living situation, prior level of function, activities and interests, occupational role performance, and individual goals. This information is important when choosing activities and treatment planning.

Sensorimotor components include information about sensation and sensory awareness, neuromusculoskeletal skills, and motor skills. Using the American Spinal Injury Association scale, key sensory areas are tested to identify the neurologic level of injury. The sensory evaluation should also include light touch, stereognosis, kinesthesia, pain and temperature, and joint proprioception. In order to prevent ulcers and irritations, it is imperative that patients with SCI understand that the insensate parts of the body are extremely vulnerable to pressure and trauma (American Spinal Injury Association, 2000).

The neuromusculoskeletal evaluation of the upper and lower extremities and the trunk includes range of motion, muscle tone, strength, endurance, and postural control. Strength is tested using manual muscle testing (Hislop & Montgomery, 2007) and the dynamometer for grip (Kendall, McCreary, & Provance, 1993). Muscle tone is tested using the *Ashworth Scale* (Haas, Bergström, Jamous, & Bennie, 1996). Gross motor coordination and fine motor coordination/dexterity are also identifiers of arm and hand function. Fine motor coordination is tested using the *Nine Hole Peg Test* (Mathiowetz, Weber, Kashman, & Volland, 1985). The information gathered from these evaluations is important, because it will affect performance on mobility skills, activities of daily living, skin care, and bowel and bladder care. It will also indicate a patient's need for adaptive equipment, a universal cuff, positioning devices, upper extremity splints, and lower extremity bracing. It is important to communicate with the physical therapist regarding the status of the lower extremities and the ambulation devices that he or she recommends.

Because of the traumatic events that cause SCI, it is not uncommon for people to suffer a head injury at the same time. It is important to evaluate cognition with assistance from the neuropsychologist. This provides important information about memory and problem solving, which are skills that contribute to a patient's ability to learn new information, to adapt to new strategies, and to direct care. The psychologist also assists with the evaluation of psychosocial skills, which contribute to a patient's ability to cope with disability and to participate in therapeutic activities.

Activities of daily living are evaluated using the *Functional Independence Measure* (FIM; Wright, 2000). This provides information about feeding, grooming, bathing, dressing, homemaking, community skills, bowel and bladder function, bed mobility, and transfers. Once baseline status is formulated, a treatment plan and goals can be established with a patient and his or her family (Wright, 2000).

## Family

An important task of rehabilitation that begins immediately is to prepare the patient and his or her family for discharge to home. In addition to an interview with the patient, it is important to conduct an interview with the family to determine a primary caregiver and family priorities. It is also necessary to consider the family's values, cultural and religious practices, and goals when establishing the treatment plan. It is important to know where and with whom the patient is going to live and what resources the family has. The social worker can assist with gathering financial information, contacting appropriate community resources, and supporting counseling. Since the length of stay for inpatient hospitalizations has decreased over the years, a bigger burden of care falls on the family of the SCI patient. A meeting between the patient, the patient's family, and all treatment team members is useful in educating the family about the present functional status as well as future needs. This is also a good time to schedule a home visit with the family in order to evaluate home accessibility and the presence of architectural barriers. Further family training sessions are scheduled to ensure that all caregivers are competent with and knowledgeable about equipment and capable of assisting the patient (Hill, 1986; Somers, 2010).

## Practice Setting

The occupational therapist provides treatment at many stages of recovery for the patient with SCI. After stabilization and/or surgery, therapy in the acute care setting occurs. Positioning, splinting, and range of motion are the focus of treatment to maintain range of motion and to prevent contractures and pressure ulcers. Once the patient is medically stable, therapy continues in a more intensive patient rehabilitative setting. After inpatient therapy, treatment continues in home care, outpatient, or worksite settings. It is very important for therapists to communicate with caregivers and other professionals along the continuum of care to ease the transition to the new environment (Hill, 1986).

## Sociopolitical

Individuals with disabilities may be devalued in society and thus subject to discrimination in a variety of ways. Architectural and transportation barriers may make it difficult for people with mobility impairments to access home, work, and community settings. A person with a disability is likely to experience discriminatory behavior related to returning to his or her prior home, work, and school. Lack of adequate medical coverage and funding sources provides another challenge for people with disabilities. The Americans With Disabilities Act of 1990 (ADA) promotes the inclusion of people with disabilities in mainstream society. ADA ensures that people with SCI have equal opportunity for employment as well as equal access to public facilities, institutions, and transportation. Modifications may need to be made to the workplace to make it more accessible, and employers are required by law to make the necessary changes to accommodate a person with a disability. ADA empowers individuals with disabilities to advocate for their rights and to take the necessary actions against institutions or facilities that deny equal opportunities or access.

Financial assistance may be needed to meet the needs of the SCI patient in returning home and to the community. The social worker at the hospital helps identify available resources at the federal, state, and local levels. The Social Security Administration determines eligibility for financial assistance based on disability. There are Veterans Administration offices located regionally to assist veterans with needed services. State Offices of Vocational Rehabilitation assist with equipment purchase, job placement, counseling, and financial assistance. The National Center for Victims of Crimes, as well as other voluntary and charitable organizations on the national, state, and local levels, can provide information about services to which the individual with a disability is entitled.

## Lifestyle/Lifespan

Individuals with SCI have the same hopes, desires, and interests as do people without a disability. The person with SCI can return to a satisfactory lifestyle. Because of the extent of losses a person encounters after SCI, a number of issues will

**Table 16.1** Issues Related to Spinal Cord Injury

| Accessibility | Financial | Medical | Family | Social |
|---|---|---|---|---|
| Home | Daily medical supplies | Skin care: prevention of decubiti | Support for daily care | Interaction with peers |
| School/work | Cost of attendant care | Orthostatic hypertension | Role interruption | Role resumption |
| Community | | | Potential role reversal | Role reconfiguration |
| Driving/transportation | Home modifications | Heterotropic bone | | |
| | Work site modifications | Bowel and bladder control | Adjustment to disability | Adaptive leisure |
| | Vehicle adaptations | Respiration | | |
| | Planning for future living arrangements | | | |
| | Durable medical equipment (DME) | | | |

be faced throughout the lifespan. The patient and family should be made aware of social, medical, accessibility, and financial concerns.

The extensive physical, functional, and personal losses that a person with SCI faces can lead to feelings of grief. Each patient progresses through the stages of grief in different ways and at different times. It may take years for a person to adjust to a disability from SCI. The functions of relationships change, and it is not uncommon to lose friends and sexual partners as a result. It is the purpose of the rehabilitative team to educate and support the patient and family as they cope with these social changes. Because of changes in body image and feelings of worthlessness, it is important to access social supports in the community, including those that offer psychological and peer support.

Primary medical issues that remain during the life of the SCI patient include respiratory, skin, bowel, and bladder problems and autonomic dysreflexia. For higher level cord injuries, respiratory complications are a threat regardless of whether mechanical ventilation is needed. Respiratory rehabilitation includes measures to manage secretions and to enhance breathing ability. The patient and his or her family need to be provided with the knowledge and skills necessary to prevent respiratory complications from the inability to effectively clear secretions and decrease vital capacity. The threat of skin breakdown in the individual with SCI is continuous, especially as aging decreases skin elasticity. A rigid pressure relief system and skin care routine is essential to the prevention of decubitus ulcers. Bowel and bladder dysfunction can lead to urinary tract dysfunction and gastrointestinal problems. Autonomic dysreflexia, an exaggerated, sympathetic response to a noxious stimulus below the level of the spinal cord lesion, can be life threatening. The causes, signs, and symptoms of, and treatment for, dysreflexia should be reiterated to the patient and family in order to prevent a serious medical emergency. The extensive set of issues that the person living with SCI will face throughout his or her lifetime is summarized in Table 16.1.

During rehabilitation, the SCI patient and his or her family must be taught the knowledge and skills necessary to remain healthy. If the patient is unable to be independent in certain skills, communication and assertiveness skills are required to facilitate the patient's ability to manage his or her care.

## Clinical Decision-Making Process

### Defining Focus for Intervention

In defining a focus of treatment for the patient with an SCI, the five most important factors are as follows:

1. level and pattern of injury
2. degree of head and upper extremity control
3. degree of wrist and hand function
4. trunk control
5. psychosocial adjustment to the disability (Hill, 1986)

The occupational therapist is most interested in which muscles and sensory systems are intact and functional.

For patients with high-level injuries (C1–C5), head and/or proximal upper extremity control will need to be harnessed and used to access environmental control systems and adaptive equipment. The degree of residual wrist and hand function present will determine the need for training alternative grasp patterns (i.e., tenodesis grasp at C6) versus the development and strengthening of more traditional grasp patterns (at C7 and below). The degree of residual trunk control will affect decisions regarding seating and positioning, wheelchair selection, and functional mobility training. Finally, the degree of adjustment to disability will affect the patient's motivation to learn adaptive strategies and participate in redesigning a productive life (Donnelly et al., 2004; Hill, 1986).

### Establishing Goals for Intervention

Goals for intervention reflect the patient's motivation, energy level, and expected level of independence. Targeted levels of independence for individuals with SCI are summarized in Table 16.2.

Close examination of the expected levels of independence illuminates the difficulty that patients with SCI may experience. Specifically, lower extremity dressing for patients with injuries at C4 through C6 takes practice, and even the most accomplished patients find it time and energy consuming. Such patients may choose to have an attendant assist with that activity during the day. This allows them to conserve time and energy for more valued work or leisure activities.

### Designing Theory-Based Intervention

An SCI affects all areas of a person's life. Therefore, a comprehensive and overarching approach such as the model of human occupation is recommended

**Table 16.2** Target Levels of Independence for Individuals With Spinal Cord Injury

| Level of injury | Level of independence |
| --- | --- |
| C1 | Respirator dependency |
| | Motorized wheelchair dependency |
| | Computer and environmental control system powered by sip/puff; tongue switch, eye gaze, or voice activation |
| | Dependent in all self-care but able to direct caregiver |
| C2–C3 | Motorized wheelchair dependency |
| | Computer and environmental control system powered by head switch or voice activation |
| | Dependent in all self-care but able to direct caregiver |
| C4–C5 | Motorized wheelchair or light manual wheelchair with quad spokes |
| | Mobile arm support and quad cuff for self-feeding |
| | Computer and environmental control system powered by adapted upper extremity switches |
| | Self-dressing with dressing loops |
| | Maximum assistance required for all self-care |
| | Able to direct caregiver |
| C6 | Tenodesis function in upper extremity may limit the need for assistive devices for self-care |
| | Tenodesis splint to support hand function |
| | Manual wheelchair with quad spokes and wheelchair gloves |
| | Sliding board transfers with supervision |
| | Can access standard controls for computer systems and environmental controls |
| C7–C8 | Same as above with increased strength and endurance noted in distal musculature of wrist and hand |
| T1 or lower | Independent manual wheelchair use |
| | Combination of braces and crutches for ambulation in home environment |
| | Independent in all transfers |
| | Independent in self-care |

(Kielhofner, 2008). In addition to the model of human occupation, the biomechanical frame of reference can be used to guide the components of the treatment plan designed to maintain range of motion, prevent deformity, and increase residual muscle strength. The rehabilitation frame of reference can also be incorporated to guide the selection of adaptive devices, such as a quad cuff, and compensatory techniques, such as the use of tenodesis grasp (Kielhofner, 2009).

## Evaluating Progress

From the perspective of the model of human occupation, progress is noted if the patient is seen to be moving toward a well-balanced life that includes the resumption of roles, occupations, and relationships that he or she deems satisfying and that contribute to an overall quality of life. From the biomechanical perspective, progress is noted if increased strength is achieved in innervated muscles and if splinting, serial casting, and positioning have decreased or prevented deformity. From the rehabilitation perspective, progress is noted if the patient no longer relies on the therapist for verbal cues, correction, or assistance in carrying out daily living activities (Kielhofner, 2008, 2009).

## Determining Change in or Termination of Treatment

Because recovery and rehabilitation of SCI is such a long process, termination of treatment is rarely a concern. It is more common for goals to be adjusted to fit the energy patterns of the life the patient is constructing. As noted earlier, lower extremity dressing may be difficult and/or time consuming for the patient. Although it may have been set as a goal in combination with other self-care tasks, that activity may be abandoned for direct care in this area so that more energy can be given to work or leisure activity. Prioritization of goals continues throughout the rehabilitation process (Donnelly et al., 2004; Hill, 1986).

### Case Study

*Description*

HR is a 21-year-old male injured in a diving accident at a family reunion. Prior to his injury, HR was living with a roommate in a third-floor apartment in a large city. He worked full-time at an auto detail shop and was studying to be a pharmacy technician at a local community college and planned to pursue a pharmacy degree in the future. HR and his roommate share simple meal preparation and homemaking. To HR, "basketball is life." He plays in a local league and is an avid fan of local NBA teams—he attends every game. HR is a member of a large, supportive family that lives in a nearby suburb. He is the oldest sibling in a family of three children. He has a girlfriend who attends college in a nearby state.

Immediately after the accident, HR was admitted to the acute care hospital that was designated as a component of the regional SCI care system. He remained in the acute care hospital for 10 days. During that time, his spine was stabilized. It was determined that HR's level of injury was C6. In acute care, HR was evaluated by an occupational therapist. The occupational therapy program included the design of bilateral resting splints to maintain HR's hand position and prevent deformity, skin care and breath control education, sitting practice to diminish dizziness when upright, and transfer training. HR has made good progress and is now in the rehabilitation hospital. Assessment in rehabilitation confirms the C6 level of injury. HR's head control, upper extremity function, and trunk control are consistent with a C6 injury. Goals and a care plan are outlined for HR in the areas of self-feeding, communication, oral/facial hygiene, dressing, bowel and bladder management, splinting, and deformity control.

In the area of self-feeding, it is anticipated that HR will be independent with equipment for drinking, utensil feeding, finger feeding, and cutting food. The equipment that he will use are a cup holder, a bicycle water bottle, a utensil cuff, a sandwich holder, and an adaptive knife. In the area of communication, it is anticipated that HR will be independent with equipment for writing, typing, page turning, and telephone and computer use. The presence of tenodesis action in HR's wrists and hands will be valuable in this area. Equipment that he may use includes a writing splint, a tenodesis training splint, a typing stick, and a phone holder with shoulder rest. For oral/facial hygiene, HR is expected to be independent in washing his face; brushing and flossing his teeth; shaving; caring for his nails; combing, brushing, washing, and drying his hair; and applying deodorant. Equipment that HR will use to support oral/facial hygiene includes a toothpaste stabilizer, a dental floss holder, an electric razor with an adapted handle, an adapted shaving cream can, an adapted brush and comb, and an adapted shampoo dispenser. In dressing, HR is expected to be independent for upper and lower extremity dressing with equipment. He will use a dressing stick or a dressing loop, Velcro shoe closures, loops on socks, a zipper pull, and a sock donner. For bowel and bladder management, HR is expected to empty a catheter bag and apply an external male catheter. He may use a suppository inserter or digital stimulator for bowel management. HR is interested in becoming as independent as possible. He is motivated to build a future for himself.

### Long- and Short-Term Goals

One long-term goal of intervention for HR is to be independent with equipment for communication skills, including writing, typing, page turning, and using the telephone and computer. The short-term goal of intervention for HR is to demonstrate tenodesis action bilaterally sufficient to manipulate 1-inch objects.

### Therapist Goals and Strategies

The therapist's goals include improving tenodesis function in HR's right upper extremity to reduce reliance on adaptive devices and techniques. The therapist's strategies include the following:

1. Fabricate a tenodesis training splint for the right hand to encourage development of a strong and functional tenodesis pattern.
2. Design and implement activities to develop more precise tenodesis control, allowing for the manipulation of progressively smaller and heavier objects.

### Activity: Velcro and Standard Checkers

Prior to beginning the session, the therapist collects a standard checkerboard with 1½-inch checker and an adapted checker game constructed of 1½-inch blocks with hook Velcro on the bottom of each checker. Each checker is fitted on top with a plastic loop. Loop Velcro is attached to each block square of the checkerboard. The Velcro surfaces provide resistance when the checkers are lifted from the board. HR is seated at the table and fitted with the tenodesis training splint. The therapist sits by his side. The checker game starts with the standard checker set. The therapist provides a demonstration and verbal cues regarding how to approach and grasp the checkers using a tenodesis grasp. The therapist describes the role of the splint in training the movement. The game is completed. As HR's tenodesis becomes more habitual, the therapist upgrades the activity by moving to the adapted set. The small plastic top loop is a smaller target than the standard checkers. This requires finer application and placement with the tenodesis grasp. Removing and placing the Velcro checker requires a stronger tenodesis than does a standard checker. By challenging HR to manipulate finer and heavier or more resistive objects, the therapist helps HR develop the most functional tenodesis possible.

It is critical for HR to focus on an activity that will systematically allow for the development of a strong and functional tenodesis in the right upper extremity. He will need to learn to coordinate wrist flexion, finger extension, wrist extension, and finger flexion patterns. This movement can be reinforced by the use of a tenodesis training splint. A functional tenodesis will reduce HR's reliance on adaptive equipment for self-care.

*Treatment Objectives*

HR will complete a competitive game of checkers using a standard checker game and a tenodesis training splint for support.

# Resources
## Internet Resources

Medline Plus on Spinal Cord Injuries: www.nlm.nih.gov/medlineplus/spinalcordinjuries .html

National Institute of Neurological Disorders and Stroke Spinal Cord Injury Information Page: http://www.ninds.nih.gov/disorders/sci/sci.htm

National Spinal Cord Injury Association: www.spinalcord.org

Spinal Cord Injury Resource Center: www.spinalinjury.net

## Print Resource

Selzer, M., & Dobkin, B. (2008). *Spinal cord injury: A guide for patients and families.* Saint Paul, MN: American Academy of Neurology Press.

# References

Altrice, M., Morrison, M., McDowell, S., & Shandalov, B. (2006). In D. Umphred (Ed.), *Neurological rehabilitation* (5th ed.). St Louis, MO: Mosby.

American Occupational Therapy Association. (2008). *Occupational therapy practice framework: Domain and process* (2nd ed.). Bethesda, MD: Author.

American Spinal Injury Association. (2000). *International standards for neurological classification of spinal injury patients.* Chicago, IL: Author.

Americans With Disabilities Act of 1990, 42 U.S.C. § 12101 et seq. (1990) (amended 2008).

Consortium for Spinal Cord Medicine. (1997). *Acute management of autonomic dysreflexia: Adults with spinal cord injury presenting to health care facilities.* Washington, DC: Paralyzed Veterans of America.

Consortium for Spinal Cord Medicine. (1998a). *Depression following spinal cord injury: Clinical practice guidelines.* Washington, DC: Paralyzed Veterans of America.

Consortium for Spinal Cord Medicine. (1998b). *Neurogenic bowel management in adults with spinal cord injury: Clinical practice guidelines.* Washington, DC: Paralyzed Veterans of America.

Donnelly, C., Eng, J., Hall, J., Alford, L., Giachino, R., Norton, K., & Kerr, D. (2004). Client centered assessment and the identification of meaningful treatment goals for individuals with spinal cord injury. *Spinal Cord, 42,* 302–307.

Ducharme, S., & Gill, K. (1997). *Sexuality after spinal cord injury.* Baltimore, MD: Paul H. Brookes.

Garland, D. (1991). A clinical perspective on common forms of acquired heterotopic calcification. *Clinical Orthopaedics and Related Research, 242,* 169–176.

Haas, B., Bergström, E., Jamous, A., & Bennie, A. (1996). The inter-rater reliability of the original and of the modified Ashworth Scale for the assessment of spasticity in patients with spinal cord injury. *Spinal Cord, 34,* 560–564.

Hill, J. (1986). *Spinal cord injury: A guide to functional outcomes in spinal cord injury.* Rockville, MD: Aspen.

Hislop, H., & Montgomery, J. (2007). *Daniels and Worthington's muscle testing: Techniques of manual muscle examination* (8th ed.). Philadelphia, PA: Saunders.

Kendall, F., McCreary, E., & Provance, P. (1993). *Muscles: Testing and function* (4th ed.). Baltimore, MD: Lippincott, Williams & Wilkins.

Kielhofner, G. (2008). *Model of human occupation.* Philadelphia, PA: Lippincott, Williams & Wilkins.

Kielhofner, G. (2009). *Conceptual foundations in occupational therapy* (3rd ed.). Philadelphia, PA: FA Davis.

Kirshblum, S., Gulati, M., O'Connor, K., & Voorman, S. (1998). Bowel care practices in chronic spinal cord injury patients. *Archives of Physical Medicine and Rehabilitation, 79,* 20–23.

Lundy-Ekman, L. (2007). *Neuroscience for rehabilitation:* Philadelphia, PA: Saunders.

Mathiowetz, V., Weber, K., Kashman, N., & Volland, G. (1985). Adult norms for the Nine Hole Peg Test of finger dexterity. *Occupational Therapy Journal of Research, 5*(1), 24–38.

National Spinal Cord Injury Information Network. (n.d.). *Anatomy and physiology.* Retrieved from http://www.spinalcord.uab.edu/show.asp?durki=21468

National Spinal Cord Injury Statistical Center. (2011). *Spinal cord injury: Facts and figures at a glance.* Birmingham: University of Alabama.

Schonherr, M., Groothoff, J., Mulder, G., & Eisma, W. (2000). Prediction of functional outcome after spinal cord injury: A task for the rehabilitation team and the patient. *Spinal Cord, 38,* 185–191.

Smith, L., Weiss, E., & Lehmkuhl, A. (1996). *Brunnstrom's clinical kinesiology* (5th ed.). Philadelphia, PA: FA Davis.

Somers, M. (2010). *Spinal cord injury: Functional rehabilitation* (3rd ed.). Upper Saddle River, NJ: Pearson.

Wright, J. (2000). *The FIM™.* Retrieved from http://www.tbims.org/combi/FIM

# Cumulative Trauma Disorders
## *Carpal Tunnel Syndrome*

*Michael J. Gerg*
*Marlene J. Morgan*

## 🌿 Synopsis of Clinical Condition

### Prevalence and Etiology

*Cumulative trauma disorder* is a term that is used to describe a number of conditions that involve soft tissue structures, such as nerves, tendons, tendon sheaths, muscles, and blood vessels. Cumulative trauma disorders (CTDs) occur from repeated physical movements. Symptoms associated with CTDs include the following:

- 🌿 tightness, discomfort, burning, or soreness in the elbows, forearms, wrists, hands, or fingers
- 🌿 coldness, paresthesia, or numbness in the hands
- 🌿 decreased strength and coordination in the hands
- 🌿 nocturnal pain that wakes the individual
- 🌿 feeling the need to massage the hands or wrists (Fast, 1995)

In addition to the symptoms outlined above, CTDs share a number of characteristics. CTDs are affected by both the intensity and duration of work or activity and symptoms, are poorly localized, are episodic, and are nonspecific. Close examination of the activity patterns of the patient may reveal a work cycle that is short and repetitive, a stressful work environment, or prolonged periods of being in less than desirable (nonneutral), static postures. The development of symptoms is slow and insidious. It may take months or years for the condition to develop, and subsequent recovery may also take months or years (Fast, 1995). CTDs may occur throughout the upper extremity. Fast (1995) included the following in a list of conditions commonly treated by occupational therapists:

- 🌿 thoracic outlet syndrome
- 🌿 lateral and medial epicondylitis
- 🌿 carpal tunnel syndrome

- de Quervain's syndrome
- trigger finger
- cubital tunnel syndrome
- bicipital tendonitis

## Common Characteristics and Symptoms

In this chapter, we use carpal tunnel syndrome (CTS) to illustrate the clinical reasoning and problem-solving approach that an occupational therapist would use to treat a patient who presents with the symptoms of CTD. CTS results from the impingement of the median nerve as it traverses through the carpal tunnel at the wrist. The carpal tunnel is formed by the arch of the carpal bones and the transverse carpal ligament. The carpal bones form the dorsal, lateral, and medial aspects, and the transverse carpal ligament forms the volar aspect. This ligament has ulnar attachments on the pisiform bone and the hook of the hamate, and radial attachments to the trapezium and scaphoid tubercle. The eight long flexor tendons of the fingers, the flexor pollicis longus tendon, and the median nerve all pass through the carpal tunnel. CTS is accepted as the most frequent entrapment neuropathy (Vender, Truppa, Ruder, & Pomerance, 1998). It is one of the diagnoses most frequently seen by occupational therapists working in outpatient orthopedic practices.

Common symptoms of CTS include paresthesia (tingling), hypoesthesia (diminished sensation), anesthesia (numbness), and pain in the hand, especially in the thumb, index, middle, and radial half of the ring fingers. Thenar sensation is preserved as it is innervated by the palmar cutaneous branch, which bifurcates from the median nerve proximal to the transverse carpal ligament. Pain may also radiate into the forearm or shoulder. Many patients experience increased pain and tingling at night and may also experience weakness and atrophy of the thenar muscles. A pattern of weakness in the muscles innervated by the terminal median nerve, distal to the carpal tunnel, may result in weak grip and limited ability to make a fist, and decreased fine motor coordination may also be apparent. The muscles innervated by the terminal median nerve include the abductor pollicis brevis, the opponens pollicis, the superficial head of the flexor pollicis brevis, and the first and second lumbricals. Individuals typically report difficulty manipulating small objects, difficulty sustaining grasp of objects, and frequent dropping of objects.

Median nerve compression and the resulting symptoms usually occur in stages. In the early compression stage, the patient typically complains of intermittent symptoms. In the moderate compression stage, the patient complains of ongoing abnormal sensation. Thenar weakness is also evident at this stage, with decreased abductor pollicis brevis and opponens pollicis strength. Sensory changes are persistent in the severe compression stage. Some degree of atrophy in the thenar muscles is observed, and electromyographic (EMG) examination by a physician shows denervation of the muscles supplied by the median nerve.

Although there is no universally accepted treatment for CTS, surgical treatment is usually preferred to nonsurgical, or conservative, treatment (Verdugo, Salinas, Castillo, & Cea, 2002).

It should be noted that differential diagnostic testing should be performed to rule out other disorders that can mimic the symptoms of CTS. These include diabetic retinopathy, cervical radiculopathy, vascular pathology, thoracic outlet syndrome, pronator syndrome, anterior interosseus nerve syndrome, and thumb carpometacarpal joint arthritis.

## Target Areas for Intervention

CTS is 3 times more likely to occur in women than in men. Patients usually begin to experience symptoms between 30 and 50 years of age, but it can occur at any age. The development of symptoms of CTS may be related to work or other activities. Repetitive and/or static activities in nonneutral postures and, specifically, activities that require forceful wrist flexion or tight gripping are thought to contribute to the development of the condition. Computer use, assembly line work, knitting, needlework, and woodworking are examples of activities that may contribute to the exacerbation of CTS symptoms. A major contributing factor to the condition is the patient's lifestyle. After treatment, many patients need to alter the way they do tasks. CTS may also be seen in patients with seemingly unrelated medical conditions, such as diabetes, rheumatoid arthritis, and obesity. CTS may also be associated with pregnancy and use of oral contraceptives.

CTS is difficult to cure. Although this condition is disabling to some people, it can usually be managed effectively through a coordinated care plan involving the physician, the therapist, and the patient.

## 🌿 Contextual Considerations

### Clinical

Occupational therapists use a combination of pathological, histological, and clinical findings to decide the course of treatment for a patient with CTS. The physician may complete a nerve conduction study to assess the status and conduction capacity of the median nerve. In addition, the physician may use an EMG examination to test for the integrity of the muscles innervated by the median nerve. The components of the clinical occupational therapy evaluation for the patient with CTS must incorporate information about the musculoskeletal status, activities of daily living (ADL), instrumental activities of daily living (IADL), and work history (Headley & Singer, 1998; J. Lisak, personal communication, December 15, 2002). Reviewing the patient's postural habits for occupational performance activities during which he or she spends long periods in the same posture (e.g., work, sleep) is an invaluable tool for focusing interventions that will incorporate body mechanics and ergonomics training. The occupational therapy assessment includes the following:

  🌿 Patient interview to determine the patient's current symptoms and the effect that CTS is having on the patient's ADL and IADL abilities. The *Canadian Occupational Performance Measure* (Law et al., 1990) provides a way to measure improvement in functional progress and to identify meaningful occupational performance activities that can later be used in intervention planning.

  🌿 Detailed work history and information about the person's job tasks and the physical requirements of the tasks.

  🌿 Subjective evaluation of the patient's pain level and location of pain. The most common method for doing this is the Borg CR-10 Scale (Borg, 1985), which asks the patient to rate his/her pain on a scale of 0 to 10.

  🌿 Musculoskeletal status, which is assessed by completing range of motion (ROM), *Manual Muscle Test* (MMT; Hislop & Montgomery, 2007), integumentary assessment of the wound site, sensory testing, and coordination testing. Grip and pinch strength may also be assessed with caution. A clinician should avoid performing dynamometric testing if the patient is already reporting a significant amount of pain. If this testing is performed, the patient should be instructed to exert him- or herself only to the threshold of pain.

The components and frequency of the data collected in the musculoskeletal component of the clinical data vary depending on whether the patient's treatment plan involves surgical or nonsurgical (conservative) treatment.

For patients receiving nonsurgical (conservative) treatment, the initial musculoskeletal assessment consists of the following:

  🌿 sensory evaluation
  🌿 active ROM (AROM) and passive ROM (PROM)
  🌿 MMT, with special emphasis on the muscles innervated by the median nerve
  🌿 grip and pinch strength testing
  🌿 coordination testing

The complete series of assessments is repeated monthly or bimonthly (depending on the setting requirements), and data are compared to detect positive or negative changes in median nerve function (J. Lisak, personal communication, June 15, 2010). For patients who are seen after surgical intervention, assessment is staged in a way that is consistent with the healing of the postsurgical wound:

  🌿 first postsurgical visit: ROM and integumentary (wound) assessment
  🌿 3 weeks after surgery: MMT
  🌿 4 weeks after surgery: sensory evaluation

## Family

Family support and encouragement are critical throughout recovery from CTS. Changes in lifestyle and activity patterns required to prevent the recurrence of this repetitive trauma will need to be reinforced and rewarded on an ongoing basis. Patients may struggle with the interruption of their work role during recovery and may fear that their vocation is in jeopardy. Family education regarding the etiology of CTS and subsequent prevention measures is also critical.

## Practice Setting

Patients with CTS typically receive occupational therapy services in an outpatient hand clinic. This is true for patients whose CTS is being treated after surgery or without surgical intervention.

## Sociopolitical

Patients with work-related CTS may have services paid for through workers' compensation funds, provided that it is deemed a work-related injury. It should be noted that some states do not recognize CTD injuries as compensable injuries. In this instance, even if the work contributed to the individual's having CTS, it will have to be funded through private sources (i.e., the person's health care). The time away from work after surgery is often up to 6 to 7 weeks. There are societal costs to this from both a micro- and a macroperspective. From the microperspective, the workplace needs to replace the absent worker during the time off. This can have an effect on the individual's work setting related to employee morale, the disruption of work, and the costs involved to replace the worker (Leigh, Markowitz, Fahs, & Landrigan, 2000). From a macro perspective, the cost of workers' compensation in the United States in 2006 was 87.6 billion dollars. A gradual and graded plan for returning to work will be required to ensure that the worker is able to return. Worksite modifications and/or job restructuring may be required to ensure that the symptoms of CTS are not exacerbated upon return to work. Both the occupational therapist and the physician use an ongoing assessment of the patient's progress to determine both the steps and the pace of a return-to-work strategy. Return to work for patients with CTS is guided in the legal arena by the employment provisions of the Americans With Disabilities Act (ADA).

## Lifestyle/Lifespan

A major factor contributing to CTS is the patient's lifestyle. Patients with CTS may experience problems with ADL (such as buttoning and fastening garments), IADL (such as driving and using the phone), work-related tasks (such as computer use and assembly line work), and leisure activities (such as digging in a garden or knitting). Activities that require repetitive wrist flexion, extension, and circumduction, as well as those requiring forceful wrist flexion, are problematic and often exacerbate the symptoms of CTS.

In addition to the physical symptoms and problems associated with CTS, patients may have psychosocial concerns. Some patients may fear that CTS will result in a permanent disability. Others may eliminate desired activities from their routine because of associated pain. Still others may fear losing a job if they are not able to return to work or require a modified workstation or schedule.

After treatment, many individuals will need to alter the way they do tasks or use specially designed or adapted tools. Tools that have larger, built-up, or padded handles and commercially available, ergonomically designed tools are recommended. In addition, patients may need to be educated to change the way they approach tasks. During task performance, patients should be encouraged to keep their wrist as straight (neutral) as possible. In this position, the carpal tunnel is at its widest, which alleviates pressure on the median nerve. Patients should be reminded not to repeat the same movement over a period of time and to take frequent rest breaks during activity. Sustained grip and pinch should be avoided if possible, and patients should be encouraged to substitute their whole hand when grasping and carrying objects rather than relying on the thumbs, index fingers, and middle fingers. Patients should be encouraged to ask for help when engaging in activities that make the symptoms worse (American Occupational Therapy Association, 2002).

## Clinical Decision-Making Process

### Defining Focus for Intervention

The clinical findings are the primary determinant of the focus of occupational therapy treatment for patients with CTS. To reduce the compressive forces on the median nerve as it passes through the carpal tunnel, the physician may choose to use either a surgical or a nonsurgical approach. Nonsurgical, or conservative, methods rely on reducing CTS symptoms by modifying the patient's workstation and activity pattern and splinting the wrist in a neutral position (J. Lisak, personal communication, June 15, 2010). These occupational therapy strategies are complimented by anti-inflammatory medications that are prescribed by the physician and possibly an injection of a corticosteroid into the carpal tunnel space to alleviate inflammation. Surgical intervention is directed at the etiology of the condition. The carpal tunnel is opened by releasing the transverse carpal ligament, allowing more space for the median nerve. After the surgical release of the carpal tunnel, the patient participates in an occupational therapy program that focuses on supporting the wrist and a systematic program to increase strength, coordination, and function in the areas of the hand supplied by the median nerve (J. Lisak, personal communication, June 15, 2010).

### Establishing Goals for Intervention

The goals for successful rehabilitation of patients with CTS are consistent, regardless of whether they are receiving nonsurgical (conservative) treatment or surgical intervention. The overarching goals for intervention are as follows:

- Reduce pain and paresthesia.
- Maintain or increase muscle strength.

ꙮ Maintain or improve hand function.

ꙮ Educate the patient on a home exercise program and postural/lifestyle changes.

## Designing Theory-Based Intervention

Patients with CTS benefit from a program designed to use a combination of the biomechanical and the rehabilitation frames of reference. The biomechanical frame of reference is the driving force behind the components of a treatment plan designed to restore function in the hand by promoting wound healing, controlling edema, increasing strength and ROM, and improving sensation and coordination. The rehabilitation frame of reference is instrumental in guiding the selection and design of the compensation techniques, adaptive equipment, ergonomic worksite modifications, and lifestyle changes that will be required to promote a symptom-free life for the patient.

Routine treatment for patients with CTS is protocol driven. It is important to note that treatment protocols for patients of this type are specific to the facility and to the physician. It is important to consult with the physician (especially after surgery) to inquire how the patient should be managed. A surgeon generally has a preferred method for the postsurgical care of a patient. For a patient being treated in a nonsurgical (conservative) way, the protocol may include all or a selection of the following:

ꙮ Provide the patient with a prefabricated soft wrist splint to wear for 6 to 8 weeks at night and for postural support during activities where wrist positioning may provoke symptoms (Moscony, 2007). The proper position of the wrist should be 0 to 2 degrees of flexion and approximately 3 degrees of ulnar deviation (Evans, 2011). As symptoms decrease, the splint should only be worn at night.

ꙮ Provide the patient with a home exercise program that includes both median nerve gliding and tendon gliding exercises (Rozmaryn et al., 1998).

ꙮ Use deep, pulsed ultrasound treatment to improve median nerve conduction and strength (Muller et al., 2004).

ꙮ Educate the patient regarding postural modification for work, leisure, and sleep positioning. Encouraging more neutral postures of the neck and upper extremity can reduce the occurrence of upper extremity pain (Evans, 2011; Juul-Kristensen, Sogaard, Stroyer, & Jensen, 2004).

ꙮ The physician prescribes nonsteroidal anti-inflammatory agents.

ꙮ Recommend that the patient use a continuous, low-level heat wrap to manage wrist/hand pain (Michlovitz, Hun, Erasala, Hengehold, & Weingand, 2004). These heat wraps are available over the counter and can be worn for 8 to 12 hours.

## Evaluating Progress

For patients who present with mild symptoms, a conservative approach is tried first. The goal of this strategy is to see if the symptoms of CTS can be relieved without surgical intervention. The conservative approach, as described previously, is deemed ineffective if the patient experiences persistent pain and paresthesia, development of or increase in atrophy of the thenar muscles, and continued loss

**Table 17.1** Carpal Tunnel Syndrome Postsurgical Protocol

| Days 1–14 | Day 15 | Day 24 | Day 28 |
|---|---|---|---|
| Wrist stabilization–neutral position | Sutures removed<br>Wrist AROM | Begin strengthening | Sensory evaluation and retraining<br>Work hardening may begin |
| AROM to all digits | AROM to all digits<br>Scar management techniques<br>Edema control<br>Desensitization, if needed | | |

*Note.* AROM = active range of motion.

of function. When conservative treatment is not found to be effective, the surgical approach is recommended. A surgical approach is also the first treatment of choice when a patient initially presents with moderate to severe symptoms. For a patient being treated after surgery, a general protocol designed in conjunction with the treating physician would include edema management, wound/scar management, pain management, wrist and hand ROM, strengthening, and return to work/ergonomic training. Table 17.1 provides a sample protocol.

## Determining Change in or Termination of Treatment

The surgical intervention is deemed to be successful if the symptoms of CTS (pain and paresthesia) are decreased and hand function (including muscle strength, sensory status, and coordination) is improved or restored.

### Case Study

*Description*

NY is a 45-year-old, right-hand-dominant woman who is employed as a medical biller. A primary task of her job involves entering patient information and records into a computer billing system. She is a single woman who lives alone in a one-story ranch house and was independent in all ADL and IADL. She takes care of her home, including mowing the lawn and completing minor home repairs. She is a gourmet cook and enjoys taking classes and cooking for her friends and family. About 3 months ago, she presented with symptoms of pain and tingling in her right (dominant) wrist and hand. An interview revealed that NY had been experiencing these symptoms for several months. Pain in her wrist was waking her up at night, and she experienced pain, tingling, and numbness during the day as she entered data at work. She reported that she frequently felt the need to "shake her hands out" in order for sensation to return.

NY filed a workers' compensation claim, which was accepted, and was referred to a physician on her employer's workers' compensation panel. Initially, her doctor decided to treat her conservatively. She was sent to an outpatient occupational therapy clinic to have a prefabricated wrist cock-up splint issued to her and received a corticosteroid injection into her carpal tunnel. The issuing therapist removed the metal support in the splint and fabricated a thermoplastic support that ensured her wrist would be maintained in neutral. She was instructed to wear her cock-up splint only when sleeping and for postural reinforcement while performing activities that seemed to exacerbate her symptoms. She was also instructed to perform median nerve gliding exercises for 5 to 10 repetitions, 3 to 4 times daily.

After 2 months of this regime of splinting, home exercises, and taking a nonsteroid, anti-inflammatory medication, NY continued to have symptoms. The physician then chose to do surgery, and NY had her carpal tunnel released. She began occupational therapy 5 days after her carpal tunnel release, and a postsurgical protocol was followed. Current research does not support the need for the use of a splint to support the wrist after surgery, unless the individual experiences nocturnal pain or is prone to resume activities too soon after surgery (Evans, 2011). In NY's case, she was planning to be away from work for 6 weeks and denied having nocturnal pain. She has been educated in edema control techniques and scar massage. Her surgical site is healing well. On the fifth day after surgery, following protocol, NY was instructed in tendon gliding and nerve gliding exercises and was encouraged to do gentle AROM at the wrist, with no resistance (Rozmaryn et al., 1998).

In anticipation of NY's return to work, the occupational therapist agreed to meet with NY at her place of employment. Permission was sought from her employer prior to performing a workstation evaluation. NY's employer agreed to an ergonomic assessment of her workstation and was interested in adapting the workstation to decrease any ergonomic risk factors. Upon evaluation, it was discovered that NY sat at a desk with an LCD monitor on the desktop. She was noted to flex her neck approximately 20 degrees to view the screen. Her keyboard was positioned on the desktop at greater than forearm's length from her, and she frequently kept the files that she would gather data from between her and the keyboard. As a result of this, she would rest her forearms on the files, and as they piled up on the desk, NY would need to flex her wrist to access the keys. She was also noted to keep her mouse at arm's length from her. To access both the keyboard and the mouse, shoulder elevation was required. After evaluating the worksite, the occupational therapist made some suggestions for NY and her employer to consider and recommended modifications that may need to be made to NY's workstation to protect against reinjury or the incidence of CTS in her other hand. Recommendations were made using standards listed by the Occupational Safety and Health Administration (2003). Some of the recommendations that NY feels will be most helpful include the following:

🖋 Acquire a keyboard tray with adjustable height that has a mouse tray extension. NY has received instruction on the proper height for the keyboard tray, which is at elbow height with the shoulder relaxed and both upper arms relaxed at her sides and her elbows bent 90 degrees.

🖋 Elevate the monitor height so that the top of the LCD screen is approximately at eyebrow level. This will eliminate the need for neck flexion to view the screen. Minimizing neck flexion has been found to effectively reduce wrist pain in computer users (Juul-Kristensen et al., 2004). The monitor can be elevated using a monitor riser that can be purchased or with objects (e.g., books, copy paper) readily available in the office.

🌿 Place patient files on a bookstand on the desktop that tilts the work toward the user anywhere from 15 to 40 degrees. This decreases the need for neck flexion to view patient files.

🌿 Periodically review performance of NY's median nerve glides during the course of her workday with both upper extremities.

🌿 Maintain the keyboard tilt close to 0 degrees to ensure a neutral wrist posture when typing to decrease pressure on the median nerve (Simoneau, Marklin, & Berman, 2003). To retrain posture, since NY had been in the habit of flexing her wrists, her therapist advised her to place two thin strips of athletic tape on the lateral and medial aspects of her dorsal hand, wrist, and distal forearm while in neutral. NY will feel the pull of the tape on her skin each time she flexes her wrist, and this will act as a tactile cue for posture.

🌿 Undergo training on proper sleep postures. Sleeping with the head and wrist in a neutral position maintains proper axoplasmic flow and promotes nerve health. Sleeping on the stomach is discouraged because it provides no way to maintain neutral head position.

🌿 Purchase bicycle gloves with vibration dampening volar gel padding to use when operating her lawnmower at home. This will decrease the likelihood of the vibration irritating her median nerve during lawn-care activities.

🌿 Remember to take rest breaks during her busy day.

### Long- and Short-Term Goals

The long-term goals of the postoperative phase of treatment for NY are to exhibit hand function (strength, sensation, endurance, and coordination) sufficient to complete ADL and IADL independently; incorporate proper wrist positioning into all self-care, work, and leisure activities; incorporate frequent rest breaks into all self-care, work, and leisure activities; and continue to monitor her wrist for symptoms of recurring CTS or the advent of it in her other hand.

NY will reach these goals in part through successfully achieving the following short-term goals:

1. Exhibit full AROM in the wrist and digits.
2. Demonstrate and describe the proper neutral position for the wrist.
3. Describe the list of symptoms related to CTS.
4. Identify times during her workday when she will be able to rest.
5. Demonstrate the ability to properly position her documents, keyboard, mouse, and monitor at her workstation.
6. Demonstrate proper technique for tendon gliding exercises.
7. Demonstrate proper technique for median nerve gliding exercises.

### Therapist Goals and Strategies

The therapist's goals include the following:

1. Provide support to the healing surgical site.
2. Reduce or prevent edema.
3. Manage scar formation.
4. Increase strength and restore hand function.
5. Teach compensation techniques and adaptive strategies to reduce stress and compression of the carpal tunnel.

6. Assess patient for adaptive devices and techniques that will provide proper wrist support and promote function.
7. Complete workstation evaluation and make recommendations for worksite modification.

The therapist's strategies include the following:

1. Teach patient edema control techniques to be incorporated into a home program.
2. Teach scar management techniques. Provide a silicone gel padding in the presence of pillar pain.
3. Provide a graded exercise program designed to increase muscle strength and restore hand function.
4. Teach patient tendon and median nerve gliding exercises to be incorporated into a home program.
5. Teach patient proper positions and approaches to activity for both home and work.
6. Complete worksite assessment and recommendations.
7. Provide patient education.

### Activity: Cream Cheese Mints

NY needs to increase strength and maintain the mobility that has been gained through the tendon gliding, nerve gliding, and active exercises. Activities that include flexion and extension of the wrist against light resistance, circumduction of the wrist, opening and closing of the hand, extension of the thumb, and opposition of the thumb and middle finger are appropriate choices during this time. The procedure for making cream cheese mints fits these criteria. As NY kneads the mixture of powdered sugar, cream cheese, and mint flavoring mixed in a Ziploc bag, the therapist observes for wrist position and reinforces rest breaks. The fact that the cream cheese mint mixture is in a Ziploc bag allows for the kneading to be stopped and started at any time. The mixture may be stored for up to a week before molding; therefore, this activity provides an appropriate context for educating the patient on wrist position, rest breaks, and splint application. For NY, making cream cheese mints is also consistent with her interest in cooking and may provide the opportunity for her to identify other cooking tasks that may be modified or adapted in the future.

### Treatment Objectives

The objective for this session is to engage the patient in an activity that provides gentle exercise to the wrist, thumb, and fingers while providing the opportunity to reinforce important patient education concepts regarding wrist position, splint application, and activity pacing.

# Resources

American Occupational Therapy Association: www.aota.org

Occupational Safety and Health Administration. (2003). *Computer workstations eTool*. Retrieved from http://www.osha.gov/SLTC/etools/computerworkstations/index.html

# References

American Occupational Therapy Association. (2002). *Carpal tunnel syndrome: A guide to daily activities*. Upper Marlboro, MD: Author.

Americans With Disabilities Act of 1990, 42 U.S.C. § 12101 *et seq.* (1990).

Borg, G. (1985). *An introduction to Borg's RPE Scale*. Ithaca, NY: Mouvement Publications.

Evans, R. B. (2011). Therapist's management of carpal tunnel syndrome. In T. Skirven, A. Osterman, J. Fedorczyk, & P. Amado (Eds.), *Rehabilitation of the hand and upper extremity* (6th ed., pp. 666–678). Philadelphia, PA: Mosby.

Fast, C. (1995). Repetitive strain injury: An overview of the condition and its implications for occupational therapy practice. *Canadian Journal of Occupational Therapy, 62*(3), 119–126.

Headley, B., & Singer, G. (1998). Carpal tunnel syndrome: Making the right diagnosis. *Advance for Occupational Therapy, 4*(14), 18–30.

Hislop, H., & Montgomery, J. (2007). *Daniels and Worthingham's muscle testing: Techniques of manual examination* (8th ed.). Philadelphia, PA: Saunders.

Juul-Kristensen, B., Sogaard, K., Stroyer, J., & Jensen, C. (2004). Computer users' risk factors for developing shoulder, elbow and back symptoms. *Scandinavian Journal of Work Environmental Health, 30*(5), 390–398.

Law, M., Baptiste, S., McColl, M., Opzoomer, A., Polatajko, H., & Pollock, N. (1990). The Canadian Occupational Performance Measure: An outcome measure for occupational therapy. *The Canadian Journal of Occupational Therapy, 5*(2), 48–53.

Leigh, J. P., Markowitz, S., Fahs, M., & Landrigan, P. (2000). *Costs of occupational injuries and illnesses*. Ann Arbor: University of Michigan Press.

Michlovitz, S., Hun, L., Erasala, G. N., Hengehold, D. A., & Weingand, K. W. (2004). Continuous low-level heat wrap therapy is effective for treating wrist pain. *Archives of Physical Medicine Rehabilitation, 85,* 1409–1416.

Moscony, A. M. B. (2007). Common peripheral nerve problems. In C. Cooper (Ed.), *Fundamentals of hand therapy* (pp. 201–250). St. Louis, MO: Mosby.

Muller, M., Tsui, D., Schnurr, R., Biddulph-Deisroth, L., Hard, J., & MacDermid, J. C. (2004). Effectiveness of hand therapy interventions in primary management of carpal tunnel syndrome: A systematic review. *Journal of Hand Therapy, 17,* 210–228.

Occupational Safety and Health Administration. (2003). *Computer workstations eTool*. Retrieved from http://www.osha.gov/SLTC/etools/computerworkstations/index.html

Rozmaryn, L. M., Dovell, S., Rothman, E. F., Gorman, K., Olvey, K. M., & Bartko, J. J. (1998). Nerve and tendon gliding exercises and the conservative management of carpal tunnel syndrome. *Journal of Hand Therapy, 11*(3), 171–179.

Simoneau, G. G., Marklin, R. W., & Berman, J. E. (2003). Effect of computer keyboard slope on wrist position and forearm electromyography of typists without musculoskeletal disorders. *Physical Therapy, 83*(9), 816–830.

Vender, M. I., Truppa, K. L., Ruder, J. R., & Pomerance, J. (1998). Upper extremity compressive neuropathies. *Physical Medicine and Rehabilitation: State of the Art Reviews, 12*(2), 243–262.

Verdugo, R. J., Salinas, R. S., Castillo, J., & Cea, J. (2002). Surgical versus non-surgical treatment for carpal tunnel syndrome. *Cochrane Database of Systematic Reviews, 2002*(4). doi: 10.1002/14651858.CD001552.pub2

# Posttraumatic Stress Disorder

*William Lambert*

## Synopsis of Clinical Condition

### Prevalence and Etiology

Posttraumatic stress disorder (PTSD) is an anxiety disorder that can develop after exposure to a terrifying event or ordeal in which grave physical harm occurred or was threatened (National Institute of Mental Health, 2010). The American Psychiatric Association (APA; 2000) accepts that PTSD develops in response to experiencing events that are threatening to life or bodily integrity, witnessing threatening or deadly events, and hearing of violence to or the unexpected or violent death of close associates. Events that could qualify as traumatic, according to the *Diagnostic and Statistical Manual of Mental Disorders–Fourth Edition, Text Revision* (*DSM-IV-TR*; APA, 2000), include combat, sexual and physical assault, being held hostage or imprisoned, terrorism, torture, natural and man-made disasters, accidents, and receiving a diagnosis of a life-threatening illness. PTSD can also develop in children who have experienced sexual molestation, even if this is not violent or life threatening. Despite its debilitating nature, the condition often goes undiagnosed (Grinage, 2003). The *DSM-IV-TR* reports lifetime prevalence for PTSD in approximately 8% of the adult population in the United States (APA, 2000). PTSD can affect anyone at any age but typically affects women (10% of the population) more often than men (5% of the population; National Center for PTSD, 2008). Prevalence rates vary across gender, culture, and experience depending on preexisting individual-based factors, features of the traumatic event, and posttrauma social support (Keane, Marshall, & Taft, 2006).

This disorder can develop in individuals without any predisposing conditions, particularly if the stressor is extreme and perpetrated by humans through actions

The editors gratefully acknowledge the contributions of Shannon Webb, Jamie Duminiak, Casey Holladay, Kathleen Marcucilli, and Brittany Murphy.

such as torture or rape (APA, 2000). The severity, duration, and proximity of an individual's exposure to the traumatic event are the most important factors affecting the likelihood of developing this disorder. Environmental factors, such as childhood trauma, injury, or a history of mental health issues, may increase the likelihood of developing PTSD. It is also important to note that personality and cognitive factors, such as optimism and pessimism, as well as the availability of social support systems appear to influence an individual's response to trauma.

## Common Characteristics and Symptoms

PTSD is uniquely distinguished from other anxiety disorders because it has an identifiable stressor or trauma and the defining symptoms are related to the traumatic event (Breslaur, Chase, & Anthony, 2002). There is a constellation of symptoms that must be present in order for a diagnosis of PTSD to be made. They are the following: reexperiencing symptoms, avoidance symptoms, and hyperarousal symptoms. Reexperiencing symptoms include visual and auditory flashbacks, bad dreams, and frightening thoughts. Avoidance symptoms include feelings of guilt, depression, worry, and emotional numbness. Individuals with PTSD may stay away from places, events, and objects that remind them of their traumatic experience, and/or they may have trouble remembering this particular experience at all. Individuals with PTSD may lose interest in the activities they once engaged in and enjoyed. Hyperarousal symptoms include feeling tense, being easily startled, experiencing angry outbursts, and having difficulty sleeping. All of these symptoms are very distressing and can cause an individual's life to be disrupted. Roles, routines, and habits are affected by the symptoms of PTSD, and an individual's quality of life can suffer (National Institute of Mental Health, 2010).

The *DSM-IV-TR* is used to diagnose and classify PTSD. The symptoms of reexperiencing the event, avoidance behaviors, and hyperarousal symptoms must all be present for 1 month for a diagnosis of PTSD to be made. The criteria for the diagnosis are (a) the person must have experienced or witnessed an event or events that involved threatened death or serious injury and (b) the person's response to this event must have involved fear, helplessness, or horror. It is important to note that diagnostic criteria are based on information gathered from an adult male population. Children may present with markedly different symptoms, such as disorganized or agitated behavior.

The traumatic event is persistently reexperienced in a variety of ways, such as recurrent thoughts, dreams, or emotions, making the person feel that he/she is experiencing the trauma again. The individual will also experience intense psychological distress at exposure to cues that symbolize or resemble part of the traumatic event. Physiological reactions can occur as well. This leads to persistent avoidance of stimuli associated with the trauma, which can result in avoidance of activities, places, and individuals as well as thoughts and feelings associated with the trauma. PTSD can cause impairments in a person's life, which interferes with his or her functioning in daily activities and can affect work and social relationships (APA, 2000).

PTSD is classified as acute if the duration of symptoms is less than 3 months. Chronic PTSD is diagnosed when the symptoms last longer than 3 months. PTSD can be specified as occurring with delayed onset if the onset of symptoms is more than 6 months after the stressor or traumatic event (APA, 2000).

## Target Areas for Intervention

Clients with PTSD may experience impairments in their occupational performance secondary to their symptoms of anxiety and fear. Occupational therapy can address anxiety and stress through identifying stress triggers and developing adaptive and positive coping skills. Relaxation techniques can be taught as a coping skill to assist clients in managing symptoms outside of therapy.

Advocacy and community education are also important areas for occupational therapy intervention to address. Clients may report isolation related to the stigma of PTSD and the inability of others to understand their circumstance. Occupational therapy may provide treatment in groups to allow for social interaction with others with similar diagnoses. It may also be beneficial to gear the occupational therapy toward family involvement to reestablish connections and understanding that may have been lost.

A diagnosis of PTSD will have an impact on life roles and routines. Occupational therapy can explore various modifications to performance patterns to support participation. Depending on the population being treated, intervention may focus on creating new life roles, as in cases of veterans and victims of domestic violence. For example, therapists working with veterans with PTSD may focus on the transition from the role of soldier to the role of civilian. Treatment may involve finding ways to feel safe in their environment, adjusting work habits, and transitioning back into social and family roles.

Acute treatment for PTSD may include various expressive therapies to facilitate recall of traumatic events and emotional recovery (Froehlich, 1992). Treatment should also focus on the client's current situation and address the specific areas of occupation that are impaired.

## Contextual Considerations

### Clinical

The type and course of clinical intervention depends on the type of PTSD (i.e., acute, chronic, or delayed) that the client is experiencing and the degree to which the experience of PTSD is affecting his or her ability to function in daily life. The disorder typically involves symptoms of (a) hyperarousal, (b) reexperiencing or intrusion, and (c) avoidance and emotional numbing. Individuals with PTSD may also have concomitant or comorbid mental health conditions, such as depression and anxiety (APA, 2000).

Considering that the disorder is unique to each individual and reflective of the traumatic event that precipitated the disorder, evaluations may be based on assessing symptomatology, obtaining a personal narrative from the client, and evaluating the degree of disruption in daily life activities.

## Family

PTSD is often the result of a personal trauma that is not initially shared by family, friends, or coworkers. It can be difficult for others to understand the trauma that the individual experienced, especially when his or her ability to function afterward affects relationships and performance of life roles. Others have difficultly being empathic, particularly when the disorder affects an individual for years, as in chronic cases of PTSD. They may perceive the individual as being weak, overreacting, or malingering.

## Practice Setting

The diagnosis of PTSD has become more prevalent as a result of the military conflicts in the Middle East (Burke, Degeneffe, & Olney, 2009). The occupational therapists most likely to treat individuals with PTSD are those who work with casualties of war, such as those working in military hospitals. In 2003, a preliminary study showed an increase in PTSD and anxiety symptoms related to the September 11th terrorist attacks on the World Trade Center in New York (Bock et al., 2003). Even though there is little evidence that occupational therapists worked with clients after 9/11, occupational therapy can play a vital role in facilitating the resumption of life roles in persons who suffer from chronic PTSD (Duminiak et al., 2010).

## Sociopolitical

Increased public awareness of the disorder and more sophisticated diagnostic techniques have contributed to societal understanding of the condition and access to compassionate, timely, and appropriate intervention and care.

## Lifestyle/Lifespan

The ramifications of PTSD are lifelong. Without treatment, resumption of pretrauma occupations and relationships may be seriously impaired.

# 🖑 Clinical Decision-Making Process

## Defining Focus for Intervention

The focus for intervention begins with an appropriate assessment. The construction of a comprehensive picture from the client's perspective, which includes the positive and negative life changes after a traumatic experience and concerns and goals for treatment, may be obtained through the use of an assessment such as the *Occupational Performance History Interview–Second Edition* (OPHI-II; Kielhofner et al., 2004).

## Establishing Goals for Intervention

Occupational therapy treatment is designed to address the symptoms of PTSD that affect activities of daily living and functional skills (Baum & Michael, 2008). Goals for intervention will depend, in part, on the unique experience of the individual. Current literature relating to occupational therapy and PTSD focuses on those who have experienced domestic violence (Javaherian, Underwood, & DeLany, 2007), natural disasters (Scaffa, Gerardi, Herzberg, & McColl, 2006), war (Burke et al., 2009), and traumatic accidents (Kirk, 2002). Target populations for the practice of occupational therapy include the following:

- veterans
- active members of the armed services
- victims of physical and sexual abuse
- survivors of natural disasters, such as hurricanes, fires, and floods
- students who have witnessed acts of violence at school and who require crisis intervention and debriefing
- the variety of individuals being treated for PTSD by doctors, psychiatrists, and psychotherapists who would benefit from referral to occupational therapy to gain or regain life skills and lead occupationally satisfying lives

The following are important concepts to consider when establishing goals for intervention:

- stigma
- lack of empathy/understanding from family, friends, and employers
- triggers, which can be any number of sensations or events (such as odors, sounds, and the physical characteristics of people, places, and things) that may trigger changes in the feelings, mood, and behavior of the individual

Although the treatment goals for individuals can vary significantly, common intervention strategies for individuals with PTSD include the following:

- stress management
- coping skills
- anxiety management
- identifying and managing triggers
- journaling, breathing, and muscle relaxation
- cognitive therapy
- exposure therapy
- group therapy
- patient education
- occupational exploration

- family education
- eye movement desensitization and reprocessing
- medication, such as antidepressants and antipsychotics
- psychotherapy
- stress inoculation training

## Designing Theory-Based Intervention

The model of human occupation addresses motivation, performance, and organization of occupational behavior in everyday life and provides a comprehensive view of the individual's domains of concern (Kielhofner et al., 2004). One effective evaluation tool that is based on and congruent with the model of human occupation is the OPHI-II. This instrument can be used to gain information about the effects of PTSD on the participant's occupational performance. The OPHI-II interview comprises three major scales: Occupational Identity, Occupational Competence, and Occupational Settings. This instrument measures change after a clear line of demarcation in a person's life, such as witnessing a traumatic event. The client's ability to perform occupations satisfactorily prior to the traumatic event can provide a baseline from which, together with the client, treatment goals can be developed based on the individual's perceived needs and desired therapy outcomes.

## Evaluating Progress

The diminished effect of the troubling symptomatology of PTSD on the performance of desired and normative daily occupations and a return to past occupations or preferred occupations for the present and future would be indicators of progress. For example, the ability to resume or function more optimally in life roles identified as important by the client and society, such as spouse, sibling, parent, friend, and worker, would indicate progress toward treatment goals.

## Determining Change In or Termination of Treatment

As in most clinical situations, a minimal response or lack of response to occupational therapy intervention would indicate the need to reassess and revisit prior treatment objectives. Termination of occupational therapy services would depend on the following:

- the treatment setting
- the client's ability to access insurance coverage and intervention services
- the client's assessment of the efficacy of treatment
- the client's satisfaction with the progress made toward treatment goals

Ideally, services would be terminated when the client is satisfied with his or her ability to function in the desired occupations that support participation in life.

# Case Study

## Description

DS is a 47-year-old computer engineer who has been diagnosed with PTSD. His workplace was within walking distance of his home, and his route from home to work brought him past a local florist and through a park. One day, when leaving work a bit later than usual, DS stopped to buy flowers for his wife at the florist and continued on through the park. Upon entering the park, he was mugged at gunpoint, robbed of all his money and personal possessions, and badly beaten. A jogger found DS, bloody and unconscious, on the side of the jogging trail.

The trauma of this violent crime left DS with flashbacks and avoidance tendencies toward the things he once loved most in life. DS became increasingly anxious, depressed, and irritable. His daily routine became disrupted, and he became increasingly withdrawn. DS's family physician referred him to a psychiatrist, who diagnosed DS with PTSD, prescribed antidepressant medication, and referred DS to a local outpatient facility for intervention.

In addition to psychological counseling sessions, DS was referred for occupational therapy intervention. The OPHI-II revealed that DS had been an avid gardener and walker and that he had enjoyed home maintenance tasks. He stated that prior to acquiring PTSD, he enjoyed planting and caring for flowers and trees, doing yard projects, such as making a flagstone patio, and expanding and creating perennial flower beds and making container gardens with seasonal annuals, especially in the spring and summer, his favorite time of year. His wife enjoyed his efforts, and they frequently spent summer evenings on the patio surrounded by his lovely plantings.

After DS developed PTSD, he lost interest in these formerly satisfying occupations. He stopped gardening, and soon the flower beds were overrun with weeds. He no longer had the motivation to garden, and all of the tasks he had formerly enjoyed seemed overwhelming. He had avoided being outdoors since the attack. He remembered that the beautiful floral display in the park inspired him to pick up flowers for his wife and some flats of annuals before the traumatic assault. The sight of flowers often triggered flashbacks, and DS began to drive to work, careful to avoid the route that passed the park, as it invoked a flight response.

## Long- and Short-Term Goals

The long-term goals for DS are (a) to participate in his identified meaningful occupation of gardening without prompting from the therapist, his family, or others and (b) to return to a satisfying and healthy lifestyle that demonstrates an ability to deal adaptively with the symptoms of PTSD.

Short-terms goals for DS are as follows:

1. DS will use a landscape design computer program to create a virtual garden.
2. DS will learn coping skills that he can use to manage his PTSD, such as identifying triggers and engaging in relaxation techniques or deep breathing exercises.

## Therapist Goals and Strategies

1. Provide DS with an indoor activity that relates to his stated interest in gardening.

2. Instruct DS to proactively use relaxation techniques and deep breathing exercises in response to triggers, such as certain flowers, scents, or garden scenes.

3. Gradually introduce opportunities to carry out more outdoor gardening activities.

### Activity: Creating a Virtual Garden

DS is provided with a computer program that allows the user to design all aspects of the home landscape, including patios, walkways, and containers. DS decides that he will start with a container garden design and designs a window box that would be suitable for his own home. Before starting on the computer, DS reviews with his therapist the deep breathing exercises that he will use if he experiences anxiety in response to any of the gardening images he encounters. Since DS is skilled at working with computers, it doesn't take him long to understand how to work the landscaping program. During the first session, DS does experience a flashback in response to a particular flower, but he practices his deep breathing exercises and persists in the activity by designing a window box that is composed of a variety of foliage plants.

On his next visit, he reports to the therapist that he has been looking through gardening catalogues and is looking forward to making his computer design a reality. DS and his wife have purchased two window boxes that will be mounted on their front windows in the spring. DS hopes to use the computer to design larger garden projects and gradually progress to engaging in the outdoor activities that give so much meaning to his life.

### Treatment Objectives

DS will increase his ability to handle the symptoms of PTSD and begin to return to the formerly gratifying occupation of gardening.

## Resources

Gateway to Posttraumatic Stress Disorder Information: http://www.ptsdinfo.org/

Gift From Within: http://www.giftfromwithin.org/

Hamblen, J. (n.d.) *Treatment of PTSD*. Retrieved from http://www.militarymental health.org/resources/treatment-of-ptsd.aspx

National Center for PTSD: http://www.ptsd.va.gov/

U.S. Department of Veterans Affairs and U.S. Department of Defense. (2010). *Management of posttraumatic stress*. Retrieved from http://www.healthquality. va.gov/Post_Traumatic_Stress_Disorder_PTSD.asp

## References

American Psychiatric Association. (2000). *Diagnostic and statistical manual of mental disorders* (4th ed., text rev.). Washington, DC: Author.

Baum, C., & Michael, E. (2008). *Testimony given to the United States House of Representatives, Committee Veterans' Affairs, Subcommittee on Health, April 1, 2008*. Retrieved from www.aota.org

Bock, B. C., Becker, B., Partridge, R., Merchant, R. C., Niaura, R., & Abrams, D. B. (2003). A prospective study of coping styles and stress symptoms after the September 11th, 2001 terrorist attack. *Medicine & Health Rhode Island, 86*(11), 340–341.

Breslaur, N., Chase, G., & Anthony, J. (2002). The uniqueness of the DSM definition of post-traumatic stress disorder: Implications for research. *Psychological Medicine, 32,* 573–576.

Burke, H., Degeneffe, C., & Olney, M. (2009). A new disability for rehabilitation counselors: Iraq war veterans with traumatic brain injury and post-traumatic stress disorder. *Journal of Rehabilitation, 73,* 5–9.

Duminiak, J., Holladay, C., Lambert, W., Marcucilli, K., Murphy, B., & Webb, S. (2010). *Changes in occupational performance for a survivor of the September 11, 2001 terrorist attacks with posttraumatic stress disorder.* Unpublished manuscript, University of Scranton, Scranton, PA.

Froelich, J. (1992). Occupational therapy interventions with survivors of sexual abuse. *Occupational Therapy in Health Care, 8*(2/3), 1–12.

Grinage, B. (2003). Diagnosis and management of posttraumatic stress disorder. *American Academy of Family Physicians, 68,* 2401–2409.

Javaherian, H., Underwood, R., & DeLany, J. (2007). Occupational therapy services for individuals who have experienced domestic violence. *The American Journal of Occupational Therapy, 61,* 704–709.

Keane, T., Marshall, A., & Taft, C. (2006). Posttraumatic stress disorder: Etiology, epidemiology, and treatment outcome. *Annual Review of Clinical Psychology, 2,* 161–197.

Kielhofner, G., Mallinson, T., Crawford, C., Nowak, M., Rigby, M., Henry, A., & Walens, D. (2004). *A user's manual for the Occupational Performance History Interview (OPHI-II).* Chicago: University of Illinois at Chicago.

Kirk, A. (2002). Prevalence of traumatic events and PTSD symptomatology among a selected sample of undergraduate students. *Journal of Social Work in Disability and Rehabilitation, 1,* 53–65.

National Institute of Mental Health. (2010). *Posttraumatic stress disorder.* Retrieved from http://www.nimh.nih.gov/health/topics/post-traumatic-stress-disorder-ptsd/index.shtml

Scaffa, M., Gerardi, S., Herzberg, G., & McColl, M. (2006). The role of occupational therapy in disaster preparedness, response, and recovery. *The American Journal of Occupational Therapy, 60,* 642–649.

# Substance Use Disorders

*Nancy Beck*
*C. Thomas North*
*Dana L. Weiss*

## 🔥 Synopsis of Clinical Condition

### Prevalence and Etiology

Substance use disorders are a complex set of problems with physiological and psychological ramifications. Individuals with a substance use disorder may require increasingly larger amounts of a substance with more frequency in order to maintain physiological homeostasis and may restructure belief systems, behaviors, and attitudes in order to maintain habitual use of the substance. The two primary classifications for substance use disorder, substance abuse and substance dependence, are based on behaviors that are routinely exhibited over a 12-month period.

Substance abuse is characterized by maladaptive patterns of substance use that lead to one or more of the following outcomes: failure to carry out role responsibilities; engagement in hazardous activity, such as driving or operating machinery while impaired; physical fights; and recurrent arrests. Substance dependence is diagnosed when the substance use results in three or more of the following outcomes: heightened tolerance of the substance, leading to increased use; withdrawal symptoms; increased use of the substance or a related substance to alleviate withdrawal symptoms; and engagement in efforts to procure the substance that eclipse more productive social, occupational, or recreational endeavors. The most frequently abused substances are alcohol (ethanol), benzodiazepines, cocaine, opiates, amphetamines, methamphetamines, and cannabis (tetrahydrocannabinol [THC]; American Psychiatric Association, 2000). In 2009, an estimated 22.5 million people (8.9% of the population ages 12 years or older) were classified with substance dependence or abuse (Substance Abuse and Mental Health Services Administration, 2010).

### Common Characteristics and Symptoms

Alcohol intoxication is characterized by animation and elevation of mood followed by reduced reaction time, impaired coordination, slurred speech, depressed affect, and, eventually, unconsciousness. Inappropriate sexual or aggressive behavior, evidence of poor judgment, and impaired social or occupational function may also occur. Individuals who have an alcohol use disorder may often have cognitive deficits in the areas of abstract reasoning, memory, and problem solving. Withdrawal may be characterized by dehydration, nausea, hypersensitivity to sound or light, and psychomotor impairment. There is a 20% fatality rate associated with untreated alcoholism (American Psychological Association, 2000; Sadock & Sadock, 2007).

Benzodiazepines are in a class of drugs called *sedative hypnotics.* Benzodiazepines may be initially prescribed by a physician, but there is a high risk of dependency associated with even short-term use. Commonly abused forms of these drugs are Ativan, Xanax, Valium, and Klonopin. These drugs may be taken orally, intranasally, or intravenously. With intravenous use, there is a risk of contracting HIV, hepatitis, methicillin-resistant *Staphylococcus aureus,* or other potentially lethal infections. Abrupt discontinuance of benzodiazepine use may lead to seizure or death. Intoxication and withdrawal symptoms are similar to those of alcohol use disorder. The detoxification process is characterized by a slow reduction of the substance (American Psychological Association, 2000; Sadock & Sadock, 2007).

Opiates (morphine, heroin, codeine, and methadone) are central nervous system depressants that precipitate dysphoria on the first use and euphoria on subsequent uses. Additional reactions are psychomotor retardation, drowsiness, impaired memory, and decreased attention. Signs of overdose include coma, pinpoint pupils, and decreased respiration. Withdrawal is characterized by fluctuations in temperature; cramps; aches; and fluid loss through diarrhea, lacrimation, and rhinorrhea. Elevated blood pressure and tachycardia may also be present. The patient under treatment for withdrawal experiences flu-like symptoms and depression.

Cocaine is classed with opiates, even though it is a stimulant. Its use is associated with a quick, euphoric high that is often followed by depression and suicidal ideation. It is highly addictive, and death from overdose is usually due to heart attack or suffocation. This drug can be ingested, inhaled, or injected. Crack is a freebase form of cocaine; it is extremely potent, and some individuals have been known to become addicted after one or two uses (Sadock & Sadock, 2007). The following diagnoses have been developed to label conditions that result from cocaine abuse: cocaine withdrawal, cocaine intoxication delirium, cocaine-induced psychotic disorder with delusions, cocaine-induced psychotic disorder with hallucinations, cocaine-induced mood disorder, cocaine-induced anxiety disorder, cocaine-induced sexual dysfunction, cocaine-induced sleep disorder, and cocaine-related disorder not otherwise specified (American Psychiatric Association, 2000). Intoxication is characterized by euphoria, increased perception of self, and increased endurance. Withdrawal from crack/cocaine is characterized by agitation and irritability. Recovery is usually within 48 hours, with depression continuing for several weeks (Sadock & Sadock, 2007).

In the United States, amphetamines (Dexedrine, Desoxyn, Adderall, and Ritalin) are the third most widely used drugs, after cannabis and cocaine. Drugs containing amphetamines have been used as stimulants, weight-loss aids, cold remedies, and treatments for attention-deficit/hyperactivity disorder and narcolepsy. Amphetamines are contraindicated for those with hypertension and are habit forming. They have been known to induce a toxic psychosis and can be fatal. Amphetamine intoxication resembles that of cocaine. The typical dependency picture is one of weight loss and paranoid ideation. Withdrawal symptoms include anxiety, tremors, dysphoric mood, lethargy, fatigue, nightmares, headache, excess perspiration, stomach cramps, muscle cramps, and ravenous appetite. Depression can be a reaction to long-term, high-dose use and can lead to suicide (Sadock & Sadock, 2007).

Cannabis (THC, marijuana, hashish, hemp, ganja, and bhang) is the most frequently used illicit substance. Although the evidence for physiological addiction is weak, a high potential for psychological addiction exists. Once tolerance has been developed, a withdrawal syndrome, including irritability, restlessness, insomnia, and anorexia, will be experienced when the drug is stopped (Preuss, Watzke, Zimmermann, Wong, & Schmidt, 2010).

Hallucinogens (natural: psilocybin from mushrooms and mescaline from peyote cactus; synthetic: lysergic acid diethylamide [LSD]) are sometimes called *psychedelics* or *psychotomimetics* because they mimic psychosis (Sadock & Sadock, 2007). Hallucinogenic intoxication includes paranoia, anxiety or depression, fear of loss of control, impaired judgment, distorted perceptions, depersonalization, derealization, and hallucinations. Physiological changes may include pupillary dilation, tachycardia profuse perspiration, palpitations, blurred vision, tremors, and/or incoordination. Approximately 10% of the American public have used a hallucinogen at least once, and more than 50% were less than 20 years of age. Relative to other illicit substances, hallucinogens are related to less morbidity and less mortality (American Psychiatric Association, 2000).

## Target Areas for Intervention

Over the long term, behaviors related to substance dependency take precedence over those associated with more productive life roles (Sadock & Sadock, 2007). The focus of occupational therapy intervention is on the facilitation of the patient's ability to choose more adaptive, substance-free methods of dealing with the stressors of daily life.

# 🌿 Contextual Considerations

## Clinical

The context of the dependency and the type of substance used will affect the tenacity of the condition and its long-term ramifications. A history of the client's substance use can alert the practitioner to the existence of substance dependence. Individuals who have a lifestyle and life history of consistent substance abuse may view sobriety as foreign and may be sufficiently uncomfortable to discourage any investment in recovery. Many long-term users may go through detoxification programs and participate in rehabilitation programs multiple times before embracing recovery. Relapses in recovery may occur because of the lure of the addictive substances and habituation of behaviors associated with substance abuse.

A study by Volkow et al. (2001) found that, compared with participants who never used drugs, methamphetamine abusers had reduced control of movement, attention, motivation, and judgment. This may explain the tendency of substance abusers to engage in risky behaviors related to their addictions without regard for the dangers that might befall them or others. Long-term substance abuse can result in permanent changes to neurological structures, causing conditions such as dementia and related short-term memory deficits, and/or permanent damage to respiratory, gastrointestinal, liver, or cardiac systems. The *Mini-Mental State Examination* (MMSE; Folstein, Folstein, & McHugh, 1975) will help identify possible dementia, but it focuses primarily on short-term memory function as an indicator. An MMSE score below 26 is a strong indicator of possible dementia.

The *Routine Task Inventory* (Allen, Earhart, & Blue, 1992) and the *Allen Cognitive Level Screen–Fifth Edition* (ACLS-5; Allen et al., 2007) are practical performance measures. The ACL assesses cognitive capacity, or an ability to learn, and it uses such landmark phenomena as error recognition, use of three-dimensional concepts, and ability to problem solve. Individuals who are agitated or depressed may score lower than their ability. Low scores, especially those below 5.0, indicate that the patient is limited in understanding cause and effect and is therefore at risk for safety.

The *Kohlman Evaluation of Living Skills* (KELS; Kohlman, 1992) is a tool used to assess the patient's instrumental activities of daily living. It is not unusual for someone with a low score on the ACL to perform moderately well on the KELS. However, it is fairly consistent that a low ACL score will accompany a poor performance on the safety measures on the KELS. The *Occupational Case Assessment and Inventory Rating Scale* (Forsyth et al., 2005) and the *Role Checklist* (Oakley, Kielhofner, & Barris, 1986) may be helpful in determining patients' perceptions of their performance of various life roles and understanding of the impact of their behavior on others.

## Family

Learning disabilities and developmental delays have been linked to maternal substance abuse during pregnancy (Zuckerman, 1985). In addition to the developmental consequences for infants who are born to substance abusers, substance use disorder often engenders a tangled constellation of dysfunctional family dynamics that is often referred to as *enmeshment* or *codependence,* which perpetuates maladaptive coping strategies and continued substance abuse. A comprehensive assessment of the social support systems available to the patient and the patient's insight regarding the family's effect on substance abuse (and vice versa) yields important information regarding the scope of intervention. The support systems available to the patient can either represent a strong barrier to rehabilitation or provide a strong impetus for recovery. If others in the household tolerate or condone the substance abuse, the enabling behaviors and codependent relationships that are engendered by these attitudes may complicate the rehabilitation effort. Conversely, family and friends who are actively engaged in reinforcing a substance-free lifestyle facilitate recovery.

Garnering primary family support may be difficult because substance abusers may frequently lie, manipulate, and distort reality in order to justify continued substance abuse. Although clients with substance use disorders may be demanding, they are frequently masking a sense of being undeserving of care. They often have difficulty recognizing and trusting success and unconsciously sabotage the successes they make in the recovery process. Habitual behaviors lead these clients to hide their feelings and hurt others before others hurt them; hence, they have few nonabusing friends. They often blame others for their problems and see life as devoid of meaning. Family education increases the understanding of the addiction phenomenon. Alcoholics Anonymous, Narcotics Anonymous, Alateen, and Al-Anon are examples of support groups for individuals with substance use disorders and their families.

## Practice Setting

An occupational therapy practitioner can expect to work with clients who are abusing or dependent on substances in any setting (e.g., schools, hospitals, community programs, assisted living centers) and in any age group (children through geriatric patients). The problem of substance abuse can occur as a result of or in addition to other problems. Individuals with substance abuse problems may be encountered in homeless shelters, prisons, and physical medicine and rehabilitation facilities.

## Sociopolitical

Treatment services for substance use disorders may be provided in free-standing facilities, hospitals, or governmental agencies. Many of these facilities are equipped to assist individuals with comorbidities, such as mental illness and substance abuse. Although government funding for these facilities and programs has diminished, the implementation of federal and state parity legislation has resulted in reimbursement for many substance use disorders, such as alcoholism, as a chronic disease.

In the mid to late 2000s, the approach to addiction-related illnesses began to change as the government-directed recovery transformation and the Mental Health Parity Act (MHPA, 2008) were introduced. Treatment approaches have become more client centered and more focused on supportive treatment and prevention. Community-based programs have begun to emphasize the development of practice supports needed for pursuing a recovery journey.

## Lifestyle/Lifespan

The norms and habits associated with substance use disorder can define the context of entire families. A culture that is built around substance abuse does not foster the acquisition of stable employment and the engagement in a healthy and meaningful lifestyle. Physical and psychological isolation is a common outcome. Support groups like Alcoholics Anonymous, Narcotics Anonymous, and Dual Recovery Anonymous offer peer-to-peer support to help addicts pursue their recovery journeys through 12-step programs.

# ▧ Clinical Decision-Making Process

## Defining Focus for Intervention

In the early stages of recovery, the focus of occupational therapy intervention is education about the recovery process and engagement in activity that rekindles a sense of self-efficacy and hope for the future. As treatment continues, the emphasis shifts to self-expression, the development of coping strategies, and the exploration of aftercare plans. While they are sober, clients need to experience feelings and activities that are related to their recovery, identify healthy ways to get support, express their feelings, have fun, find excitement in living, cope with stress, and find peace within themselves. Ongoing treatment in the community focuses on applying this new knowledge when returning to the home environment, finding or continuing employment, building relationships, engaging in recreational and stress reduction skills, and building healthy support systems.

Prisons and other correctional or forensic facilities are sites where occupational therapy practitioners may work with substance abusers. The goals and expectations of treatment are not always geared toward discharge but are paced in accordance with the stressors present in the facility and the lengths of the sentences of the clients. A goal may be to help the prisoner establish strategies for functioning safely and effectively without substances within the correctional facility.

## Establishing Goals for Intervention

The goals for treatment need to be practical and understandable to the client. When clients are part of goal planning, they feel a stronger sense of control in their treatment. The treatment becomes meaningful to them, which can increase their level of participation. Common issues around which goals are developed are anger management, stress management and outlets for feelings, effective self-expression and communication, building of support systems, awareness of self and values, spirituality, relational skills, education on symptoms of relapse, relapse prevention, wellness, and self-care. Each of these issues becomes a meaningful goal when it is coupled with particular events or personal stressors.

## Designing Theory-Based Intervention

Theoretical frameworks with a basis in learning theories, such as a developmental model or one that addresses roles and values, like the model of human occupation, effectively guide the occupational therapist in developing interventions for treatment of substance abusers. The habituated process of developing a dependence on substances and the associated roles and distorted values developed through an addiction require a major life change as the client works toward recovery. Each of these theoretical models guides the occupational therapist in understanding the development of the aberrant behaviors and the enduring process of changing the ingrained habits that the substance-dependent client has developed. The intervention often commences with instruments such as the *Occupational Performance History Interview–Second Edition* (Kielhofner et al., 2004), which engages the client's perspective and helps form a basis for self-discovery and goal planning. In a psychiatric hospital or a psychiatric unit in a general hospital, patients may have co-occurring disorders, a combination of substance abuse and a mental illness, like schizoaffective disorder or depression. An assessment of cognitive abilities may be needed to inform the development of meaningful intervention strategies that are geared to the functional level of the client (Allen et al., 1992).

## Evaluating Progress

Long-term effects of treatment are difficult to evaluate because of the high incidence of recidivism among substance abusers. The occupational therapist assesses the clients' progress in treatment by listening to what they say and observing their approach to tasks and activities. The use of self-actualization techniques, like motivational interviewing, helps facilitate the client's understanding of the need for change (Rollnick, Miller, & Butler, 2008). In concert with other members of the rehabilitation team, the occupational therapist ascertains the congruency and consistency of the clients' words and actions.

## Determining Change in or Termination of Treatment

The move from one phase of recovery to the next and, finally, to discharge is determined by the client's progressive and consistent application of adaptive coping strategies. Engagement in community-based support groups may aid in the transition to aftercare. Termination occurs when the client has abstained from substances for a specified period of time, has realistic plans for postdischarge, and has arranged to follow up with a supporting organization.

# Case Study

*Description*

SC is a 33-year-old attorney, wife, and mother of three who has a history of using substances such as alcohol and amphetamines that extends back to her college and law school days. SC states that she needed to use these substances to deal with the stresses associated with a rigorous academic program. For the past 4 years, SC has been abusing cocaine. After her second child was born, SC decided to put her career on hold and stay at home to raise her three children, who are 5, 6, and 9 years old. Her husband works quite a distance from home and stays near the office 3 nights per week. Over time, SC has become increasingly more isolated and does not feel that she has any friends, except for her brother, who also abuses cocaine and procures the drug for SC. She frequently uses alcohol as well, to increase the high or when she runs out of cocaine. SC has attempted to hide her addiction from her family by using when the children are at school and her husband is at work. However, her children and husband have noticed that SC has gone from being stylish, outgoing, and communicative to being slovenly, distant, and secretive. A neighbor finally alerted SC's husband that SC had been routinely forgetting to pick her children up from school.

At her husband's insistence, SC tried outpatient treatment and Cocaine Anonymous, but her attendance was sporadic because she insisted that she did not have a problem and could quit anytime on her own. One day, when her children were visiting their grandparents, her husband found her unconscious on the kitchen floor when he came home for a weekend. After having her stomach pumped at a local hospital, she was diagnosed with major depressive disorder and substance abuse disorder and admitted to a psychiatric hospital co-occurring disorder unit. Denying her problem, she angrily blamed her brother "for getting [her] into this." Trying to rationalize her addiction, she complained of being bored and lonely at home. Recognizing the effect of her addiction on her family, she expresses feelings of shame for hurting the people she loves, saying, "I don't deserve their love." The *Role Checklist* (Oakely, Kielhofner, & Barris, 1986) shows she highly values her family, home, productivity at work and hobbies, spiritual life, and friendships. Her depression has left her feeling hopeless, as she is unable to identify roles she has in the present or could have in the future. She has doubts that she will ever be able to live without using cocaine.

SC feels worthless and is doubtful that she can gain a sense of control over her addiction and relationships with her family. SC's habituated lifestyle does not include a feeling of productivity in any area, although being productive is very important to her. Her addiction has consumed her leisure and reduced her ability to relate effectively to her family and friends. She has become neglectful of herself and her responsibilities. She has a history of successful functioning and a caring and potentially supportive family. The addiction coupled with the depression has distorted her self-concept and her ability to recognize and address problems effectively. She is bright, well educated, and able to engage in logical, sequential thought processes if given a rational basis for processing.

SC, like many addicts, denies or rationalizes the extent of her habit and the hypnotic lure of the cocaine. The change in lifestyle that recovery demands is overwhelming and frightening for SC. Her impulsive actions and thoughts make it difficult for her to accept that there are no quick cures for her addictions. The lack of spiritual energy in her life makes the ordinariness of everyday living seem boring. She will need to make strong connections with her healthy values and roles while in treatment in order to embrace a future without cocaine that seems worth living to her.

### Long- and Short-Term Goals

The long-term goal of intervention for SC is to participate in an intensive outpatient program and to identify and pursue meaningfully satisfying activities that are healthy and practical alternatives to using cocaine. This short-term goal is to identify meaningful activities she can engage in with her family.

### Therapist Goals and Strategies

The therapist's goals include the following:

1. Stimulate SC to think about her role in the family.
2. Rekindle SC's interests in doing activities without using cocaine.
3. Facilitate SC's recognition of her self-worth.

The therapist's strategies include the following:

1. Provide concrete evidence of SC's interests and roles in the family through activity.
2. Facilitate SC's self-reflection through group process and direct, honest feedback.

### Activity: Self-Discovery Tapestry

Using a life review instrument, such as the *Self-Discovery Tapestry* (Meltzer, 2001), SC will be able to rediscover the positive aspects of her life, establish how critical events in her life facilitated or hampered her progress toward her life goals, and redefine and expand her life goals for the future. In a group setting, SC will complete the survey and then complete the Tapestry Form with various colored markers. The completed Tapestry Form will yield a graphic representation of SC's valued occupations and motivating elements, like family and career, and provide a picture of her future goals and aspirations.

The group members are asked to share their Tapestry Forms with each other. Through a facilitated discussion, they will help each other identify adaptive or maladaptive coping strategies that they have used in their various life transitions, discuss ways to overcome obstacles that prevent them from achieving their goals, and suggest strategies for effective utilization of support systems. Tapestry Forms can be referred to during subsequent group sessions to gauge progress toward goals and reflect on successful application of newly learned coping strategies.

### Treatment Objectives

SC will identify at least two activities that will facilitate progress toward her life goals and accept feedback from her peers about her choices.

## Resources

Alcoholics Anonymous: www.alcoholics-anonymous.org

Al-Anon Family Groups: www.al-anon.alateen.org

Narcotics Anonymous: www.na.org

National Institute on Alcohol Abuse and Alcoholism: www.niaaa.nih.gov

National Institute on Drug Abuse: http://www.drugabuse.gov/nidahome.html

Substance Abuse and Mental Health Services Administration: http://www.samhsa .gov/

# References

Allen, C., Austin, S., David, S., Earhart, C., McCraith, D., & Riska-Williams, L. (2007). *Manual for the Allen Cognitive Level Screen-5 (ACLS-5) and Large Allen Cognitive Level Screen-5 (LACLS-5)*. Camarillo, CA: ACLS and LACLS Committee.

Allen, C. K., Earhart, C. A., & Blue, T. (1992). *Occupational therapy treatment goals for the physically and cognitively disabled*. Rockville, MD: The American Occupational Therapy Association.

American Psychiatric Association. (2000). *Diagnostic and statistical manual of mental disorders* (4th ed., text revision). Washington, DC: Author.

Folstein, M. F., Folstein, S., & McHugh, P. R. (1975). Mini-mental state: A practical method for grading the cognitive state of patients for the clinician. *Journal of Psychiatric Research, 12,* 189.

Forsyth, K., Deshpande, S., Kielhofner, G., Henriksson, C., Haglund, L., Olson, L., Skinner, S., & Kulkarmi, S. (2005). *The occupational circumstances assessment interview and rating scale* (Version 4.0). Chicago: Model of Human Occupation Clearinghouse, University of Illinois.

Kielhofner, G., Mallinson, T., Crawford, E., Nowak, M., Rigby, M., Henry, A., & Walens, D. (2004). *Occupational performance history interview* (Version 2.1). Chicago: Model of Human Occupation Clearinghouse, University of Illinois.

Kohlman, L. T. (1992). *Kohlman evaluation of living skills*. Rockville, MD: American Occupational Therapy Association.

Meltzer, P. (2001). Using the Self-Discovery Tapestry to explore occupational careers. *Journal of Occupational Science, 8*(2), 16–24.

Oakley, F., Kielhofner, G., & Barris, R. (1986). The role checklist. *Occupational Therapy Journal of Research, 6,* 157–170.

Paul Wellstone and Pete Domenici Mental Health Parity and Addiction Equity Act of 2008, 29 C.F.R. § 2590 *et seq.* (2008).

Preuss, U. W., Watzke, A. B., Zimmermann, J., Wong, W. M., & Schmidt, C. O. (2010). Cannabis withdrawal severity and short-term course among cannabis-dependent adolescent and young adult inpatients. *Drug and Alcohol Dependence, 106*(2), 133–141.

Rollnick, S., Miller, W., & Butler, C. (2008). *Motivational interviewing in health care: Helping patients change behavior*. New York, NY: Guilford Press.

Sadock, B. J., & Sadock, V. A. (2007). *Kaplan and Sadock's synopsis of psychiatry: Behavioral sciences/clinical psychiatry* (10th ed.). Philadelphia, PA: Lippincott, Williams & Wilkins.

Substance Abuse and Mental Health Services Administration. (2010). *Results from the 2009 National Survey on Drug Use and Health: Volume I. Summary of national findings* (Office of Applied Studies, NSDUH Series H-38A, HHS Publication No. SMA 10-4586 Findings). Rockville, MD: Author.

Volkow, N., Chang, L., Wang, G.-J., Fowler, J. S., Leonido-Yee, M., Franceschi, D., . . . Miller, E. N. (2001) Association of dopamine transporter reduction with psycho-motor impairment in methamphetamine abusers. *American Journal of Psychiatry, 158*, 377–382.

Zuckerman, B. (1985). Developmental consequences of maternal drug use during pregnancy. *National Institute on Drug Abuse Research, 59*, 96–107.

# Schizophrenia and Related Disorders

*C. Thomas North*

*Nancy Beck*

##  Synopsis of Clinical Condition

### Prevalence and Etiology

Thought disorders, which include schizophrenia and psychoses, represent some of the most serious mental disorders. The typical disease course is a relatively early onset (late teens for men, early 20s for women), followed by a lifelong illness that can severely impact the patient's functioning and participation (Sadock & Sadock, 2007). Worldwide, the prevalence of schizophrenia is between 0.5% and 1.5% of the population. Onset may be insidious or abrupt. There is typically a prodromal phase, which is characterized by a decrease in hygiene, social withdrawal, and loss of interest in school or work. Some individuals may remain chronically ill, while others may experience remissions and exacerbations. Full recovery is uncommon.

The disorders in this grouping are characterized by a predominance of psychotic symptoms. Psychotic symptoms may be present as secondary features in other disorders, such as mood disorders and dementias. The following disorders will be discussed in this chapter:

- schizophrenia
- schizophreniform disorder
- schizoaffective disorder
- delusional disorder
- brief psychotic disorder
- shared psychotic disorder

### Common Characteristics and Symptoms

Symptoms of schizophrenia are described as *positive* or *negative*. Positive symptoms include delusions, hallucinations, and agitation, whereas negative symptoms include flattened or dulled affect, poverty of speech, apathy, anhedonia, withdrawal, and inattentiveness. If delusions are bizarre, no other symptoms are necessary for the diagnosis of schizophrenia (American Psychiatric Association, 2000). Similarly, if the hallucinations are auditory and consist of a running commentary of the patient's thoughts or behaviors, or are a conversation between two or more voices, no other symptoms are necessary. Auditory hallucinations are by far the most frequent type of hallucinatory symptoms. Gustatory, olfactory, or tactile hallucinations may have a neurological or physical cause (Sadock & Sadock, 2007).

There are five subtypes of schizophrenia. Paranoid type is characterized by a predominance of delusions, paranoia, and possibly hallucinations, with minimum disturbance of speech, thought, or affect and little disorganized or catatonic behavior. A diagnosis of disorganized type is made if the patient's predominant symptoms are disorganized speech, disorganized behavior, and disturbed affect. A third subtype is catatonic type. A patient with this diagnosis can exhibit motoric immobility or stupor, excessive or purposeless activity, extreme negativism or muteness, peculiar posturing, stereotyped movements, peculiar mannerisms, grimacing, echolalia, or echopraxia.

At least two symptoms from this list are necessary to make the diagnosis. The most typical manifestation of schizophrenia is the undifferentiated type. This label is applied if most of the criteria for schizophrenia are present but none are sufficiently prominent to label the schizophrenia as catatonic type, paranoid type, or disorganized type. Residual type schizophrenia differs from the others in that there is a preponderance of negative symptoms, whereas positive symptoms are virtually absent (American Psychiatric Association, 2000).

The major differences between schizophreniform disorder and schizophrenia are the duration of symptoms and the level of impairment. In schizophreniform disorder, the duration exceeds 1 month but is less than 6 months and does not usually precipitate a significant change in social, occupational, or self-care function (American Psychiatric Association, 2000). Between 60% and 80% of individuals diagnosed with schizophreniform disorder will progress to schizophrenia (Sadock & Sadock, 2007).

The diagnosis of schizoaffective disorder is somewhat complex. The patient must display symptoms of schizophrenia and, at some point, concurrently experience a depressive episode, a manic episode, or a mixed episode. Delusions or hallucinations must be present, and they must be in the absence of the mood symptoms. In both instances, substance use and medical causes must be ruled out (American Psychiatric Association, 2000).

Delusional disorder, which is also known as *paranoia*, *paranoid psychosis*, or *paranoid state*, is characterized by the presence of nonbizarre delusions for at least 1 month, the possible presence of delusion-congruent tactile or olfactory hallucinations (other schizophrenic symptoms are absent), and minimal impairment of functioning. Mood episodes, if present, are brief relative to delusional periods (American Psychiatric Association, 2000).

Brief psychotic disorder lasts from 1 day to 1 month. With a rapid onset, it is frequently in response to a major life event. Symptoms are similar to that of schizophrenia, but only one of the symptoms need be present (American Psychiatric Association, 2000). Negative symptoms are absent.

Shared psychotic disorder, which is also known as *shared paranoid disorder*, *induced psychotic disorder*, *folie à deux*, *folie impose*, and *dual insanity*, usually involves two individuals living together in relative isolation. One, the primary case, is chronically ill and delusional. The other person, the secondary case, is typically dependent and may be passive, suggestible, and less intelligent than the primary case. The secondary case eventually embraces the same delusions as the primary case. If and when the primary case is removed from the situation, the secondary case has a spontaneous remission (Sadock & Sadock, 2007).

Among those factors associated with a better prognosis are good premorbid adjustment, acute onset, later onset, retention of insight, precipitating events, presence of mood disorder symptoms, good family support, education beyond high school, and marriage. Factors associated with poor prognosis include early onset, no precipitating factors, insidious onset, poor premorbid adjustment, history of negative symptoms prior to diagnosis, lack of meaningful social relationships, family history of schizophrenia, poor support systems, no remissions within 3 years, numerous relapses, and limited education (Sadock & Sadock, 2007).

The causes of schizophrenia are unknown. Recent research suggests that schizophrenia is not one disease but possibly several different diseases with different causes that manifest as similar disorders. It has been speculated that factors such as dopamine processing, serotonin imbalance, viral infection, trauma, and stress may be linked to schizophrenia (Sadock & Sadock, 2007). Schizophrenia is a complex disorder that is the result of a combination of biomedical and psychosocial factors. A combined approach to treatment, which includes antipsychotic medications along with nonpharmacological approaches, including occupational therapy, is most frequently used with this population (Sadock & Sadock, 2007).

The occupational therapist should be aware of the side effects of the pharmacological treatments used with this population. Antipsychotic medications fall into two major groups: the dopamine receptor agonists, and the serotonin–dopamine antagonists. Dopamine receptor agonists (e.g., Thorazine, Stelazine, Prolixin, Mellaril, Serentil, Navane, Loxitane, Moban, Haldol) were formulated to control the positive symptoms of psychosis, such as delusions and hallucinations. These medications have unpleasant and serious side effects.

The most widely used medications are serotonin–dopamine antagonists (e.g., Clozaril [clozapine], Risperdal [risperidone], Zyprexa [olanzapine]), which treat the positive and negative symptoms of psychosis and have fewer and less serious side effects. Patients on serotonin–dopamine antagonists have fewer relapses and fewer hospitalizations than patients who are not. The adverse effects of clozapine include dizziness, sedation, tachycardia, hypotension, electrocardiogram changes, nausea, sialorrhea (excessive salivation), anticholinergic effects, and muscle weakness. At high doses, there is a 4% risk of seizures. Blood disorders (leukopenia, granulocytopenia, agranulocytosis) occur in less than 1% of these patients but are potentially lethal (Sadock & Sadock, 2007).

## Target Areas for Intervention

Foci for occupational therapy intervention include working with the client to identify personal goals and develop functional interactive and self-care skills, reality orientation, and task modification to compensate for disorders in judgment and organization.

# ⚘ Contextual Considerations

## Clinical

Individuals with schizophrenia have difficulty with social interaction, new learning, and comprehending causality. The *Allen Cognitive Levels Test* (ACL; Allen et al., 2007) provides information regarding the patient's capacity for learning unfamiliar tasks (Leung & Man, 2007). The *Routine Task Inventory* (Allen, Earhart, & Blue, 1992) and the *Kohlman Evaluation of Living Skills* (KELS; Kohlman, 1992) are performance-based tests that employ familiar instrumental activities of daily living. Typically, the person who does poorly on the ACL will not do well on the safety tasks in the KELS because the latter require an understanding of cause and effect. The *Occupational Circumstances Assessment Interview and Rating Scale* (OCAIRS; Forsyth et al., 2005) is useful in that it provides an indication of the patient's insight into the personal and familial impact of his or her illness. In addition to assessments of function and insight, the occupational therapist should conduct an interest inventory and a leisure assessment to inform the design of an occupational therapy program that is motivating and engaging for the patient. The client must be involved in decision making and goal setting in order to develop a recovery plan that is meaningful (Pollard & Olin, 2005).

## Family

The emotional and financial cost of caring for the patient with schizophrenia can be burdensome to the family. These factors, in combination with the disordered social and communication patterns of the patient, can be very challenging to family interactions, and the patient may become alienated. The primary support system may comprise fellow residents of a group home or community rehabilitative residence. Education regarding the maintenance of a structured, supportive environment that fosters independence is important for the patient and the members of his or her support system (Pollard, 2007).

## Practice Setting

Although individuals who are severely impaired remain in long-term, structured residences, the U.S. Department of Health and Human Services Substance Abuse and Mental Health Services Administration advocates for consumers' living in the least restrictive setting that is agreeable to them. Community reintegration and reduced dependence on institutional living is the desired outcome of inpatient treatment. Inpatient occupational therapy treatment focuses on engaging the patient in interests, generating hope for recovery, recognizing symptoms, and identifying practical coping strategies.

Partial hospital programs allow the patient to live in the community while he or she attends a daily treatment program. Partial programs emphasize the development of skills needed to engage in meaningful life occupations, such as social interactions, self-care, community mobility, work, and symptom recognition and management. Although occupational therapy is indicated in this aspect of treatment, reimbursement for this type of intervention may be limited.

The "clubhouse" format is an example of a peer-managed, community-based day program. Although few professional staff members are present, this venue provides clients with the opportunity to develop a social network and work skills and to engage in productive activity. Locally funded drop-in centers provide clients who have ongoing psychiatric needs with a safe environment in which to engage in productive activity and develop community living skills. Peer support groups, such as Dual Recovery Anonymous and the National Alliance on Mental Illness, provide support for sustaining productive and meaningful community living.

## Sociopolitical

The U.S. Department of Health and Human Services Substance Abuse and Mental Health Services Administration implemented the recovery model noted in the previous section by launching major advances in advocacy and actions to address the stigma of mental illness and offer dignity to all individuals who have a mental illness. The focus on advocacy, client empowerment, and community-based recovery strategies facilitated significant improvements in the reimbursement for mental health services.

## Lifestyle/Lifespan

Delusions may result in the patient not taking prescribed medication. The dosages, timing, and number of different medications may confuse the patient who is cognitively involved. Inconsistent management or cessation of a medication regimen may cause repeated hospitalizations. The maladaptive behaviors associated with this condition, if not mitigated, may put the patient at risk for lifelong social isolation.

The devastating and enduring effects of the illness create a lifelong need for support for clients and their caregivers (Pollard, 2007). Local chapters of organizations like the National Association on Mental Illness provide ongoing support for individuals and families who live with schizophrenia and other psychotic disorders.

## 🖉 Clinical Decision-Making Process

### Defining Focus for Intervention

Using data gathered from referral documentation, the medical history, patient and caregiver interviews, and assessment tools such as the OCAIRS and the KELS, the occupational therapist assesses the client's habits, roles, and capabilities. Consultation with the client, in concert with a history and description of the client's routines, gives an indication of the client's goals and aspirations, the barriers to those goals, and the potential for productive participation in the client's chosen life tasks (Kielhofner et al., 2004).

The focus for occupational therapy intervention is usually reduction of the barriers to the client's active participation in life tasks. For instance, if diminished cognitive abilities and/or distracting hallucinations impair the client's ability to consistently manage his or her medication routine, then reality orientation and task simplification may become the focus for occupational therapy. If maladaptive communication skills hinder the client's social interaction, then activities that provide practice in differentiating passive, assertive, and aggressive communication patterns may be the focus for intervention.

### Establishing Goals for Intervention

In an inpatient setting, the primary goal is reduction of symptoms so they do not interfere with function and the safety of the client and others. Specific goals are informed by the needs that are expressed by the client and may include the mitigation of delusional thoughts, the reduction of impulsive behaviors, and the improvement of concentration and attention through the use of activity. In a community setting, intervention will be focused on public demeanor, family and peer relationships, self-care, and employment. Both the patient and the family should be educated in the nature of the disease and symptom recognition. As clients and caregivers become more skillful in recognizing the signs of impending exacerbations, they will be able to seek professional assistance before a crisis results.

### Designing Theory-Based Intervention

The model of human occupation, occupational behavior theory, and the tenets of the recovery model are key sources for the development of intervention strategies. By using a client-centered, occupation-based perspective, the therapist, in concert with the client, can frame interventions that will facilitate successful engagement in the life tasks that are consistent with the client's personal identity. Assessments like the *Role Checklist* (Oakley, Kielhofner, & Barris, 1986) and OCAIRS provide a method for the therapist to assist the client in prioritizing life tasks and occupations, identifying barriers to successful engagement in these occupations, and designing strategies for overcoming these barriers. Activities that are designed to elicit coping behaviors form the core of occupational therapy intervention, while educational sessions and group discussion are employed to relate the activity experience to daily life and stimulate internalization of newly learned coping skills. In addition to engagement in structured therapy activities and discussion groups, occupational therapists may encourage client interest in leisure and/or exercise activities that can foster self-reliance and self-efficacy and can be continued after discharge. For example, the patient, though limited in some areas, may express the need to assume the role of parent, child, sibling, student, or worker. The occupational therapist can assist in the process through analysis of the patient's skills and the skills necessary for the successful execution of the life tasks that are inherent to the roles that have been identified. The focus of intervention may be on the identification, modification, and/or adaptation of the tasks or environment in which they are performed.

The cognitive disabilities framework (Allen, Earhart, & Blue, 1992) helps to define the client's cognitive abilities and limitations based on observation of performance on a series of unfamiliar tasks. The cognitive disabilities that often accompany schizophrenia are frequently manifested in an inability to manage medication routines. Occupational therapists may often simplify tasks by reducing the number of decisions or steps required for successful task completion. For instance, to simplify the management of many daily medications, the therapist might construct a partitioned pillbox and place a picture of each pill in each of the partitions. This strategy would provide the patient with visual and physical cues as he or she fills the pillbox daily. The recapitulation of ontogenesis frame of reference (Mosey, 1986) focuses on the developmental nature of interaction. A patient who suffers from irritability, agitation, and withdrawal because of paranoid ideation may be treated in a series of activity sessions that require progressive levels of interaction (solitary, parallel, dyadic, and group) in order to increase social interaction skills.

## Evaluating Progress

Functional activity is evidence of mastery for the client and an essential ongoing evaluation tool for the practitioner. A completed task (e.g., craft, picture, written exercise) provides tangible evidence of functionality. The manner in which the client approaches a task, the level of support the client requires for successful completion of a task, and the reaction of the client to task completion are all indicators of progress. Through the analysis of the client's performance on the activity, the practitioner can measure improvement and assess to what extent the client is progressing toward the goals of treatment.

# Determining Change in or Termination of Treatment

Clinical observation helps the practitioner assess the client's reality orientation, attention span, social interaction, safety awareness, and other skills that will be required in the discharge environment. At times it may be necessary to terminate a client from a group or session because behavior, peer interaction, verbal outbursts, or sudden paranoid response compromises the safety of the patient or others.

## Case Study

### Description

JM is a 55-year-old man who was diagnosed with schizophrenia when he was 21 years old. JM has been in and out of hospitals for most of his adult life. Before the onset of his illness, he graduated from high school and successfully held a series of clerical positions of which he was very proud. After the onset of his illness, which included auditory hallucinations, he attempted to work but was fired from several jobs. He applied for state-funded medical assistance. He now lives with his four brothers and his mother, who are supportive caregivers. They are a little confused about how to handle his periodic irrational thoughts and outbursts but are basically good supports for him. He is ambulatory and in good physical health. JM frequently engages in long, boisterous harangues and vehemently denies that he has any problems. When he started attending occupational therapy groups in a partial hospitalization program, he would loudly proclaim, "Hi, I'm fine. I don't have any problems. Let me help you. How are you?" JM has good memories of working and takes pride in the service he provided through work. He is clean and well dressed and eager to help his peers and the staff. He enjoys doing many of the activities provided in the program. He follows through with the responsibilities he is given but needs direction to get started.

JM takes pride in working with and helping others. He has a boisterous voice and a friendly, helpful demeanor. He needs to do concrete tasks and be in a supportive atmosphere with reduced stimuli in order to be an effective worker, and he no longer requires the partial hospitalization environment. He is anxious about leaving the partial program with which he has become familiar and comfortable. He doesn't want to change and asks, "Why can't I just be picked up by the van, come to partial, and work in ceramics, instead of attending groups?" Although he is resistant to taking public transportation, he is capable of independently negotiating the bus routes. He is capable of caring for himself with guidance and support from his family. Although he is not a self-starter, he is reliable in independently completing tasks that are given to him. He requires regular, supportive, and encouraging feedback to gain a sense of satisfaction in his work and feels whole and "normal" when he is able to help others.

His family makes sure that he is clean and dressed. He has been attending the partial hospitalization program 5 days per week and is transported to and from the program by city-funded transportation for individuals with handicapping conditions who cannot negotiate public transportation.

### Long- and Short-Term Goals

JM has expressed that he is very interested in helping others through volunteering. The long-term goal of intervention for JM is to independently use public transportation to commute to volunteer activities. This goal will be reached in part through successfully achieving the short-term goal of negotiating bus travel with the assistance of his brother.

### Therapist Goals and Strategies

The therapist's goals include the following:

1. Increase organizational skills.
2. Increase self-confidence.
3. Increase independence.

The therapist's strategies include the following:

1. Provide family/caregiver education and engage JM's brother to mentor JM as he learns and practices the bus route to and from the hospital.
2. Provide maps that clearly delineate the bus route and walking route from the bus stop to home and to the hospital. Include significant landmarks.
3. Provide training to family so they can assist JM by practicing the route from home to the hospital using maps and identifying landmarks.
4. Gradually reduce partial program days and use of assisted travel.
5. Gradually withdraw assistance and accompany each independently achieved milestone with praise.

### Activity: Assisted Travel on Public Transportation

The therapist will provide family/caregiver education in order to prepare JM's brother to help JM learn the bus schedule and bus route and plan the trip from home to the hospital. The first trip will be on a weekend, when there are few travelers. The family will receive training regarding how to encourage JM to talk about his experience, and the family and therapist will use praise to encourage his continued use of public transportation.

JM wants to help others but is not interested in a full-time job. He has expressed some curiosity and interest in ceramics. The therapist explains to JM that one way to achieve this goal is to transition from his status in the partial program to a volunteer program in the ceramics room. However, at this suggestion, JM appears anxious and resistant. At a meeting with his family and the therapist, it is suggested that this transition from partial hospitalization to volunteerism needs to be gradual to avoid stress-induced exacerbation of his illness. JM agrees that the gradual change will give him a chance to gain mastery over his responsibilities as a volunteer and an independent commuter. The continued support of the treatment program helps him process the feelings that arise as he makes the transition. His family's involvement helps them learn what JM is doing, understand the problems he might face using public transportation, and proactively process solutions that will bring him closer to his ultimate goal of being an independent and productive volunteer.

### Treatment Objectives

JM will be able to independently plan and complete the trip from home to the hospital on public transportation.

# Resources

American Occupational Therapy Association: www.aota.org

National Alliance on Mental Illness: www.nami.org

National Institute of Mental Health: www.nimh.nih.gov

World Fellowship for Schizophrenia and Allied Disorders: www.world-schizophrenia.org

# References

Allen, C., Austin, S., David, S., Earhart, C., McCraith, D., & Riska-Williams, L. (2007). *Manual for the Allen Cognitive Level Screen-5 (ACLS-5) and Large Allen Cognitive Level Screen-5 (LACLS-5)*. Camarillo, CA: ACLS and LACLS Committee.

Allen, C. K., Earhart, C. A., & Blue, T. (1992). *Occupational therapy treatment goals for the physically and cognitively disabled*. Rockville, MD: The American Occupational Therapy Association.

American Psychiatric Association. (2000). *Diagnostic and statistical manual of mental disorders* (4th ed., text revision). Washington, DC: Author.

Forsyth, K., Deshpande, S., Kielhofner, G., Henriksson, C., Haglund, L., Olson, L., Skinner, S., & Kulkarmi, S. (2005). *The occupational circumstances assessment interview and rating scale* (Version 4.0). Chicago: Model of Human Occupation Clearinghouse, University of Illinois.

Kielhofner, G., Mallinson, T., Crawford, E., Nowak, M., Rigby, M., Henry, A., & Walens, D. (2004). *Occupational performance history interview* (Version 2.1). Chicago: Model of Human Occupation Clearinghouse, University of Illinois.

Kohlman, L. T. (1992). *Kohlman evaluation of living skills*. Rockville, MD: American Occupational Therapy Association.

Leung, S. B., & Man, D. (2007). Validity of the Chinese version of the Allen Cognitive Level Screen Assessment for individuals with schizophrenia. *Occupational Therapy Journal of Research: Occupation, Participation and Health, 27*(1) 31–40.

Mosey, A. C. (1986). *Psychosocial components of occupational therapy*. New York, NY: Raven Press.

Oakley, F., Kielhofner, G., & Barris, R. (1986). The role checklist. *Occupational Therapy Journal of Research, 6,* 157–170.

Pollard, D. (2007). *Empowering caregivers: Relevant lifestyle profiles* (2nd ed.). Monoma, WI: Selectone Rehab.

Pollard, D., & Olin, D. (2005). *Allen's cognitive levels: Meeting the challenges of client focused services*. Monoma, WI: Selectone Rehab.

Sadock, B. J., & Sadock, V. A. (2007). *Kaplan and Sadock's synopsis of psychiatry: Behavioral sciences/clinical psychiatry* (10th ed.). Philadelphia, PA: Lippincott, Williams & Wilkins.

# Mood Disorders

*C. Thomas North*
*Nancy Beck*

## 🍃 Synopsis of Clinical Condition

### Prevalence and Etiology

*Mood disorders* is a classification for multiple behavioral health conditions. Depression and bipolar disorder are two of the most prevalent mood disorders that an occupational therapist may encounter in practice. There are three basic elements to all mood disorders: emotional, behavioral, and physical. For mood disorders to be diagnosed, the distress must be clinically significant and cannot be accounted for by another disorder or physical ailment. Mood disorders often develop in the early adult years and greatly affect an individual's level of functioning. The severity of the impact is generally reflected in the length of time one has been suffering with the mood disorder and the types of symptoms he or she is having.

Depression is a serious medical illness that affects 5% to 8% of the U.S. population in any 12-month period. An estimated 15 million people in the United States have a depressive episode each year. Major depressive disorder most typically develops in adolescence or early adulthood and is prevalent in the population at rates of about 5% to 12% for men and twice that for women. There seem to be no significant differences in prevalence related to ethnicity, education, income, or marital status. As many as 15% of individuals diagnosed with major depressive disorder die of suicide. The death rate among those over 55 years of age with major depressive disorder is 4 times that of the general population (American Psychiatric Association, 2000).

### Common Characteristics and Symptoms

Individuals with depression may experience profound sadness or irritability lasting 2 weeks or more, accompanied by changes in sleep and appetite, decreased energy, decreased concentration and memory, a lack of interest in usual activities, and decreased ability to experience pleasure. Frequently, there are feelings of helplessness, worthlessness, shame, and guilt. Psychomotor retardation may also be observed.

The clinical manifestation of depression in children and adolescents differs from that of adults. Grade school children are more likely to complain of generalized aches and pains than they are to report feelings of helplessness and hopelessness. Depression may be observed in adolescents who act out, run away, perform poorly in school, and use drugs and alcohol. Suicide is the third leading cause of death in children between the ages of 15 and 19 years. It is imperative that children and adolescents be fully evaluated and treated when they are experiencing these symptoms.

Individuals with bipolar disorder experience unusually intense emotional states that occur during distinct periods called *mood episodes*. This emotional dysregulation is a core characteristic of the disorder. The mood episode can go from extremely low (depression) to extremely high (mania). Bipolar disorder is often misdiagnosed because individuals who are in a depressed mood episode appear to have the same symptoms as someone with depression, and these individuals are less likely to go to the doctor when they are experiencing the elation associated with a manic episode.

In a manic mood episode, an individual will display increased goal-directed activity, excessive involvement in high-risk activities, decreased need for sleep, increased talkativeness, pressured speech, grandiose delusions or inflated self-worth, flight of ideas or racing thoughts, and extreme distractibility. Typically, these symptoms last more than 1 week, and they often require hospitalization. There is a less intense manic mood episode called *hypomania*, which typically only lasts about 4 days and seldom requires hospitalization.

Symptoms of bipolar disorder may present differently in children and adolescents. Children and adolescents experiencing a depressive episode may feel very sad, have somatic complaints, experience sleep and appetite disturbances, have reduced energy, be apathetic, and have increased suicidal ideation. Children and adolescents during a manic mood episode may act unusually elated or silly, appear agitated, have decreased attention span, and speak very fast with a flight of ideas. They may also have difficulty sleeping but not feel tired and demonstrate an increased participation in risky behaviors.

Commonly prescribed medications for the treatment of depression are called *selective serotonin reuptake inhibitors* (SSRIs). They are generally safe and have limited side effects that may diminish over time (Sadock & Sadock, 2007). For bipolar disorder, the use of antidepressants such as SSRIs is contraindicated, as they may cause an increase in manic and hypomanic behaviors. Individuals with bipolar disorder are often prescribed mood stabilizers such as lithium and Depakote, which require levels to be obtained via blood tests as well as close monitoring by the prescribing physician.

Electroconvulsive therapy (ECT) is an effective treatment for depression and bipolar disorders; however, it is not a first line of treatment. It may be considered in cases for which multiple trials of medications and different therapeutic approaches have not worked. During a course of ECT, an individual is put under anesthesia and electrical impulses are administered. Treatments last from 30 to 90 seconds, and individuals usually recover within 5 to 15 minutes. ECT may cause some short-term side effects, including confusion, disorientation, and memory loss (Pandya, Pozuelo, & Malone, 2007).

## Target Areas for Intervention

The profound sadness and sense of hopelessness that are experienced by individuals who are diagnosed with major depressive disorder or other mood disorders lead to isolation, helplessness, and disengagement from all the activity that supports self-efficacy and gives meaning to life. Occupational therapy focuses on the reestablishment of self-efficacy through engagement in structured activity that is designed to help the client develop a broad repertoire of strategies for coping with the stressors of daily life and resume engagement in life roles.

# 🌾 Contextual Considerations

## Clinical

Clients with mood disorders experience a feeling of hopelessness and helplessness, and suicide or homicide may seem the only way out. They have lost their ability to cope with the stresses in their lives, have become disconnected from their support systems, and have no energy and/or ability to concentrate on engaging in daily activities. Posture, gait, level of alertness, and affect are frequently good indicators of mood. Most mood disorders are cyclical and characterized by manic, hypomanic, and/or depressive cycles punctuated by remission periods in which the patient is fully functional.

The *Role Checklist* (Oakley, Kielhofner, & Barris, 1986) and the *Occupational Circumstances Assessment Interview and Rating Scale* (OCAIRS; Forsyth et al., 2005) provide data regarding the impact of the illness on the patient as well as the patient's perception of others' understanding of the illness. The *Occupational Performance History Interview–Second Edition* (Kielhofner et al., 2004) provides information about support systems and capacity for recovery. The *Canadian Occupational Performance Measure–Fourth Edition* (Law et al., 2005) creates measures for the patient's perception of performance over time.

## Family

A family history of mood disorders, maladaptive behaviors, or depressive episodes is usually present in individuals with mood disorders. Family education and training can facilitate the development of insight into the nature of the illness and strategies for coping with the patient. Both client and family should be trained to recognize the signs of impending manic or depressive episodes.

## Practice Setting

Clients with mood disorders may be seen in acute psychiatric hospitals if they are so debilitated that survival without supervision is unlikely or if they pose a suicide risk. In this setting, the goals for occupational therapy are as follows:

1. Reduce stress and increase receptiveness to treatment.
2. Identify and practice functional coping strategies.
3. Gain insight into solving life issues (Belmont Center for Comprehensive Treatment, 2001).

In a rehabilitation program, partial hospitalization program, or intensive outpatient program, occupational therapy goals focus on gaining independence and consistency in the identification and practice of coping skills and life management. In outpatient settings, goals may focus on coping with work problems, relational problems, parenting, pain management, and depression due to medical problems. Community-based programs include support groups and self-help groups. These approaches work best for those who fully understand their illness and benefit from offering and accepting support from others with similar experiences.

Recovery from a depressive episode is gradual. Frequently, clients participate in individual and group therapy in a partial hospitalization setting coupled with community-based groups and are discharged as soon as the risks are mitigated. In all settings, the client is an active participant in establishing meaningful and practical treatment goals. Goal attainment is dependent on the clients' commitment to and participation in their own recovery. Treatment can be a process of the clients' rekindling or relearning coping strategies that they have used in the past and expanding their repertoire of skills to be able to manage their daily stressors in a more satisfying and productive way.

## Sociopolitical

With the advent of federal and state parity legislation, depression is viewed as a chronic illness and is reimbursed accordingly, typically without any limit to the amount of treatment days required. However, the continued stigma of mental health disorders may cause some individuals to be less likely to seek out services because they are ashamed or embarrassed.

The social stigma of mental illness has ramifications in treatment and recovery. Although legal protection for individuals with mental illness has been ensured by civil rights legislation, lack of public understanding and acceptance of the mentally ill may present barriers to community integration. Advocacy groups, such as the National Alliance on Mental Illness, offer hope with dignity to all individuals who have a mental illness. The Substance Abuse and Mental Health Services Administration and the Center for Mental Health Services promote evidence-based practices in mental health that focus on illness management and recovery, community treatment, family education, and supported employment and housing and facilitate major advances in treatment for mental health disorders.

## Lifestyle/Lifespan

Any disorder that impairs function will have a negative effect on emotional, social, occupational, relational, and financial resources. Medications are a costly, lifelong need. The cyclical nature of mood disorders allows the patient to be productive in periods of remission. The successful patient will learn to recognize the cycles as natural phenomena and can learn to use coping skills and the support of family and friends.

## 🕊 Clinical Decision-Making Process

### Defining Focus for Intervention

Consulting the client's record, conferring with other members of the intervention team, and conducting an initial interview with the client will provide a perspective on family relationships, support systems, interests, work/school issues, pain and medical issues, psychiatric history, living arrangements, precipitating factors leading to treatment, anticipated length of stay in the practice setting, and discharge options, which helps inform the development of occupational therapy intervention.

### Establishing Goals for Intervention

The first step in the treatment process is to assist the client in identifying how the illness has affected the roles, routines, and habits inherent in functional daily living. Once the therapist, in concert with the client, has established the life tasks that are most meaningful to the client, the general goals for intervention are focused on increased awareness of more adaptive coping strategies, assisted engagement in structured activities that require the repeated employment of these strategies, and the progressively independent deployment of these strategies for use in everyday life.

### Designing Theory-Based Intervention

The model of human occupation and occupational behavior theory inform the development of intervention strategies. By using an occupation-based perspective, the therapist can frame interventions that will facilitate successful engagement in the life tasks that define personal identity. Assessments like the *Role Checklist* (Oakley, Kielhofner, & Barris, 1986) and OCAIRS (Forsyth et al., 2005) provide a method by which the therapist and the client can prioritize life tasks and occupations, identify barriers to successful engagement in these occupations, and design strategies for overcoming these barriers.

Activities that are designed to elicit coping behaviors form the core of occupational therapy intervention, and educational sessions and group discussion are used to relate the activity experience to daily life and to stimulate internalization of newly learned coping skills. In addition to engagement in structured therapy activities and discussion groups, an occupational therapist may encourage the client's interest in leisure and/or exercise activities that can foster self-reliance and self-efficacy and be continued after discharge.

Numerous sources are available that can be used to promote and educate clients on a wide variety of coping skills. *Life Management Skills VI* (Korb-Khalsa, Azok, & Leutenberg, 2002) provides excellent resources for group sessions. Board games, paper-and-pencil exercises, role-playing, relaxation exercises, discussion, and sports or physical activity are examples of approaches that can be taken to address most coping skills.

## Evaluating Progress

Diminished lability, reduction of suicidal ideation, increased initiative, increased reflectivity, active engagement, and planning for the future are all indications of progress.

## Determining Change in or Termination of Treatment

If a client shows either no signs or diminished signs of progress after 1 to 2 weeks, it is important to assess the course of treatment. A history of treatment resistance (noncompliance with medications, prolonged depressive episodes, personality disorder with chronic suicidal ideation, chronically dependent personality traits, or chronically obsessive or racing thoughts) may indicate that more time in treatment is needed. It also may indicate that the client has a baseline of diminished function that will not change substantially before discharge. The safety of the client is most important. Discharge plans should include an intensive "step down" from hospitalization, like a partial hospitalization program or a rigorous outpatient regimen.

Support systems become very important when considering discharge and are an ongoing issue addressed in almost all treatment interventions. Depression does not suddenly appear, and it does not suddenly go away. The recovery process continues after discharge from all settings. The clients' support network can strengthen the process, adding increased stability for the transition from discharge to quality lifestyle. It is helpful to meet with the family or other support network before discharge to provide education about the illness or facilitate communication between the client and his or her supports. Discharge readiness occurs when the client is stable enough to safely move on to the next level of care or is able to resume daily functions using the support of outpatient services, medication, family, or significant others.

### Case Study

*Description*

BT is a 28-year-old second-year medical student who attends school in the Northeast. He admitted himself to the hospital for the second time in a year, after taking an overdose of his psychiatric medication. He lives alone and has minimal contact with his family, who live in the West. He has casual friends from class but no close friends or relatives in the area. In the initial assessment interview, he was quiet and somewhat reluctant to talk but admitted that he had stopped going to classes for about 2 weeks, had stopped eating, and was sleeping a lot. He was having difficulty concentrating and had been refusing to answer the phone. His limited interests included studying, running by himself, and occasionally going to the park to watch the boat races. He admitted spending a lot of time alone in his apartment. His psychiatric history revealed that he had been seeing a psychiatrist at school for the past year. He appeared in an occupational therapy group for the first time with sad affect and quiet demeanor, clean, conservatively dressed, and sitting somewhat stiffly by himself, not talking to his peers.

Upon further assessment via interview, BT talked about his family life, saying abruptly with a slight edge in his tone, "My parents aren't affectionate. They only tell me what I do wrong. Sometimes my mom encourages me but not too often. We live in a small town, where everyone knows about me going to school in the Northeast and don't think that I'll make it." The *Role Checklist* revealed that of his roles in life, he valued being a family member and a student and had some interest in friendship, but he did not define family member or friend as a role he held presently. He pictured his future as being a student. He indicated that he used to like going places and doing things with his friends and wanted his family to be more supportive.

The results of the assessments indicated that BT is a shy person who has difficulty expressing his feelings effectively. He also seems to have difficulty expressing anger in a satisfying way, turning his anger inward toward himself. His view of the future is sparse and limited to the immediate future, with student being the only role he envisions. He may be feeling an overwhelming fear and pressure to prove to his hometown that he can succeed. He has marginal confidence in his psychiatrist but is fearful of changing to a new psychiatrist. BT has a limited repertoire of activity and seems unable to expand his interests. His supports are limited to his psychiatrist and a casual female friend, whom he only sees in class. He has pervasive hopelessness about the future and is unable to cope with his relational and school stressors. He has difficulty seeing the relevance of leisure outlets and has extreme difficulty expressing his feelings. He seems to lack role models and methods for feeling expression; hence, his thoughts are internalized, without the benefit of others' perspectives. His goal is to return to school and not be so lonely. Through treatment, he can learn to use activities to communicate his thoughts and feelings in a productive way that helps him relate to peers, develop friendships, and release anger/feelings in ways that are comfortable for him and help him achieve his social and career goals.

### Long- and Short-Term Goals

The long-term goal of intervention for BT is to resume his classroom studies, communicate his needs to others, and continue seeing a psychiatrist for aftercare support. This goal will be reached in part through successfully achieving the short-term goal of identifying ways to express anger and other feelings through healthy outlets.

### Therapist Goals and Strategies

The therapist's goals include the following:

1. Provide activities to express feelings.
2. Facilitate integration of experience and knowledge.

The therapist's strategies include the following:

1. Educate BT about how to express feelings.
2. Provide experiences to practice expressing feelings through activity participation.
3. Process the activity through facilitated discussion, to help client relate the experience to his life.

*Activity: Stress Ball Activity and Discussion*

The activity begins with each participant in a group of six quickly identifying a personal stressor in order to compile a list of stressors. The group will then participate in an activity that generates a discussion about ways to reduce stress. The activity is interactive and challenges the participants to practice various stress-relieving actions. Each participant is asked, in turn, to catch a stress ball that has stress management techniques printed on it. Each participant is asked to act out the techniques printed under the right thumb as it is caught. The techniques could be to say something positive to someone, massage your neck, take five deep breaths, or make a funny face, among others. Occasionally, all participants are asked to try the suggested activity. Many stress relievers produce laughter and spontaneous stress relief.

The activity is followed by a discussion about the activity and its relevance to the topic of stress relief and communication. The therapist encourages and facilitates discussion about stress-relief activities that clients have tried, the reactions they experienced during the activity, ideas about stress relief the participants have in common with each other, and how they might use what they learned in their home, social, and work environments. Clients are encouraged to talk about their roles in the activity, the things they said to encourage each other, and the feelings they experienced during the activity. Other activities might include yoga, writing, volleyball, themed collages, and trust walks.

*Treatment Objectives*

1. BT will experience stress relief during the activity.
2. BT will identify three outlets for feelings.
3. BT will identify one person with whom he can do activities.

# Resources

American Occupational Therapy Association: www.aota.org

Depression and Bipolar Support Alliance: www.dbsalliance.org

National Alliance on Mental Illness: www.nami.org

National Institute of Mental Health: www.nimh.nih.gov

Substance Abuse and Mental Health Services Administration: www.samhsa.gov

# References

American Psychiatric Association. (2000). *Diagnostic and statistical manual of mental disorders* (4th ed., text revision). Washington, DC: Author.

Belmont Center for Comprehensive Treatment. (2001). *Rehabilitative services department manual*. Philadelphia, PA: Author.

Forsyth, K., Deshpande, S., Kielhofner, G., Henriksson, C., Haglund, L., Olseon, L., Skinner, S., & Kulkarmi, S. (2005). *The occupational circumstances assessment interview and rating scale* (Version 4.0). Chicago: Model of Human Occupation Clearinghouse, University of Illinois.

Kielhofner, G., Mallinson, T., Crawford, E., Nowak, M., Rigby, M., Henry, A., & Walens, D. (2004). *Occupational performance history interview* (Version 2.1). Chicago: Model of Human Occupation Clearinghouse, University of Illinois.

Korb-Khalsa, K., Azok, S. D., & Leutenberg, E. (2002). *Life management skills VI*. Beachwood, OH: Wellness Productions.

Law, M., Baptiste, S., Carswell, A., McColl, M. A., Polatojko, H., & Pollock, N. (2005). *Canadian occupational performance measure* (4th ed.). Bethesda, MD: AOTA.

Oakley, F., Kielhofner, G., & Barris, R. (1986). The role checklist. *Occupational Therapy Journal of Research, 6,* 157–170.

Pandya, M., Pozuelo, L., & Malone, D. (2007). Electroconvulsive therapy: What the internist needs to know. *Cleveland Clinic Journal of Medicine, 74*(9), 679–685.

Sadock, B. J., & Sadock, V. A. (2007). *Kaplan and Sadock's synopsis of psychiatry: Behavioral sciences/clinical psychiatry* (10th ed.). Philadelphia, PA: Lippincott, Williams & Wilkins.

# Osteoarthritis and Rheumatoid Arthritis

*Rosalyn Lipsitt*

## 🌿 Synopsis of Clinical Condition

### Prevalence and Etiology

Osteoarthritis and rheumatoid arthritis are chronic conditions characterized by painful joints. Osteoarthritis, which develops because of a breakdown of the cartilage between joints, is a diagnosis commonly associated with adults and older adults. Rheumatoid arthritis, on the other hand, is a systemic disease caused by an autoimmune attack on the synovium, the thin membrane that lines and lubricates the joints, ultimately causing a breakdown of the joints' supporting structures. In addition, rheumatoid arthritis may involve an individual's internal organs, eyes, and skin and may be diagnosed in children (as juvenile rheumatoid arthritis) as well as adults. Both types of arthritis result in joint pain and decreased physical functioning.

There are four types of drugs currently used to treat the major forms of arthritis: analgesics, biologics, nonsteroidal anti-inflammatory drugs (NSAIDs), and disease-modifying antirheumatic drugs (DMARDs). Analgesics are purely for pain, with the most commonly prescribed being acetaminophen. For severe pain, drugs containing opioids are used, such as codeine, hydrocodone, and transdermal patches. The second type, biologics, are engineered vaccine medications made from a living organism, such as a virus, gene, or protein. The third form of medication, NSAIDs, includes COX-2 inhibitors and salicylates and is safer for the stomach. The fourth group of drugs, DMARDs, is prescribed primarily for rheumatoid arthritis and works to decrease permanent damage to joints.

People with arthritis are challenged to come to terms with issues relating to mobility, vocation, occupational satisfaction, competence in activities of daily living, body image, and ability to cope. Although this challenge may result in anxiety and depression for many people with arthritis, it is not universal. According to Robinson, Kennedy, and Harmon (2011), occupational therapy treatment for individuals with chronic pain today includes psychosocial as well as rehabilitative interventions, such as stress management, assertiveness training, facilitation of a peer-support network, and psychotherapeutic approaches. It is important for occupational therapists to understand the condition and its repercussions, treat each person as an individual, and take a holistic approach by including psychosocial issues in practice.

According to the Centers for Disease Control and Prevention, as of 2005, osteoarthritis has affected 26.9 million American adults (Lawrence et al., 2008). More than 100 different forms of arthritis have been identified, and these are divided into eight categories (Hansen & Atchison, 2000). Some form of arthritis is evident in most individuals over the age of 50 years. As the population ages, more cases are expected to be diagnosed. According to Hunter, Schneider, Mackin, and Callahan (1990), arthritis is one of the leading causes of work disabilities, second only to cardiac conditions.

## Common Characteristics and Symptoms

The following are the most common types of arthritis:

- ankylosing spondylitis
- bursitis
- cervical arthritis
- gout
- infectious arthritis
- juvenile rheumatoid arthritis
- osteoarthritis
- osteonecrosis
- psoriatic arthritis
- reactive arthritis (formerly Reiter's syndrome)
- fibromyalgia
- rheumatoid arthritis
- lumbosacral arthritis
- rheumatoid foot and ankle
- tendonitis

All of the following are autoimmune connective tissue diseases that can cause arthritis:

- lupus erythematosus
- systemic lupus erythematosus
- scleroderma
- polymyositis
- dermatomyositis

Osteoarthritis is the primary example of degenerative arthritis. It is primarily an adult condition and, in the older age groups, is more prevalent among women than men. It affects the weight-bearing joints (knees, hips, and spine) and the distal interphalangeal (DIP) joints of the hands or metatarsophalangeal joints of the feet (Hunter et al., 1990). It is believed to be related to age and genetics. In osteoarthritis, also referred to as *degenerative joint disease*, the thinning or other damage to cartilage creates a rough, or eroded, surface. As opposing bones attempt to glide in the absence of "cushioning," inflammation develops, contributing to the formation of bony ridges and spurs. These bony malformations, and the inability of the opposing bones to meet uniformly, cause deformity and pain during activity or rest.

Some etiologies of osteoarthritis are less common than the process just described. Because cartilage naturally breaks down with age, due to wear and tear of the joint, it is believed that in some cases, arthritis may develop as a result of, or secondary to, other physiological conditions, such as congenital defects and obesity. Some of the other risk factors associated with arthritis are bowed legs, dislocated hips, genetic defects, overuse or injury to a joint as a result of an accident, diabetes, and certain hormonal disorders, such as gout and poor posture.

Early in the disease process, an individual will experience morning stiffness in the joints, which subsides during the course of the day, and possibly a crackling sound (crepitus) with movement of the joint. As the disease progresses, movement will be accompanied by increasing pain and swelling, caused by synovitis; increased amounts of synovial fluid; or changes in bone or cartilage, such as the formation of marginal osteophytes protruding into the joint space (Hunter et al., 1990). These are observable on the DIP joints and are referred to as *Heberden's nodes*, and those at the proximal interphalangeal (PIP) joints are known as *Bouchard's nodes*. Ulnar deviation of the wrists, also known as a *zigzag deformity*, is also a common manifestation of rheumatoid arthritis as well as osteoarthritis.

Rheumatoid arthritis is a chronic and systemic (vs. localized) disease and is the most common form of inflammatory arthritis. There are actually more than 100 different types of rheumatoid arthritis. In this form of the disease, an unknown event triggers the immune system to produce chemicals, which stimulate an inflammatory reaction. This reaction causes inflammation of the synovium (the thin membrane that lines and lubricates the joint), which then proliferates, creating pannus (an overgrowth of synovial tissue), which results in swelling. Eventually, the pannus, a rough, grainy tissue, invades the joint cavity and destroys the components of the joint, namely, the capsule, ligaments, and tendons. Unlike osteoarthritis, which is localized, rheumatoid arthritis may involve body systems other than joints, such as the blood, lungs, and heart.

The symptomology of rheumatoid arthritis differs somewhat from osteoarthritis. Rheumatoid arthritis usually affects joints bilaterally. Symptoms may be constant or may present with intermittent "flares" and remissions. Pain may be present as may other symptoms, such as fatigue; low-grade fever; weight loss; dryness of the eyes and mouth; color changes in fingers and toes; inflammation of the eyes, heart, lungs, skin, and nerves; and the appearance of rheumatoid nodules, most often seen near a joint. Other manifestations of rheumatoid arthritis as well as their descriptions are as follows:

1. Fusiform swelling: Digits become spindle-shaped because of swelling in the PIP joints.
2. Boutonniere deformity: The PIP joint is flexed because of a detached central slip. This causes the DIP joint to hyperextend.
3. Swan neck deformity: metacarpal phalangeal (MCP) joint exhibits a flexion contracture, which in turn creates hyperextension of the PIP joint and flexion of the DIP joint. The processes that result in these abnormal positions of the interphalangeal joints are set into motion as a result of contractures of the interosseous and flexor muscles and tendons.
4. Thumb deformities, which include the following:
   - boutonniere-type deformity
   - volar subluxation of the thumb
   - exaggerated adduction of the thumb, flexion of the MCP joint, and hyperextension of the DIP joint (Nalebuff, 1990)

## Target Areas for Intervention

Occupational therapy intervention focuses on patient education in the following areas: coping skills, joint protection, energy conservation, pain management, safe exercise, adaptive strategies, assistive devices, splinting, and self-empowerment in seeking information and social support in the community.

# Contextual Considerations

## Clinical

Occupational therapists typically use several assessments to evaluate the physical manifestations, psychosocial aspects, and functional challenges of the condition. Many assessments are available that address each of these aspects of diagnosis and treatment; however, for the purposes of this text, an example of each type has been chosen. The types of assessments that will prove most helpful in determining goals and interventions for this diagnosis are an interview, a physical examination of all joints and systems of the hand, a functional assessment, and a semistructured, client-centered interview to help prioritize focus for treatment. The initial interview provides key data when determining priorities for goals and intervention. It is during the interview that the therapist gains rapport with the patient and learns about his or her physical and social environment, cognition, affect, experience of the illness, and priorities for treatment.

The hands and wrists are evaluated by observation, palpation, goniometry, and manual muscle testing. Each hand is inspected for trophic changes (e.g., condition of skin, degree of warmth, redness). Palpation is used to determine structural abnormalities of the joints and crepitus. Active range of motion will reveal any limitations due to stiffness, pain, tenderness, or locking of the tendon (trigger finger). Active and passive range of motion is measured with the goniometer, respecting any pain that may be present. Manual muscle testing may also be performed, unless the patient is in an acute stage and in pain. If the patient complains of nerve pain or if the examination suggests deficits, sensory testing is also performed. Some patients with rheumatoid arthritis experience neuropathies or carpal tunnel syndrome as a result of tenosynovitis of the digital flexors. Functional evaluations are also important. A self-care assessment is very valuable in determining the degree of function and will reveal compensatory techniques used by the patient. The *Occupational Performance History Interview* (Kielhofner, 2004) is a semistructured interview that allows for a more in-depth observation of the individual and an occupational history.

The *Canadian Occupational Performance Measure* (COPM; Law et al., 2005) is another interview-based instrument that allows the patient to report personal perceptions of self-care and leisure function and productivity. The patient is able to rate the degree of difficulty for each type of task and how important each of those tasks is to him or her. This assessment assists with collaborative goal setting.

## Family

The diagnosis of arthritis impacts the lives of individuals and their families in different ways. Some individuals may experience anxiety, depression, or anger if they are faced with increasing dependency on others and limitations in their ability to carry out the tasks that are associated with roles such as spouse, parent, worker, or student.

## Practice Setting

Individuals with a diagnosis of arthritis may be encountered in long-term care facilities, assisted living, rehabilitation hospitals, adult day care, community programs, outpatient facilities, and home care settings.

## Sociopolitical

Most managed care systems require arthritis patients to be managed by a primary care physician (PCP), who may not possess the specialized knowledge of a rheumatologist and may not be aware of the special needs of the patient with arthritis and the benefits that occupational and physical therapy may provide. The capitation system imposed by some managed care systems may actually discourage PCPs from referring patients to rheumatologists. Therapists will need to stress patient education to empower individuals to become active participants in developing a healthy and productive lifestyle and managing their health care needs.

The development of measurable, functional goals for occupational therapy is of paramount importance because current cost containment strategies call for shorter medical treatment sessions and evidence of the value of services prior to reimbursement (Melvin & Jensen, 1998).

## Lifestyle/Lifespan

According to Livneh and Antonak (1997), there is extensive variability in psychological responses related to adaptation to arthritis. Fatigue, pain, limited flexibility, and neuropathies will influence the level of participation in many life tasks. Some common responses to a diagnosis of rheumatoid arthritis are initial disbelief, denial, anxiety, and depression. Some people experience anger, which may be internalized or externalized. These emotions are in response to the patient's changing lifestyle, to which many adaptations may need to be made because of loss of function. Medical costs and home, community, and workplace accessibility are a few of the challenges persons with arthritis must face over the course of his or her lifetime.

Many individuals will benefit from using special devices, such as a raised toilet seat, grab bars, special scissors, hand splints, and special eating equipment, some of which may not be covered under insurance and will add to living expenses. Depending on the severity of the symptoms, some individuals may need environmental adaptations to the workplace to reduce overuse of joints, such as waist-level filing drawers, built-up writing implements and other tools, and an ergonomically correct chair. For others, an adjusted work schedule or vocational change may be required.

# ⚕️ Clinical Decision-Making Process

## Defining Focus for Intervention

In defining the focus for intervention, the therapist is guided by the type of arthritis with which the patient presents, the results of the physical assessment (range of motion, sensation, deformities, and functional abilities), how they impact the patient's life roles (assessed by the *Occupational Performance History Interview*), and their perception of the impact of the condition on their independence (assessed by the COPM). Comorbidities, such as cardiac conditions, and medications that may affect cognition or motor functioning are taken into consideration, to ensure that the interventions will be appropriate and safe for the patient. Most commonly, occupational therapists intervene with this diagnosis, in any or all of the following focus areas:

1. Preparatory or enabling activities to prepare the patient for treatment (e.g., paraffin baths, active and passive range of motion, heat)
2. Patient education regarding work simplification, joint protection, energy conservation, exercise programs, use of assistive devices, and resources for support in the community (Hurkmans et al., 2009; Tuntland et al., 2009)

3. Activities of daily living and instrumental activities of daily living training (e.g., use of assistive devices for cooking)

4. Exploration of leisure activities, which includes adapting an existing activity, if needed, or learning a new activity

5. Work or productive activities, including instruction in how to perform the required tasks using joint protection and energy conservation and adapting the environment, if needed (Steultjens et al., 2004)

6. Splinting to rest painful joints or to slow the process of deformities (Wallen & Gillies, 2006)

7. Coping strategies, which require occupational therapists to address patients' concerns and anxieties regarding the progressive nature of the condition

Intervention in each of these areas assists with increasing a sense of self-efficacy and serves to decrease anxiety and depression in the patient.

## Establishing Goals for Intervention

Occupational therapy goals for individuals who present with arthritis are determined by several factors, including the physician's referral, the setting, the results of the initial evaluations, and the insurance coverage defining the length of treatment. Informed by these factors, the occupational therapist analyzes data collected from interviews and assessments and collaborates with the patient in the establishment and prioritization of long- and short-term goals for treatment.

## Designing Theory-Based Intervention

The complex nature of arthritis warrants the employment of more than one frame of reference. For example, issues of joint deformity and weakness may be addressed by the biomechanical and rehabilitation frames of reference. Splinting to prevent further deformity, the institution of an exercise program to maintain and increase muscle strength, and the use of modalities such as paraffin for pain relief represent the biomechanical frame of reference. Training in the use of adaptive devices and the incorporation of energy-conservation techniques and work-simplification strategies represent the rehabilitation frame of reference. Additionally, the model of human occupation provides the therapist with a holistic view of the patient that incorporates the physical ramifications of the conditions within the context of the patient's personal values, needs, and life roles (Kielhofner, 1997).

Precautions that should be taken during assessment and intervention are as follows:

1. During acute exacerbation, when patients present with joint swelling, redness, and pain, manual muscle testing and passive range of motion should be avoided.

2. Patients using heat at home to relieve pain and stiffness should be advised to use the heat for no more than 20- or 30-minute intervals and to avoid the use of heating pads overnight.

3. For patients on blood thinners, care should be taken not to offer activities or tasks that require sharp objects (e.g., using sewing needles, handling flowers with thorns).
4. Sharp objects should also be avoided with patients who have peripheral neuropathy in the hands.
5. Activities requiring excessive pinching and gripping should be avoided. Tools and implements should be built up with padding whenever possible.

## Evaluating Progress

Progress is demonstrated by an increase in, or stabilization of, passive and active ranges of motion and strength, a reduction in pain, and an increase in the ability to integrate adaptive techniques and equipment into activities of daily living with progressively less cuing from the therapist.

## Determining Change in or Termination of Treatment

The level and speed with which the patient assumes or resumes active participation in life roles associated with work, leisure, and/or self-care activities will help guide changes in or termination of treatment.

## Case Study

### Description

MT is a 65-year-old widow who has been referred for outpatient treatment, presenting with a diagnosis of rheumatoid arthritis that has affected the joints in both hands. She lives alone in a newly built apartment building in the center of a large northeastern city. Her one-bedroom apartment is accessible by elevator and is equipped with a bathroom grab bar next to the tub. The kitchen is modern and fully equipped, with a refrigerator, microwave, and dishwasher. All kitchen appliances and handles are standard. MT has always been productive, and she was an avid knitter until 3 years ago, when arthritis pain became more frequent and severe in both hands. In addition, MT has found it necessary to limit her writing, despite the fact that she enjoys writing notes to her grandchildren and exchanging original recipes with her friends, with the latter requiring her to pen recipes onto her personalized recipe cards. She has continued to cook and bake, despite her discomfort, in preparation for holiday meals, which she enjoys preparing for her two adult children and three grandchildren.

### Long- and Short-Term Goals

The long-term goal of intervention for MT is to complete light meal preparation incorporating adaptive equipment and energy-conservation techniques. This goal will be reached in part through successfully achieving the short-term goal of independently demonstrating safe and proper use of selected adaptive cooking equipment (e.g., cutting board, jar opener, electric knife, rocker knife, large-handled utensils) during simple cold-meal preparation.

## Therapist Goals and Strategies

The therapist's goals include the following:

1. Increase patient's knowledge regarding adaptive equipment.
2. Increase patient's ability to use selected adaptive equipment safely and appropriately.
3. Increase patient's awareness of resources for medical information, social support, community mobility (transportation), and sources for adaptive equipment/devices.

The therapist's strategies include the following:

1. Avoid manual muscle testing and passive range of motion during acute exacerbation of arthritis symptoms (e.g., joint swelling, redness, pain).
2. Provide bilateral resting hand splints to prevent deformity and reduce pain.
3. Provide large-handled fork, spoon, and rocker knife to facilitate self-feeding and reduce stress on joints.
4. As symptoms subside, institute a graded exercise program to maintain/increase upper extremity strength.
5. Provide written materials, direct verbal instruction, and modeling of the use of assistive devices, to increase patient's knowledge regarding concepts of energy conservation and joint protection (avoidance of excessive grip, pinch, or ulnar deviation of the wrist).

## Activity: Making Turkey Sandwiches

In preparation for this activity, the therapist assembles the following adaptive equipment: an adapted cutting board, which is fitted with nails to stabilize large items; a rubber or under-cabinet jar opener; an electric knife; a rocker knife; a knife with a built-up handle; and a rolling cart. The patient uses the rolling cart to retrieve a turkey breast, butter, lettuce, and mayonnaise from the refrigerator and transport them to the counter. The patient retrieves the bread from the counter and the necessary adaptive equipment from the drawers located at waist level. Using the rolling cart and placing the bread and utensils in a convenient location are examples of effective use of energy-conservation techniques. The patient is instructed to place the turkey breast on the adapted cutting board and use the electric knife to cut several slices. The step represents the integration of a piece of adaptive equipment (cutting board) with an energy-conservation technique (electric knife usage). The patient uses the knife with the built-up handle to butter the bread and the jar opener to open the jar of mayonnaise. After spreading the mayonnaise with a large-handled knife, the patient assembles the sandwich and cuts it using the rocker knife. These steps represent the use of adaptive equipment. The patient places the sandwich on lightweight plates. The cart is used to return items to the refrigerator, counters, and drawers, and the patient is instructed to rinse dishes in warm water and gently squeeze a large sponge during and after cleanup.

As the symptoms subside, the focus for MT's program shifts to instrumental activities of daily living. The therapist then collaborates with the client to identify and prioritize meaningful activities, which will be incorporated into therapy. Energy-conservation and joint protection strategies are taught to the client so that the strategies may be implemented now and in the future, as needed. This will require her to generalize concepts of energy conservation and joint conservation to meal preparation.

### Treatment Objectives

MT will be able to safely and successfully manipulate adapted tools and equipment in the preparation of a simple meal.

## Resources

About Arthritis: www.arthritis.about.com

American Occupational Therapy Association: www.aota.org

Arthritis.com: www.arthritis.com

Arthritis Foundation: www.arthritis.org

Fibromyalgia Information Foundation: www.myalgia.com

Johns Hopkins Health Alerts: http://www.johnshopkinshealthalerts.com/

Scleroderma Foundation: www.scleroderma.org

SeniorShops.com: www.seniorshops.com

Spondylitis Association of America: www.spondylitis.org

UC Berkeley Wellness Letter: www.wellnessletter.com

## References

Hansen, A., & Atchison, B. (2000). *Conditions in occupational therapy: Effect on occupational performance* (2nd ed.). Philadelphia, PA: Lippincott, Williams & Wilkins.

Hunter, J., Mackin, E., & Callahan, A. (Eds.). (2002). *Rehabilitation of the hand and upper extremity* (5th ed.). St. Louis, MO: Mosby.

Hunter, J., Schneider, L., Mackin, E., & Callahan, A. (1990). *Rehabilitation of the hand: Surgery and therapy* (3rd ed.). St. Louis, MO: Mosby.

Hurkmans, E., van der Giesen, F. J., Vliet Vlieland, T. P. M., Schoones, J., & van den Ende, E. C. H. M. (2009). Dynamic exercise programs (aerobic capacity and/or muscle strength training) in patients with rheumatoid arthritis. *Cochrane Database of Systematic Reviews, 4.* doi: 10.1002/14651858.CD006853.pub2

Kielhofner, G. (1997). *Conceptual foundations of occupational therapy* (2nd ed.). Philadelphia, PA: FA Davis.

Kielhofner, G., Mallinson, T., Crawford, E., Nowak, M., Rigby, M., Henry, A., & Walens, D. (2004). *Occupational performance history interview* (Version 2.1). Chicago: Model of Human Occupation Clearinghouse, University of Illinois.

Law, M., Baptiste, S., Carswell, A., McColl, M. A., Polatojko, H., & Pollock, N. (2005). *Canadian occupational performance measure* (4th ed.). Bethesda, MD: American Occupational Therapy Association, Inc.

Lawrence, R. C., Felson, D. T., Helmick, C. G., Arnold, L. M., Choi, H., Deyo, R. A., . . . Arthritis Data Workgroup. (2008). Estimates of the prevalence of arthritis and other rheumatic conditions in the United States. Part II. *Arthritis & Rheumatism, 58(1),* 26–35.

Livneh, H., & Antonak, R. (1997). *Psychosocial adaptation to chronic illness and disability.* Austin, TX: PRO-ED, Inc.

Melvin, J., & Jensen, G. (Eds.). (1998). *Rheumatologic rehabilitation: Assessment and management.* Bethesda, MD: American Occupational Therapy Association, Inc.

Nalebuff, E. (1990). The rheumatic thumb. In J. Hunter, E. Mackin, & A. Callahan (Eds.), *Rehabilitation of the hand: Surgery and therapy* (3rd ed.). Philadelphia, PA: Mosby.

Robinson, K., Kennedy, N., & Harmon, D. (2011). The issue is—is occupational therapy adequately meeting the needs of people with chronic pain? *American Journal of Occupational Therapy, 65,* 106–113. doi: 10.5014/ajot.2011.09160

Steultjens, E. E. M. J., Dekker, J. J., Bouter, L. M., Schaardenburg, D. D., Kuyk, M.-A. M. A. H., & van den Ende, E. C. H. M. (2004). Occupational therapy for rheumatoid arthritis. *Cochrane Database of Systematic Reviews, 1.* doi: 10.1002/14651858.CD003114.pub2

Tuntland, H., Kjeken, I., Nordheim, L. V., Falzon, L., Jamtvedt, G., & Hagen, K. B. (2009). Assistive technology for rheumatoid arthritis. *Cochrane Database of Systematic Reviews, 4.* doi: 10.1002/14651858.CD006729.pub2

Wallen, M. M., & Gillies, D. (2006). Intra-articular steroids and splints/rest for children with juvenile idiopathic arthritis and adults with rheumatoid arthritis. *Cochrane Database of Systematic Reviews, 1.* doi: 10.1002/14651858.CD002824 .pub2

# Diabetes | *Rosalyn Lipsitt*

## 🌿 Synopsis of Clinical Condition

### Prevalence and Etiology

Diabetes mellitus is a disorder of the endocrine system. There are three types, all characterized by increased glucose in the bloodstream (known as *hyperglycemia*). Hyperglycemia is due to the body's inability to produce sufficient insulin or the body's cells' inability to respond to available insulin.

### Common Characteristics and Symptoms

#### Types of Diabetes

*Type I Diabetes*

In the past, Type I diabetes was called *juvenile diabetes*; however, individuals over age 40 years have been known to contract this type, and therefore the term is less common today. Type I diabetes is known to appear suddenly before age 30 years (Saudek & Margolis, 2006). This type is characterized as an autoimmune disease. The body produces antibodies that attack and damage the beta cells in the pancreas, the cells responsible for producing insulin. At first, beta cells may just be impaired; however, in less than a year, they are likely to produce little or no insulin, which results in the need for the patient with diabetes to regularly inject insulin. The exact etiology is unknown; however, possible causes are exposure to common viruses or other substances early in life and genetics, although most patients with this type have no family history.

*Type II Diabetes*

This type, which is the most common form of the disease, is known as *non–insulin dependent diabetes mellitus*. Type II diabetes usually develops in adults over the age of 40 years, most of whom are overweight. Those at greatest risk for this type are African Americans, Native Americans, and Hispanic Americans

(Margolis & Saudek, 2002). In Type II diabetes, the pancreas usually produces insulin; however, receptors on cell surfaces, which interact with the insulin, are unable to create passageways for the insulin to enter the blood cells. Therefore, glucose builds up in the bloodstream, rather than being transported as fuel to other body structures. As a result, the body is forced to break down lipids and muscle tissue to create glucose for use by the body's cells. Possible causes for Type II diabetes are genetics, pancreatic diseases, surgical removal of the pancreas, tumors in endocrine organs, corticosteroid use in treatment of asthma and arthritis, and use of niacin for treatment of high cholesterol. Symptoms for this type result from poor utilization of glucose by the cells. It is important to note that not all patients experience every symptom, and some symptoms may occur in a very mild form. Symptoms for Type II diabetes include the following:

- feeling ill
- thirst
- weight loss
- blurred vision
- frequent infections
- slow healing of skin lesions
- hunger
- fatigue
- numbness or tingling
- impotence

### Gestational Diabetes

This type of diabetes develops or is discovered during pregnancy, usually appearing at 24 to 28 weeks gestation. With gestational diabetes, the placenta produces hormones that interfere with the body's response to insulin. It typically recedes at the conclusion of pregnancy; however, women with this diagnosis are at higher risk for developing diabetes later in life (Sammarco, 1991). Because symptoms are rare in these cases, routine screening for elevated blood sugar takes place between the 24th and 28th week of pregnancy. If the tests are positive, the mother is instructed to maintain a low-calorie, low-sugar diet and begin a monitored exercise program. Blood sugar will be monitored throughout the pregnancy (Burrow, Duffy, & Copel, 2004). Poorly controlled diabetes before conception and during the first trimester of pregnancy can cause major birth defects in 5% to 10% of pregnancies and spontaneous abortions in 15% to 20% of pregnancies. During the second and third trimesters of pregnancy, poorly controlled diabetes may result in excessively large babies, which poses risks to both the mother and the child (National Diabetes Information Clearinghouse, 2008).

## Complications of Diabetes

Acute complications from diabetes include the following:

1. Diabetic ketoacidosis (hyperglycemia): This response requires immediate medical attention. Symptoms include abdominal pain, vomiting, rapid breathing, extreme fatigue, drowsiness, and sweet breath odor.

2. Hypoglycemia (low blood sugar): This condition may occur when too much insulin is administered, when there has been a delay in administering insulin, when the patient has missed a meal, or when the patient exercises without eating first. The symptoms patients may experience are crankiness, confusion, excessive perspiration, and hunger. For these symptoms, it is necessary to administer a sweetened drink, a high-sugar snack, or glucose tablets or gels. In the event of loss of consciousness or seizure, it is vital to seek immediate emergency medical attention.

Non-acute complications from diabetes include the following:

1. Retinopathy (microvascular disease)
2. Glaucoma and cataracts
3. Nephropathy (kidney disease)
4. Coronary heart disease, high blood pressure, and stroke
5. Peripheral vascular disease
6. Neuropathy (nerve damage): Neuropathy is the most frequent complication of patients with Type II diabetes. Of those who have had diabetes for 25 years, there is a 50% prevalence of peripheral neuropathy (Zuberi & Miller, 2000). The three types of neuropathies include peripheral, mononeuropathy, and autonomic neuropathy. Peripheral neuropathy is the most common, characterized by a progressive loss of function of the sensory nerves in the limbs. The patient may experience numbness, tingling, and pain in the bilateral extremities (Landry, 2006). Mononeuropathy leads to pain and weakness in areas supplied by a nerve, or nerves, whose blood supplies have been disrupted. These symptoms may improve gradually, without any treatment; however, nerve damage from peripheral neuropathy responds slowly, if at all, with diabetic control (Saudek & Margolis, 2006).
7. Amputation: Diabetic foot problems, which arise from peripheral vascular disease, neuropathies, and slow healing of wounds and infections, sometimes lead to limb amputation.

## Target Areas for Intervention

Occupational therapy intervention focuses on the assessment of sensation in the limbs and related performance in activities of daily living (ADL) and instrumental activities of daily living (IADL).

# 🌿 Contextual Considerations

## Clinical

An initial interview is essential for obtaining information about the patient's physical and social environments, prior self-care abilities, and productive and leisure activities. It allows the therapist to establish rapport and form an initial impression regarding the patient's cognitive status and affords the patient the opportunity to communicate personal concerns and perceptions regarding the illness.

In addition to the interview, functional assessments, such as those described below, are useful in evaluating a patient who exhibits the complications of diabetes that may interfere with his or her ability to safely conduct daily life activities. The *Occupational Performance History Interview–Second Edition* (OPHI-II; Kielhofner et al., 2004) is a semistructured interview that allows for a more in-depth observation of the individual and a picture of the person's occupational history over time. The *Functional Independence Measure* (Uniform Data System for Medical Rehabilitation, 2009) is a measure of disability that functionally assesses ADL communication and cognitive function. The patient is rated on 18 critical tasks, on a 7-point scale, from *independent* to *dependent*. The *Semmes-Weinstein Calibrated Monofilament Test* (Semmes, 1960) is used to determine the extent of neuropathies in the hands or to determine if any sensory loss in the hands exists. The various microfilaments measure degrees of light touch. Information from this instrument is important because it helps the occupational therapist address safety issues with the patient when planning ADL or leisure activities. An inability to accurately judge sharp and dull sensations may be dangerous. Other sensory testing should include the ability to feel temperature, tactile localization, stereognosis, and two-point discrimination. Manual muscle testing, in the absence of acute arthritis or other contraindications, is important in choosing an exercise program or other functional activities.

## Family

The dietary requirements of an individual with diabetes may impact his or her household. Families must be sensitive to these requirements when making food and menu choices. Medication and dietary requirements may necessitate adaptations in social activities. Spouses may require education regarding the effects of diabetes on sexual intimacy. Environmental adaptations and adaptive utensils may be required for the person with diabetes, depending on the extent of complications, such as visual and other sensory deficits as well as mobility restrictions resulting from amputations. Life insurance is particularly costly for persons with diabetes and their families. The American Diabetes Association provides information on policies designed to accommodate this population.

## Practice Setting

Treatment of an individual with diabetes involves a team of professionals: diabetes nurse educators, endocrinologists, primary care physicians, registered dieticians, exercise physiologists, mental health professionals, ophthalmologists, podiatrists, occupational therapists, and physical therapists (Saudek & Margolis, 2006). Occupational therapists most likely treat individuals with diabetes who have undergone surgery for amputation or who have been hospitalized for other reasons in a rehabilitation setting. In addition to the rehabilitation setting, the occupational therapist may encounter a patient with diabetes in a community setting, a nursing home, or home care.

## Sociopolitical

The major sociopolitical issue related to patients diagnosed with diabetes is medical insurance coverage. Individuals with diabetes incur many expenses related to medications, testing equipment, supplies, and shoe gear. Medicare coverage is discussed in Table 23.1.

## Lifestyle/Lifespan

Lifelong adjustments in self-care habits include glucose monitoring, administration of insulin, weight management/dietary restrictions, and skin management. Community mobility may be affected for individuals who live in states that require a doctor's certification confirming the ability of the individual with diabetes to be a safe driver. Coping issues related to possible role loss, management of chronic illness, and other lifestyle changes may leave individuals with diabetes at risk for depression. Diabetes may have an impact on vocational choices and the work environment. Individuals with diabetes may require workplace accommodations in the form of flexible scheduling to allow for meals and medication. The American Diabetes Association provides advocacy and an attorney's network for cases of employment discrimination.

**Table 23.1** Medicare Coverage for Patients With Diabetes

| Supplies/services | Individuals covered under Medicare |
| --- | --- |
| Self-testing equipment and supplies | Individuals with diabetes who have Medicare coverage. Limits on supplies and how often they can be purchased. Not restricted to insulin users. Medicare pays 80% of the cost of test strips. |
| Depth-inlay shoes Custom-molded shoes Shoe inserts | Individuals with diabetes who qualify under Medicare Part B must have one or more of these conditions in one or both feet:<br>■ history of partial or complete foot amputation<br>■ history of previous foot ulcers<br>■ history of callus that could lead to ulcers<br>■ peripheral neuropathy with signs of problems with calluses<br>■ poor circulation<br>■ foot deformity<br>Individuals being treated under a comprehensive diabetes care plan who need therapeutic shoes and/or inserts because of diabetes. |
| Medical nutrition therapy services | Individuals are covered by Medicare when referred by a physician. Patients pay 20% of Medicare-approved amount after the yearly Part B deductible. |
| Flu and pneumococcal vaccines | Individuals with diabetes covered by Medicare can get the following:<br>■ flu shot once a year<br>■ pneumonia vaccine |
| Glaucoma screening | For individuals with diabetes, once every 12 months under Medicare. Also available for anyone at high risk for glaucoma or with a family history for glaucoma. Patient pays 20% of the Medicare-approved amount after the yearly Part B deductible (see www.medicare.gov). |

## ✳ Clinical Decision-Making Process

### Defining Focus for Intervention

The focus of an occupational therapy program may be preventative or restorative or a combination of both. Working in collaboration with the nurse, diabetes educator, or dietician, the occupational therapist plans patient education related to diet. The occupational therapist will plan and set up a cooking activity with one or more patients, to cook appropriate meals or snacks while at the same time addressing safety in the kitchen and safe functional mobility for those with walkers, prostheses, or wheelchairs. The occupational therapist will address proper stump management for patients who have undergone an amputation, as well as foot care for all patients with diabetes. Patients are issued long-handled mirrors to perform daily skin inspections of a residual limb and unaffected foot and are taught to notice any sores or abrasions and to report these to their physicians. The occupational therapist will assist the patient with any issues related to his or her work environment or work schedule. Organizational skills may need to be improved in order to plan glucose testing and self-medication into the workday. The therapist will also educate the patient regarding energy conservation, if needed. In addition, patients with low vision may need adapted workplace environments. Safety education in light of sensory deficits is an important occupational therapy intervention. Patients with diabetes must be educated about wearing shoes at all times, both indoors and out, because of decreased sensation in the feet. Patients are also advised to test bathwater with their elbows or have a family member assist with this task, to avoid scalding their hands and feet. Individuals with compromised sensory systems are also advised to avoid using sharp objects during leisure activities or in the kitchen. The occupational therapist will offer the patient alternatives for kitchen tasks, as well as help him or her explore safe leisure activities.

Occupational therapists will also address patients' concerns and anxieties about the condition itself. Many patients with chronic or progressive illness may experience anxiety and depression. Assistive devices and proper education regarding self-care and safety serve to relieve many concerns. However, the occupational therapist will need to be aware of supportive services in the community, such as volunteers, paratransit services, and support groups, to address patients' psychosocial issues.

### Establishing Goals for Intervention

Occupational therapy goals for individuals with diabetes are determined by several factors, including the physician's referral, the setting, the results of the initial evaluations, and the insurance coverage defining the length of treatment. Informed by these factors, the occupational therapist analyzes data collected from interview and assessments and collaborates with the patient in the establishment and prioritization of long- and short-term goals for treatment.

## Designing Theory-Based Intervention

It is important for the patient with diabetes to adapt to the chronic, progressive nature of this condition. The occupational adaptation frame of reference assists the therapist in constructing an intervention process that facilitates internalized adaptation on the part of the patient (Schkade & Schultz, 1992). In order for the process to take place, the therapist must empower the patient to be his or her own advocate and give the patient the tools to adapt to the chronic condition. This frame of reference is holistic, and its use ensures that the intervention is relevant to the patient's context.

## Evaluating Progress

Because occupational therapy intervention for patients is largely guided by an adaptation model, progress is noted when the patient demonstrates consistency in incorporating adaptive strategies into daily activities. Examples of such progress would be evident in a patient who uses a skin inspection mirror as part of a morning self-care routine or who consistently plans and prepares meals that meet nutritional guidelines.

## Determining Change in or Termination of Treatment

Termination of treatment is recommended if either the allotted time for therapy has been reached or therapy goals have been attained. Goals may be modified if the patient does not show signs of improvement or movement toward goals.

## Case Study

*Description*

RS is a 73-year-old, cognitively intact widow, with a past medical history of cerebral vascular accident and insulin-dependent diabetes mellitus. During her routinely scheduled doctor visit, RS related that she was feeling weakness in her arms and legs and found herself fumbling more as she handled smooth objects. She felt that the combination of the weakness and decreased dexterity was compromising her ability to safely complete ADL. The doctor scheduled a series of neurological tests for RS, to determine the etiology of her symptoms. It was determined that the decrease in strength was a result of deconditioning secondary to a sedentary lifestyle after the stroke and that the decrease in fine motor function was the result of a peripheral neuropathy. RS was referred to a skilled nursing facility for a short stay to participate in a rehabilitation program.

RS has been living in a two-story home with her single daughter for 3 years, since she was discharged from the hospital after a stroke. Prior to this admission, RS was independent with ADL, light meal preparation, and light household tasks. She was able to self-monitor her glucose levels and administer insulin. She did not drive. RS's daughter, GS, is 50 years old and works full time as an administrative assistant in a large insurance company. Once a year, GS takes RS on a 1-week vacation; however, most of the time, RS is alone in the house watching television, playing solitaire, or talking on the phone with friends. She enjoys needlepoint but has found it increasingly difficult.

The occupational therapy initial evaluation included an interview to determine the details of the patient's physical and social environments, her productive activities, her overall cognitive ability, her experience of the recent setback, and her priorities for treatment. The OPHI-II was also administered. Manual muscle testing was applied to determine the extent of weakness in the extremities, and a functional assessment of self-care tasks was conducted to observe the degree of functional independence and need for assistive devices. Sensation testing was performed to assess any sensory deficits in the patient's hands. The initial evaluation revealed that RS exhibited fair to good upper extremity and lower extremity strength. She required moderate to minimum assistance with morning self-care tasks. The *Semmes-Weinstein Calibrated Monofilament Test* showed that RS had diminished sensation for light touch and for feelings of sharp/dull and hot/cold in both hands because of peripheral neuropathy.

Results of RS's initial evaluation were discussed with her. In addition, possible interventions for ameliorating some of her declining abilities were offered. Collaboration with the patient resulted in setting priorities for treatment. During the course of the discussion, RS emphasized the importance of her maintaining independence with self-care. Because she valued her sense of independence, she was agreeable to accepting assistive devices for dressing and bathing while participating in functional activities designed to gradually build strength. Equally important to RS was exploration of leisure activities for the purpose of finding a satisfying occupation in which to engage during long hours at home while her daughter was at work. RS was a creative person and was interested in discovering an outlet for her creativity. Ultimately, goals and interventions for RS focused on ADL and strengthening and leisure activities.

### Long- and Short-Term Goals

The long-term goal of intervention for RS is to demonstrate the ability to incorporate principles of safety awareness for sensory deficits into all ADL, IADL, and leisure activities. This goal will be reached in part through successfully achieving the short-term goal of demonstrating the ability to incorporate safety awareness strategies into leisure activities.

### Therapist Goals and Strategies

The therapist's goals are to provide education and demonstration of adaptive equipment and strategies that will promote safety awareness of sensory deficits during ADL, IADL, and leisure activities. The therapist's strategies include the following:

1. Educate patient in foot and nail care.
2. Reinforce importance of keeping skin protected and clean.
3. Provide assistive devices, such as skin inspection mirror, buttonhooks, and zipper pulls.
4. Suggest the use of shoes with Velcro closures.
5. Advise patient to seek assistance with toenail and fingernail care.

6. Demonstrate how to compensate for decreased temperature sensation in fingers with techniques such as testing water in sink or tub with elbows.

7. Provide simulations of daily activities in which the patient will have the opportunity to develop safe methods for approaching daily living activities. The therapist will provide intermittent correction or verbal cues as reminders, as needed.

### Activity: Rubber Stamps

RS was introduced to the craft of rubber-stamping, which provided a creative, safe hobby that does not require fine motor skill or the use of sharp tools. Rubber stamps are available in different sizes and in myriad designs, ranging from children's themes to designs that would appeal to adults, such as flowers, border designs, and decorative alphabets. Ink pads are also available in many colors and sizes. The stamp is pressed onto the ink pad and then applied to paper, cardboard, or any other surface for decoration. The design may be colored in or left as is.

In addressing RS's goals, a large piece of shelf paper, approximately 20 × 20 inches, was mounted on a slant board, placed in front of her, and tilted away from her at approximately 120 degrees. Stamps were placed in front of her, and the ink pad was placed at midline. This configuration incorporated shoulder flexion and elbow extension into the leisure activity of creating a decorative piece of wrapping paper. Use of bilateral wrist weights could be incorporated into the activity to build upper extremity strength and endurance.

Block printing is a leisure activity that might substitute for the needlepoint that RS had to abandon because of diminished sensation and vision. Block printing is safe for a person with diabetes because it does not require sharp objects, which pose a danger to individuals with peripheral neuropathies and low vision, and will help to increase upper extremity strength. Since RS is artistic and creative, block printing is a good choice.

### Treatment Objectives

Treatment objectives are to increase the patient's awareness of how a particular activity might satisfy the need to be creative in a safe manner and support the patient's need to maintain upper extremity strength and coordination.

## Resources

American Association of Diabetes Educators: www.aadenet.org

American Diabetes Association: www.diabetes.org

American Dietetic Association: www.eatright.org

Children With Diabetes Online Community: www.childrenwithdiabetes.com

DocGuide: www.docguide.com

International Diabetes Center at Park Nicollet Health Services: www.parknicollet.com/diabetes

International Society for Pediatric and Adolescent Diabetes: www.ispad.org

Medicare: www.medicare.gov

# References

Burrow, G., Duffy, T., & Copel, J. (2004). *Medical complications during pregnancy.* Philadelphia, PA: Saunders.

Kielhofner, G., Mallinson, T., Crawford, E., Nowak, M., Rigby, M., Henry, A., & Walens, D. (2004). *Occupational performance history interview* (Version 2.1). Chicago: Model of Human Occupation Clearinghouse, University of Illinois.

Landry, M. (2006). Peripheral nerve disorders. In L. Levy & V. Hetherington (Eds.), *Principles and practice of podiatric medicine* (2nd ed.). New York, NY: Churchill Livingstone.

Margolis, S., & Saudek, C. (2002). *Diabetes.* New York, NY: Medletter Associates, Inc.

Sammarco, G. (1991). *The foot in diabetes.* Philadelphia, PA: Lea & Febiger.

Saudek, C., & Margolis, S. (2006). *Johns Hopkins white papers: Diabetes.* Redding, CT: Medletter Associates, Inc.

Schkade, J., & Schultz, S. (1992). Occupational adaptation: Toward a holistic approach to contemporary practice. Part 1. *American Journal of Occupational Therapy, 46,* 917–925.

Semmes, J. (1960). *Somatosensory changes after penetrating brain wounds in man.* Cambridge, MA: Harvard University Press.

Uniform Data System for Medical Rehabilitation. (2009). *Guide for the uniform data set for medical rehabilitation (adult FIM), version 5.0.* Amherst, NY: UB Foundation Activities.

Zuberi, L., & Miller, J. (2000). Metabolic and endocrine disorders. In S. Mandel & J. Willis (Eds.), *Handbook of lower extremity neurology* (pp. 91–95). Philadelphia, PA: Churchill Livingstone.

# Low Vision and Perceptual Visual Impairment

*Stephen G. Whittaker*

## 🌿 Synopsis of Clinical Condition

### Prevalence and Etiology

About 2% of the population has low vision, which denotes an inability to read newsprint with glasses or worse. Most causes of visual impairment are age related (Scheiman, Scheiman, & Whittaker, 2006). Yet, as discussed in the next section, all of these symptoms may also result from a visual disability that has never been addressed. Only about 50% of older people with a visual disability are referred for vision rehabilitation services by their optometrist or ophthalmologist (Massof & Lidoff, 2000). In addition, many individuals in their 80s with normal, age-related vision loss become visually disabled because of environmental factors. This chapter will describe how an occupational therapist might screen for vision disability and address normal, age-related vision disabilities in various pediatric and adult settings.

### Common Characteristics and Symptoms

#### Aspects of Visual Impairment

There are several aspects of visual impairment, as indicated in Table 24.1: impaired visual acuity, impaired contrast sensitivity, central field loss, peripheral field loss, oculomotor problems, and perceptual problems. These aspects of visual impairment are not independent of one another. For example, people with central field loss always have impaired acuity and usually have impaired contrast sensitivity as well.

*Impaired Visual Acuity.* Visual acuity is the ability to see high-contrast detail, such as the letters on a doctor's eye chart. The most obvious symptom of impaired acuity in older adults is an inability to read, or difficulty reading, newspaper print.

**Table 24.1** Five Tests That Evaluate Sensory Visual Function

| Test | Indications | Common causes | Intervention |
|---|---|---|---|
| 1. Functional visual acuity threshold: the smallest high-contrast shape someone can see | ■ Difficulty reading<br>■ Holds material close<br>■ Difficulty seeing television | ■ Needs new glasses<br>■ Macular degeneration<br>■ Untreated or advanced diabetic retinopathy<br>■ Advanced glaucoma<br>■ Optic atrophy | 1. Enlarge the shape being viewed.<br>2. Use an optical or electronic magnification device.[a]<br>3. Move object closer. |
| 2. Functional contrast sensitivity: the lowest contrast shape someone can see. The shape is at least twice as large as visual acuity threshold. | ■ Difficulty seeing spilled water<br>■ Light sensitivity<br>■ Difficulty seeing faded print or print on colored backgrounds | ■ Macular degeneration<br>■ Diabetic retinopathy<br>■ Advanced glaucoma<br>■ Optic atrophy<br>■ Optic neuritis<br>■ Multiple sclerosis | 1. Enhance the contrast of shapes using color or light.<br>2. Change light so that it is from the side or above. Eliminate glare.<br>3. Adjust light intensity according to person's preference.<br>4 Use an electronic contrast enhancement device or tinted lenses.[a] |
| 3. Functional peripheral visual field: vision to the side of, above, or below where someone is looking | ■ Hesitation when reaching for objects<br>■ Trips and bumps into objects to side<br>■ Hesitation walking | ■ Optic atrophy<br>■ Treated diabetic retinopathy<br>■ Advanced glaucoma<br>■ Stroke, pituitary tumor, or other brain injury | 1. Teach the person visual scanning strategies to compensate for field defects.<br>2. Have person adopt head positions to compensate for field defects.[a]<br>3. Use prism glasses that might compensate for field defects.[a] |
| 4. Functional central visual field: blind areas where someone is trying to look | ■ Missing words and letters<br>■ Difficulty finding place when scanning<br>■ Frustration | ■ Macular degeneration<br>■ Untreated diabetic retinopathy | 1. Teach person to use side vision (advanced technique).[a]<br>2. Use magnification.<br>3. Use nonsighted techniques. |
| 5. Functional eye movements and binocular fusion: range of eye movement and eye positions of clearest vision | ■ Atypical head positions<br>■ Double vision | ■ Traumatic brain injury, especially closed-head trauma<br>■ Stroke | 1. Teach the person to adopt a head position that allows him or her to look straight ahead without double vision and/or minimal eye motion (nystagmus). This is a temporary fix.<br>2. If the problem is double vision, patch one eye, but only during a specific task in adults.[a]<br>3. Use of prism and/or visual training.[a] |

[a]Intervention requires special training in low vision rehabilitation methods and the supervision of an optometrist or ophthalmologist.

Children and younger adults who can focus at near distances and have impaired acuity will hold reading material closer than usual to their eyes in order to read and will also have difficulty seeing smaller print at a distance. In addition, someone with poor acuity will have difficulty watching television or recognizing faces at a distance. Squinting with both eyes when trying to see something indicates poor acuity and the need for corrective lenses. Squinting may indicate different problems under different conditions, as discussed later. Interestingly, even people with severe loss in visual acuity may see well enough for safe mobility or to recognize people at a distance. The most reliable hallmark of impaired acuity is a reading problem.

*Impaired Contrast Sensitivity.* Clinical tests of contrast sensitivity assess the ability to see larger, low-contrast objects. A good simulation of impaired contrast sensitivity is driving at night with a foggy windshield. A person with impaired contrast sensitivity will also have impaired visual acuity and glare sensitivity. Symptoms of impaired contrast sensitivity include the inability to see low-contrast shapes, like water on the floor, the last step of poorly lit carpeted steps, pets, or smaller pieces of furniture that match the color or the pattern of a carpet. Glare occurs when a light or the reflection of a light is in front of a person so that it shines directly into the eyes. Squinting both eyes in bright light even when not trying to see something indicates glare sensitivity. People with impaired contrast sensitivity will have difficulty seeing facial expressions or the television if there is a lot of light in the room. Normal aging involves mild reduction in contrast sensitivity and acuity, especially under lower light conditions. The hallmark of impaired contrast sensitivity is sensitivity to bright lights and glare.

*Central Field Loss.* Central field loss is the most common cause of visual impairment and visual disability in the elderly (Berger, Fine, & Maguire, 1999; Scheiman et al., 2006). Generally, our best visual acuity is in the center of our visual field in a region known as the *macula* (Figure 24.1). The drop-off in acuity from the center of our visual field can be easily demonstrated by looking at a single letter in the middle of this line. While looking at the letter, you will notice that letters above and below and to the right and left become less distinct the farther the letter is from the letter on which you are fixating. Certain diseases discussed in this chapter attack the macular region, resulting in a blind spot in the center and reduced visual acuity.

Unlike most simulations of this condition, blind spots (scotomas) do not appear as dark or gray spots; the visual system tends to fill in these holes in a person's vision. This "filling in" can be demonstrated using the following exercise. Close your left eye and look at the first letter of this line with your right eye. If you are about 40 centimeters (16 inches) from the page, you can find a blind spot by moving the tip of a pen about 8 to 9 centimeters (3 to 3.5 inches) to the right of where you are looking. The tip of the pen will disappear as it enters the blind spot. If you move the pen around and make sure your left eye is covered, you will find your blind spot because everyone has a physiological blind spot in the temporal

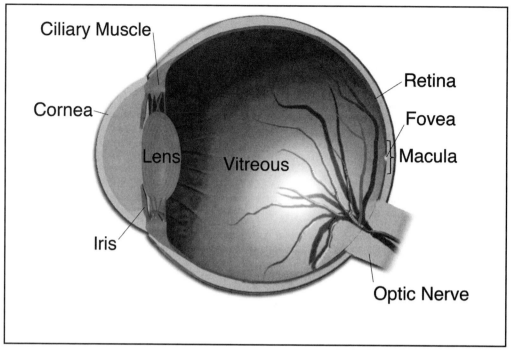

**Figure 24.1.** Illustration of a frontal (top) view of the right eye. From *Low Vision Rehabilitation: A Practical Guide for Occupational Therapists*, by M. Scheiman, M Scheiman, and S. G. Whittaker, 2007, Thorofare, NJ: SLACK Incorporated. Copyright 2007 by SLACK Incorporated. Reprinted with permission.

field of each eye, created where the optic nerve enters the eye. Notice that this blind spot does not appear as a dark spot; the brain just fills in that space. This occurs with central and often with peripheral field loss as well.

Individuals with macular degeneration have reduced acuity, can't recognize faces, and have a great deal of difficulty reading even large print. People with macular scotomas will complain of things appearing and disappearing and will often miss words or parts of words when reading enlarged text. In some cases, the brain fills in the scotoma with visual hallucinations, a phenomenon known as *Charles Bonnet syndrome*. An older adult with even mild cognitive deficits could find these symptoms disorienting and confusing. The limitations placed on familiar social and intellectual pursuits can cause emotional distress. Approximately one in four people with central field loss have stopped activities because of major depression (Rovner & Ganguli, 1998; Rovner & Shmuely-Dulitzki, 1997).

*Peripheral Field Loss.* The occupational therapist who works with people who have brain injury often encounters patients with peripheral vision loss, also called *field cuts*. A field loss that affects the same region in both eyes is *homonymous*. A field loss that affects different regions in the visual fields of each eye is called a *heteronymous field defect*. A *homonymous hemianopsia* affects half of the visual field in both eyes: the temporal field in one eye and nasal field in the other eye. A common stroke, affecting the middle cerebral artery, often will result in loss of vision on the affected side, but this usually affects only one quarter of the visual field, a *homonymous quadranopsia*, or less. In addition, some retinal diseases, discussed later, will also cause overall reduction in visual field, or *tunnel vision*. Symptoms of peripheral field loss involve bumping into objects or not seeing people approach on the affected side. These individuals might have problems looking for objects and might skip lines when reading. People with significant peripheral field loss underestimate and sometimes deny vision loss. Most cases of unilateral field loss involve central sparing, which means a person can see on both sides in the center of the visual field, such as whole words or a whole face. More debilitating is a unilateral field loss, which splits the central field so that the person sees only one half of an object. Children with developmental disabilities, brain injury, or cortical dysfunction may have peripheral field loss, often referred to under the idiopathic diagnosis of *cortical blindness*.

*Oculomotor Problems.* In adults, recent onset eye movement problems are associated with brain injury (Leigh & Zee, 2006). In children, eye movement disorders emerge during visual development (Scheiman, 2002). Problems with eye movements are often difficult to detect by just observing a person's behavior. Normally, both eyes look at the same point, called *conjugate gaze*. Even if there is a problem with only one eye, the result is a nonconjugate eye position, where the eyes are looking in different directions, a condition called *strabismus*. If the onset of strabismus has been recent, especially in adults with brain injury, the person often complains of double vision or visual confusion because each eye is looking at something different. Double vision, or diplopia, is intermittent and, after time, the double vision and visual confusion tend to become less frequent and often disappear. The visual system might adapt to eliminate the diplopia by suppressing vision in one eye, or the person might simply close one eye. For this reason, a symptom of strabismus is squinting one eye when trying to look at something. Sometimes, people with a smaller angle of deviation will have difficulty reading with two eyes because of impaired acuity from diplopia, a problem that is relieved by closing or patching one eye. Even if the eyes are conjugate, strabismus is not present because the person can overcome an incipient tendency for the eyes to become nonconjugate. This person might have difficulty reading because of eye strain.

If a person has nystagmus, the eyes will tend to shake uncontrollably. Nystagmus, which can often be seen by carefully looking at the eyes, will result in reduced visual acuity. Nystagmus often has a null point, a range of eye positions where the nystagmus quells. Visual–motor mislocalization (overreaching targets), headaches related to vision or reading, postural problems (especially head tilts), and difficulty scanning and reading are also symptoms of ocular motility problems.

Strabismus or any suspected vision problem in an infant warrants immediate referral to a pediatric optometrist or ophthalmologist because visual development is affected and permanent vision loss can result. In adults, a referral is not urgent, but visual problems are more easily managed if the referral is made sooner rather than later.

*Perceptual Problems.* Brain injury to the temporal or parietal lobes or developmental disabilities will result in a higher order perceptual impairment, such as trouble recognizing shapes or objects (object agnosia), trouble recognizing words (alexia), or various problems locating objects (visual–spatial agnosia and constructional apraxia). A common higher order deficit associated with brain injury and other perceptual disorders is neglect, or inattention. A common example would be a person with a right-hemisphere stroke who develops left inattention, or left neglect. These individuals lose awareness of an area in space (Trobe, 2001; Zoltan, 2007). When asked to look for something, these individuals will not look into the area of the neglect. For example, someone with left neglect will tend to skip the first letters of words or the first words of each line, and when the text does not make sense, the person will not think to look for the missing letters or words unless cued. A person with left neglect will tend not to notice obstacles on the left and will often bump into them. A severe neglect can be confused with a peripheral field loss. Sometimes a person will have both neglect and a peripheral field loss from brain injury.

## Interaction of Sensory and Perceptual Processes

One must test for and compensate for sensory vision impairment before testing for perceptual problems. For example, a person who exhibits a problem with object, word, or shape recognition may have impaired acuity or contrast sensitivity but otherwise normal perceptual function. One must not assume, however, that the sensory impairment necessarily limits perceptual function in some hierarchical fashion (i.e., that a person with impaired acuity necessarily has perceptual problems). With practice, people with impaired acuity, for example, learn to recognize people by their form or how they walk, rather than relying on detailed facial features, just as people with typical vision learn to navigate a familiar room with reduced vision resulting from dim light.

On the other hand, impaired perceptual function may be confused with impaired sensory function. A person who cannot recognize words (alexia) or objects (object agnosia) because of a brain injury will have difficulty reading a standard eye chart, typically missing less common words or objects. The eye movements of these individuals will also look abnormal because the person is searching for familiarity even though nothing is wrong with the basic oculomotor control system.

## Congenital Causes of Vision Loss

There are many congenital causes of vision loss (Jose, 1983). The more common pathogeneses of impaired vision affect older adults and are described in this section.

*Refractive Error.* Refractive error occurs when objects being viewed do not focus on the retina. Refractive error can be corrected by eyeglasses, contact lenses, or refractive surgery, but sometimes a therapist must work with a patient who does not have the correct eyeglasses. While this problem is being remedied, the therapist must somehow compensate for the reduced vision. There are three types of refractive error: myopia, hyperopia, and astigmatism. With myopia, or nearsightedness, a person can focus and see better at close range than he or she can at a distance. With high myopia, the distance at which objects come into focus can be very close. Individuals with hyperopia, or farsightedness, can focus better on things that are farther away, and for individuals who have high refractive error, things might never focus correctly. Likewise, with astigmatism, the lens is out of shape and out of focus at all distances.

*Development of Vision Loss and Vision Loss With Aging.* Using measurement techniques that do not require verbal responses or letter recognition, vision researchers found that visual acuity and contrast sensitivity increases throughout the first 36 months of life (Teller & Mavshon, 1986). The testing methods used in this research have been adapted and validated for clinical use with neonates and infants (Mash & Dobson, 1998) and may be used with individuals with brain injuries or developmental disabilities. Practitioners must be able to evaluate vision even in neonates because normal neurophysiological visual development requires normal visual stimulation. An infant deprived of normal vision by a need for eyeglasses (refractive error), strabismus, or short durations of occlusion often develops a permanent vision loss called *amblyopia* (Levi, 1992).

Later in adulthood, several aspects of vision change. The lens loses elasticity, and the pupil clouds and yellows and its range of dilation decreases. Accompanying neural changes result in loss of contrast sensitivity and acuity. The hardening of the lens results in presbyopia, which limits the ability to focus from far to near. Most people older than 40 years of age require reading glasses because of presbyopia. As people age, the pupil tends not to dilate as much and remain smaller in diameter, a condition called *senile miosis.* Consequently, about one third less light passes through the pupils of a 60-year-old than through those of a 20-year-old (Schwartz, 2004). As a result, an older person needs more light and stronger reading glasses. Even if an older person has near 20/20 (normal) visual acuity in the doctor's office, where light is optimal, his or her visual acuity will decline dramatically in settings with less light or lower print contrast (Enoch, Werner, Haegerstrom-Portnoy, Lakshminarayanan, & Rynders, 1999). As a result, a typical person in his or her 80s who has no eye pathology would have difficulty reading under the light levels in an average living room. This disability is easily remedied with a directional table or floor lamp positioned to minimize glare, as well as slightly stronger reading glasses that should be prescribed by an optometrist or ophthalmologist. People with normal, age-related vision loss also may benefit from the weaker handheld chest or lamp magnifiers that are widely available in department and sewing stores.

*Cataracts.* If the clouding of the lens is worse than normal, a person is diagnosed with a cataract (Scheiman et al., 2006). An opacification, or clouding, of the lens has an effect similar to a cloudy window or windshield; the major effect is to increase glare sensitivity. More dense cataracts also reduce the amount of light striking the retina. Since cataracts can usually be removed and replaced by a clear artificial lens, cataracts rarely lead to low vision. Cataracts result in impaired acuity, contrast sensitivity, and glare sensitivity, especially with night driving.

*Macular Degeneration.* The macula lutea is a small patch of retina in the center of the vision. Diseases that attack the macula result in macular degeneration and reduce vision in the center of the visual field or lead to central scotoma or blind areas, as discussed previously (Berger, Fine, & Maguire, 1999; Scheiman et al., 2006). Macular degeneration is the leading cause of low vision among the elderly. With atrophic, or "dry," macular degeneration, tiny yellow globs called *drusen* form on the retina pales, and atrophic macular degeneration slowly progresses from reduced central vision to relative scotoma, to absolute scotoma, giving the patient time to adapt. Increased light intensity seems to shrink or eliminate the central scotoma (Lei & Schuchard, 1997). With the less common exudative, or "wet," type of macular degeneration, blood vessels rupture and the blood damages the retina and clouds the vitreous, leading to an abrupt, substantial, and often traumatic loss in central vision. If diagnosed early, the wet type of macular degeneration can be treated with medications and laser treatment, reducing or avoiding the hemorrhage (Scheiman et al., 2006). One of the early signs of formation of those tiny blood vessels is a distortion in vision that causes straight lines to appear wavy. Recent onset of such symptoms warrants an immediate referral to an ophthalmologist specializing in retinal disease. Macular degeneration always results in impaired visual acuity and usually results in impaired contrast sensitivity, glare sensitivity, and central field loss.

*Diabetes.* Diabetes can cause cataracts, central neuropathies and related vision loss, and proliferative diabetic retinopathy (PDR). Even with treatment, PDR often results in "Swiss cheese vision," patchy vision loss throughout the visual field. If successfully treated, central vision is spared. The risk of PDR can be reduced by careful control of blood sugar. A patient with long-standing diabetes should schedule periodic visual examinations with an eye doctor who can monitor the health of the eye, even if the patient has no vision problems. Another transient vision effect of diabetes is that refractive error and vision can change with changes in blood sugar level (Scheiman et al., 2006).

*Glaucoma.* Technically, glaucoma is a neural vision loss. In the more common forms of glaucoma, the flow of fluid out of the eye is blocked and pressure builds up. This increase in pressure herniates the globe at the weakest point around the optic nerve, and the herniation strangles the optic nerve, causing nerve damage (Scheiman et al., 2006). Like cataracts, glaucoma can be treated and vision loss avoided. For those who are socioeconomically disadvantaged and cannot afford medication and regular eye examinations, those who tend to be noncompliant with medication, and those with very long standing glaucoma, vision loss occurs. The vision loss occurs in an arc around the macular region, progressing to overall peripheral vision loss that first restricts the peripheral visual field and then causes total blindness. Those experiencing visual field loss often have glare sensitivity and experience visual acuity loss only at the later stages of the disease.

*Brain Injury.* A cerebral vascular accident or head trauma results in injury to the central nervous system. The most common functional effects of brain injury are field loss, oculomotor problems, and perceptual dysfunction (Leigh & Zee, 2006). Nystagmus from brain injury, damage to the optic nerve, or loss of central visual field may lead to impaired acuity as well. Diseases that damage the optic nerve or tracks, such as multiple sclerosis, produce optic atrophy and contrast sensitivity impairments as well as field loss (Trobe, 2001). Figure 24.2 illustrates the projection of visual information from the visual field to the visual cortex. The type of field loss depends on where in this pathway the damage occurs. Damage to the visual pathway from the optic tract, optic radiations, origin of the optic radiation, the lateral geniculate nucleus, and primary visual cortex will cause homonymous field defects, or defects to similar regions in both eyes. For example, a stroke that affects the right middle cerebral artery and damages part of the optic radiations will result in loss in part of the left visual field, the nasal visual field of the right eye, and the temporal visual field of the left eye. Insult to the optic

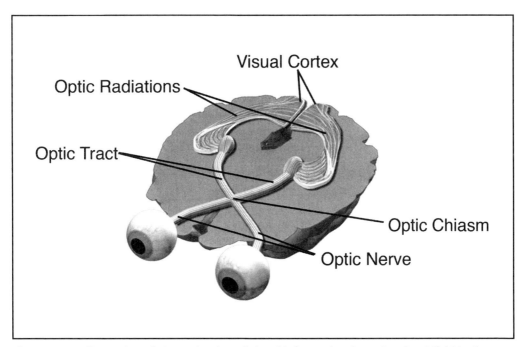

**Figure 24.2.** Illustration of the projection of visual information from the visual field to the primary visual cortex. From *Low Vision Rehabilitation: A Practical Guide for Occupational Therapists*, by M. Scheiman, M Scheiman, and S. G. Whittaker, 2007, Thorofare, NJ: SLACK Incorporated. Copyright 2007 by SLACK Incorporated. Reprinted with permission.

chiasm, where the nerve fibers cross, results in more diffuse damage. Damage to the occipital parietal cortex will affect attention on the contralateral side, with damage to the right parietal cortex usually leading to left field visual inattention or neglect. Damage to the temporal occipital regions often results in object agnosia and alexia. In addition, severe parietal damage leads to other perceptual problems (Trobe, 2001).

## Target Areas for Intervention

Comprehensive occupational therapy for low vision rehabilitation requires advanced education and additional certification. However, with some additional training, any occupational therapist should be able to identify disability and provide first response interventions. First response interventions involve patient education and use of commercially available materials that provide some relief from visual disability and that may supplement the services of certified low vision and blindness professionals. The best service delivery model for complete low vision rehabilitation includes a certified rehabilitation professional (e.g., an occupational therapist with advanced certification) and an optometrist or ophthalmologist, preferably one with some advanced training in low vision rehabilitation (Scheiman et al., 2006).

Three general interventions and strategies address visual disability with different service delivery systems. Low vision rehabilitation (Goodrich & Bailey, 2000; Scheiman et al., 2006; Warren, 2001) emphasizes visual methods to compensate for vision loss, such as optimization of lighting or use of optical devices. Another approach that predates low vision rehabilitation, blind rehabilitation, emphasizes use of nonvisual methods to compensate for vision loss, such as Braille and the use of touch and hearing (Ponchillia, Dewey, & Cymerant, 1988). Private and state agencies often employ blind rehabilitation therapists or orientation and mobility specialists to provide blind rehabilitation services. The third approach addresses visual disability from the standpoint of oculomotor problems (Scheiman, 2002) and perceptual problems (Warren, 2001; Zoltan, 2007) and is administered by occupational therapists and/or optometrists specializing in pediatric or neurological disorders. These services are provided by occupational therapists in medical rehabilitation settings and optometrists in private practice settings who specialize in binocular vision and perceptual problems. Occupational therapists who provide specialized treatment for visual disability are able to obtain certification as low vision or blindness professionals as well.

## 🍃 Contextual Considerations

### Clinical

A therapist working in an acute or subacute rehabilitation setting with older adults will often encounter comorbid visual disability as well as vision disabilities associated with a primary neurological diagnosis. Although the focus of the occupational therapy would relate to the primary disability, an occupational therapist considers all client and contextual factors in organizing a treatment plan. The therapist would, therefore, need to compensate for the vision loss in order to enable someone to recover occupational performance. For example, a person with memory loss associated with neurological complications of diabetes is likely also to have vision loss associated with diabetes. In implementing the use of written notes to compensate for memory loss, the therapist would also need to compensate for impaired acuity and contrast sensitivity by teaching the client to write larger and optimize lighting.

Clinical service delivery models of low vision rehabilitation that involve occupational therapists include home-based care; outpatient settings, often including an optometrist who specializes in low vision; and services provided in the Veterans Administration, a distinct blind rehabilitation service. An emerging model of service delivery integrates blindness and medical rehabilitation with occupational therapy services (funded by Medicare, Medicaid, and medical insurance).

When a vision disability is discovered, the occupational therapist takes two equally important actions. First, an evaluation is performed and appropriate first response interventions are initiated. Second, the patient is referred to advanced low vision and blindness rehabilitation services. If the patient has partial vision, advanced services should involve collaboration between an eye doctor, usually an optometrist, and a therapist with training in low vision rehabilitation. Advanced treatment involves a careful investigation of occupational history, cognitive and physical strengths and weaknesses, and contextual considerations (Scheiman, Scheiman, & Whittaker, 2007).

The Academy for Certification of Vision Rehabilitation and Education Professionals (ACVREP) has developed basic competency standards for professionals in the areas of orientation and mobility, low vision therapy, and vision rehabilitation therapy. ACVREP certifies basic competency, the minimum required for practice. ACVREP certification is widely recognized by many professions and agencies and is required by an increasing number of agencies that provide low vision and blindness rehabilitation services.

The American Occupational Therapy Association also provides specialty certification in low vision rehabilitation for occupational therapists and occupational therapy assistants who have 5 or more years' experience in clinical practice. For occupational therapists, this could be considered an advanced competency.

## Family

Unlike total blindness, low vision is often a hidden impairment because others cannot quickly recognize it. Without education, family and friends can be confused by someone who claims to be blind but has inconsistencies in seeing objects and is observed navigating a room. Frequently, the depression associated with loss of vision later in life is confused with cognitive impairment and leads others to treat the individual with low vision as if he or she had a cognitive impairment. Low vision also affects a person's ability to recognize faces, read facial expressions, and eat neatly. As a result, vision impairment often leads to social withdrawal and isolation.

Once low vision is identified, care must be taken to educate the person with low vision and address the need for others to know about the disability. The person's friends and acquaintances must learn to take the initiative to greet the individual when passing him or her or to use proper sighted guide technique as well as some basic accommodations and courtesies, such as not walking away from someone who cannot see without telling the person and also not speaking loudly or with condescension (Horowitz & Reinhardt, 2000; Scheiman et al., 2006). These basic skills and courtesies should be taught as part of a first response intervention.

## Practice Setting

Environmental factors can exacerbate or ameliorate the effects of visual acuity; thus, treatment of low vision places a heavy emphasis on environmental modifications, which may include optimizing lighting, using large-print bingo or playing cards, or bringing a person closer to a television set. Many interventions for visual disability involve environmental modifications or use of assistive devices that are specific to a person's home or workplace (Hall-Lueck, 2004; Scheiman et al., 2006). Effective low vision rehabilitation requires home- or work-based treatments where clients are taught how to optimize lighting or label and mark their food items, dials and controls, medications, and so forth. With older adults, the use of many devices requires careful consideration of where a person habitually sits to perform a task in order to optimize ergonomics. Often, schools, state agencies for the blind, and visually impaired or private organizations offer home- or work-based treatments provided by itinerant vision rehabilitation therapists or, in the case of schools, teachers for the visually impaired.

## Sociopolitical

There are several rehabilitation service delivery systems for people who are blind and visually impaired. The federally mandated educational services for students with special needs include students with visual impairment. Under the Individuals With Disabilities Education Improvement Act of 2004, schools must teach students compensatory techniques for visual impairment and provide needed equipment for a variety of compensatory strategies. Teachers of students who are visually impaired are special educators who have advanced training in the educational techniques necessary for these students.

Historically, services for adults with vision disability have been provided by state agencies and private organizations. These private agencies provide services and resources for transportation, equipment, and rehabilitation instruction. In addition, the Department of Veterans Affairs offers extensive services for veterans who are visually impaired.

Optometrists have been providing low vision rehabilitation services under medical eye care and, more recently, rehabilitation diagnostic codes, but optometrists who employ low vision therapists and rehabilitation instructors have not consistently received reimbursement for their services, limiting optometric-based services to dispensing and a little training with devices. In the 1990s, occupational therapists began to provide low vision rehabilitation as a service reimbursable by Medicare, Medicaid, and most medical insurance. Low vision rehabilitation has unique diagnostic codes that can be used by occupational therapists and optometrists. A financially viable and effective service delivery system involves optometrists and occupational therapists working together, often in private practice settings. Insurance pays for services but generally not equipment. Thus, the occupational therapist providing low vision rehabilitation must coordinate services with the other agencies to provide patients with all of the available resources.

Current certification standards allow occupational therapists, educators, and other health services professionals with a college degree to obtain certification as a certified vision rehabilitation teacher or a certified low vision therapist. Occupational therapists who are interested in evaluating and developing interventions for individuals with low vision must not only be mindful of these certification standards but also understand the unique specialization and certification standards of other experts in low vision and blindness, such as optometrists and certified orientation and mobility specialists (Orr & Huebner, 2001).

Blind people (as many prefer to be called) have formed a unique and very supportive culture in the United States and around the world. They have their own written language (Braille) and a history of separate education (schools for the blind), inculcating them into their own culture. Their culture, of course, emphasizes nonvisual community and leisure activities, with social activities uncluttered by cars and television. The organizations supporting this culture in the United States include the National Federation for the Blind and the American Council for the Blind. Threats to the integrity of their culture and lifestyle include inclusion education, a tendency to encourage reading print versus Braille in children with partial vision, and low vision rehabilitation techniques that emphasize use of vision.

## Lifestyle/Lifespan

An occupational therapist working with older adults with recent vision loss will often need to help his or her clients maintain familiar, "sighted" lifestyle roles and occupations, as visual methods to perform tasks are often preferred. Nonvisual techniques (e.g., recorded books, tactual markers and labeling devices, organizational skills, talking clocks), which often are much more practical, must be introduced, but often older, previously sighted people will resist these changes. For instance, many people with macular degeneration, who can comfortably understand a recorded book at a speed of 250 words per minute (Hensil & Whittaker, 2000), prefer to struggle with visual reading at speeds of less than 100 words per minute. A skilled occupational therapist will follow the lead of his or her client but should gently introduce alternative, less familiar techniques, which, over time and with repeated exposure, are often adopted.

For children and adults who are more adaptable, an introduction to the lifestyle and culture of the blind can be of great benefit, in addition to appropriate vision rehabilitation techniques. A person who is totally blind and knows the correct techniques (Duffy, 2002; Ponchillia et al., 1988; Scheiman et al., 2006; Wiener, Welsh, & Blasch, 2010a, 2010b) can independently navigate the streets or public transportation, use a computer to surf the Internet, read any published book or magazine, live alone, shop, play certain video games, play or listen to sports, ski, sail, perform or enjoy theater, enjoy music, and otherwise live, work, get married, and enjoy life.

## 🖾 Clinical Decision-Making Process
### Defining Focus for Intervention

Clinically, the occupational therapist uses a top-down approach, where clinical reasoning starts with goals that are meaningful to the client, such as enjoying a novel. The therapist then defines what specific tasks, such as visual reading, using recorded books, or Braille reading, may be used to engage in these tasks. Using the evidence base, the developed theories of visual function, and evaluation results, the therapist identifies what specific processes, social environmental demands, physical environmental demands, and task demands prevent achievement of the goal tasks; these are known as *performance-limiting factors*. For example, for the client whose goal is to enjoy a novel, the occupational therapist must know the visual requirements for visual reading (Whittaker & Lovie-Kitchin, 1993). The evaluation then assesses both contextual/environmental factors (available print size) and client factors (visual acuity) to determine if the requirements for this task can be met, and, if not, the visual process becomes a performance-limiting factor.

### Establishing Goals for Intervention

To treat vision disability effectively, the practitioner must think of each performance-limiting factor as including both client and contextual elements. For example, a person's ability to read print depends on acuity reserve, the difference between the print size being read (a contextual factor) and the smallest print someone can see (visual acuity, a client factor). One can enable reading by enlarging print or improving acuity (e.g., by optimizing lighting), or both. Performance-limiting factors include psychosocial factors, such as limited resources to purchase devices or lack of available helpers, as well as visual factors. In low vision rehabilitation, the focus is usually on compensatory interventions, such as the use of magnification devices or adaptive scanning strategies.

## Visual Acuity and Contrast Sensitivity Limitations

Optimizing light often maximizes acuity and contrast sensitivity. Light is optimized by adjusting light intensity and avoiding glare. Light intensity is best controlled by the distance of the light source. Glare is avoided by positioning a shaded light to the side to ensure the light sources and reflections of the light are minimized. One compensates for impaired acuity by increasing size magnification and relative distance magnification, for example, bringing a person closer to a television. Advanced treatment by certified low vision therapists working with optometrists involves a plethora of optical and electronic magnification devices. Electronic devices enhance contrast as well.

## Central and Peripheral Field Limitations

The disability associated with central or peripheral field loss depends on the size and position of a person's intact visual field and the size of the objects or print being used. For example, a person with an overall reduction in visual field will have more difficulty seeing larger print or objects. The general approach is to teach compensatory scanning, or looking in the direction of the field loss so that intact areas of vision are used. For example, a person with a right field loss learns to look far to the right so that the intact left field can be used to see objects to the right of midline. A person with overall field loss must scan in all directions to view larger objects or a large area. People with central vision loss learn to look above or below something rather than directly at it, which is called *eccentric viewing*. Sometimes optical devices, or prisms, may be used; for example, an individual may use a rearview mirror to facilitate compensatory scanning.

## Oculomotor and Perceptual Limitations

In adults and in children with developmental disabilities, oculomotor and perceptual impairment often results from brain dysfunction. Treatment to correct eye movement disorders involves several specialized therapeutic instruments and training in close collaboration with an ophthalmologist or optometrist specializing in eye movement disorders. The typical first intervention is using an eye patch to eliminate the symptoms of binocular dysfunction, and, often, visual pursuit and scanning exercises will be used to increase the eye's range of motion.

Occupational therapists often treat perceptual impairment. With visual neglect, the treatment involves explicitly teaching new scanning patterns to the neglected side, using increased and multimodal stimulation on the neglected side, and reducing stimulation on the unaffected side (Marshall, 2009; Zoltan, 2007). Having people with left neglect adapt to a prism that optically shifts the visual scene to the right has been shown to have long-term effects (Marshall, 2009). There are several methods for treating spatial, object, and word recognition disorders (Zoltan, 2007). In general, we have found that using activities that most closely resemble goal activities is the best way to generalize to goal occupations. For example, if a person wishes to recover cooking skills, therapeutic activities should involve cooking items or scanning in a kitchen, rather than pen-and-pencil activities. Start with easily recognized or performed discrimination tasks, and, through repetition, the individual's performance will improve. The tasks are graded from activities that are more familiar to the person being treated to less familiar activities and objects. It is important to carefully consider the premorbid activities of the individual; for example, a cook will recognize kitchen items more easily than will a woodworker.

## Designing Theory-Based Intervention

Research on low vision has grown exponentially to more than 13,000 publications (Goodrich & Arditi, 2004). Moreover, there is an enormous amount of research on the physical and neurological basis of sensory and visual processes at the National Eye Institute, a branch of the National Institutes of Health dedicated to funding vision research. With validated evaluation instruments and an understanding of optics and visual processes, the analytical evaluation should enable the occupational therapist to hone in on specific impediments to a particular activity or goal occupation, such as reading (Legge, 2007; Scheiman et al., 2006; Whittaker & Lovie-Kitchin, 1993).

There are hundreds of nontechnical adaptive devices, such as clothing markers, devices that signal when a cup is full, tactual dial markers, talking watches, and writing aids. A home visit is often involved. The therapist also teaches the patient how to use his or her remaining vision; for example, for a patient with central or peripheral field loss, the therapist would encourage the use of compensatory scanning. The therapist, with the help of an optometrist, selects appropriate devices that will help compensate for vision loss, and the therapist trains the patient to perform goal activities with these devices. Such compensatory devices include many optical devices, such as handheld magnifiers, special high-powered reading glasses, spectacle-mounted telescopes, and handheld telescopes. Electronic devices include electronic magnifiers, computer screen magnifiers, text-to-speech systems that read print and computer displays aloud, and a variety of electronic navigation notebook and recording devices. An important part of this intervention is connecting the patient with the variety of services that are available for people with vision disability, including free telephone directory services, state services for the blind, transportation services, and free recordings for the blind and physically handicapped.

## Evaluating Progress

Typically, goals are specified and progress is measured as observable and measurable task performance (Scheiman, Scheiman, & Whittaker, 2007). One must be careful to not assume that a goal activity is performed visually. For example, a goal to "read medication labels" should be specified as "identify medications" because a person may be able to easily and accurately use tactual markers to tag and identify medication. Another common goal is to "read novels." For fluent reading, the goal might be stated as "read or enjoy a novel visually, using text-to-speech or recordings for the blind." This allows for other modalities to be used to successfully accomplish the goal.

For people who physically can perform an activity, progress is measured in terms of frequency of cuing, performance accuracy, and rate or speed of performance. Reading rate (words per minute) and accuracy (e.g., 8/10 correct word identifications) are excellent measures of reading performance. For other than reading, identification accuracy (e.g., recognize faces on the TV with 3/4 accuracy) is used. Standardized tests are available for the advanced practitioner, but performance is best measured with the material a client wishes to work with or read. One must be careful to use material of comparable difficulty when evaluating progress in tasks that were assessed in earlier evaluations. If a person wishes to read the sports page of a newspaper and pay bills, then these materials should be used for the initial and subsequent tests to evaluate progress. Performance-based methods for measuring change may be quickly measured in a treatment session by, for example, counting the number of words read correctly in a 1-minute timed interval, or the number of correct identifications of an object or label divided by the number of attempts.

## Determining Change in or Termination of Treatment

Most medical insurance or individual treatment or education plans require that performance-based measures show improvement with repeated skilled therapy, or the therapy must be changed or terminated. Standardized tests such as the *Pepper Visual Skills for Reading* test (Scheiman, Scheiman, & Whittaker, 2007) have published confidence intervals that indicate what change is statistically significant. Otherwise, measured changes are descriptive, and a therapist determines if progress is reliable by repeating measurements for each treatment session and looking for trends over several sessions.

### Case Study

*Description*

JW is an 88-year-old retired nurse who enjoys needlework, cooking, sewing, and reading. She lives with her husband in a fully accessible apartment with supportive family nearby. JW has excellent social support and economic resources, and her physical and cognitive abilities are within functional limits for her goals. At the time of the evaluation, she had limited cooking to the heating of prepared foods and was independent with all aspects of self-care, except applying makeup. She had given away her sewing and needlework materials and struggled with reading large-print books. Her physical and cognitive functioning was within functional limits for all desired leisure and homemaking activities, and performance was limited primarily by visual impairment from a slowly progressing form of macular degeneration.

JW reports missing the pleasure she derived from cooking for her family and participating in a needlecraft group with her friends. She is becoming increasingly frustrated by her difficulties with reading the newspaper and books. Her ultimate goal is to resume premorbid roles and occupations.

Her pattern of reading errors, her response to changing print size, and careful field-testing revealed that JW had an area of better visual acuity (20/60 equivalent) that was flanked by regions of reduced acuity, restricting her field of view. JW's field of view and acuity were significantly improved with very intense lighting (a 75-watt directional bulb at 4–6 inches), which required JW to use yellow sunglasses and careful shading and positioning of the light to the side to minimize glare. She had a moderate loss in contrast sensitivity. With this lighting, her reading acuity was 1.2 M[1] (10–12 points) in her left eye at 40 centimeters (16 inches) and significantly worse in her right eye. Because of the field restriction, as print magnification increased, her reading first increased and then decreased, as she was only able to see a few letters, rather than whole words.

JW was taught to use the magnifier she owned to help with spot reading, such as reading cooking directions and medication bottles. Two pairs of spectacle magnifiers were recommended to the prescribing optometrist, one for regular print and fine needlework and another for larger print. All devices were evaluated wth her goal activities in the clinic and in the home in mind before recommendations were made. Follow-up instruction with the devices was performed as needed.

### Long- and Short-Term Goals

JW's long-term goals are as follows:

1. JW will be able to read newspapers and books at a rate of 100 words per minute, using adaptive equipment.
2. JW will be able to perform all aspects of meal preparation using adaptive equipment.
3. JW will be able to resume leisure activities of needlework and sewing using adaptive equipment.

JW's short-term goals are as follows:

1. JW will identify 10 large-print words correctly using lighting-control techniques and an optical device.
2. JW will identify and correct glare and optimize lighting to detect blemishes on fruits and vegetables.
3. JW will be able to thread a large tapestry needle with yarn using a spectacle magnifier.

### Therapist's Goals and Strategies

1. Evaluate occupational history, social roles, and activity patterns.
2. Perform an analytical functional visual evaluation in the clinic and in the home in order to identify performance-limiting visual factors.

---

[1]M is the metric standard for print size. M is the distance in meters at which the letter subtends 5 minutes of arc and is barely visible by someone with typical vision.

3. Educate JW regarding the specific aspects of her vision loss and adaptive strategies, such as identifying glare sources and positioning body and task lights to optimize vision.

4. Recommend lighting for preferred sitting areas.

5. Recommend adjusting the television position to avoid glare and positioning seats closer to television.

6. Apply tactile markers to stove, oven dials, and microwave controls.

7. Provide instruction and practice with eccentric viewing techniques (looking above targets) in order to maximize field of view.

*Activity: Bean Soup*

During a home visit, JW is asked to read a recipe using a spectacle magnifier and to sort the dried beans using an eccentric viewing position technique. Using techniques that have been demonstrated in the clinic, she is asked to identify glare sources and position her body in relation to task lights in order to maximize her vision and ability to use utensils and appliance controls.

*Treatment Objectives*

JW will be able to identify and adjust lighting and body position in order to maximize vision and safely carry out kitchen tasks.

# Resources

## Internet Resources

Academy for Certification of Vision Rehabilitation & Education Professionals: www.acvrep.org

American Council of the Blind: www.acb.org

American Foundation for the Blind: www.afb.org

American Occupational Therapy Association: www.aota.org

Association for Education and Rehabilitation of the Blind and Visually Impaired: www.aerbvi.org

Learning, Sight and Sound: www.lssproducts.com

National Federation of the Blind: www.nfb.org

National Library Service for the Blind and Physically Handicapped: www.loc.gov/nls/

Precision Vision LTD: www.precisionvision.com

ShopLowVision.com: www.shoplowvision.com

U.S. Department of Veterans Affairs Blind Rehabilitation Service: www.va.gov/blindrehab

Vision Education Seminars: www.visionedseminars.com

## Print Resources

Jernigan, K. (Ed.). (1994). *If blindness comes*. Baltimore, MD: National Federation for the Blind.

# References

Berger, J. W., Fine, S. L., & Maguire, M. G. (Eds.). (1999). *Age-related macular degeneration*. Philadelphia, PA: Mosby.

Duffy, M. (2002). *Making life more livable*. New York, NY: American Foundation for the Blind Press.

Enoch, J. M., Werner, J. S., Haegerstrom-Portnoy, G., Lakshminarayanan, V., & Rynders, M. (1999). Forever young: Visual functions not affected or minimally affected by aging: A review. *Journals of Gerontology: Biological Sciences, 54A*(8), B336–B351.

Goodrich, G. L., & Arditi, A. (2004). A trend analysis of the low-vision literature. *The British Journal of Visual Impairment, 22*, 105–106.

Goodrich, G. L., & Bailey, I. L. (2000). A history of the field of vision rehabilitation from the perspective of low vision. In B. Silverstone, M. A. Lang, B. Rosenthal, & E. Faye (Eds.), *The lighthouse handbook on visual impairment and vision rehabilitation* (Vol. 2). Oxford, England: Oxford University Press.

Hall-Lueck, A. (2004). *Functional vision: A practitioner's guide to evaluation and intervention*. New York, NY: American Foundation for the Blind Press.

Hensil, J., & Whittaker, S. G. (2000). Comparing visual reading versus auditory reading by sighted persons and persons with low vision. *Journal of Visual Impairment and Blindness, 94*(12), 762–770.

Horowitz, A., & Reinhardt, J. P. (2000). Mental health issues in vision impairment: Research in depression, disability and rehabilitation. In B. Silverstone, M. A. Lang, B. P. Rosenthal, & E. E. Faye (Eds.), *The lighthouse handbook on vision impairment and vision rehabilitation* (Vol. 2, pp. 1089–1109). Oxford, England: Oxford University Press.

Jose, R. T. (Ed.). (1983). *Understanding low vision*. New York, NY: American Foundation for the Blind Press.

Legge, G. E. (2007). *Psychophysics of reading in normal and low vision*. Mahwah, NJ: Lawrence Erlbaum Associates.

Lei, H., & Schuchard, R. A. (1997). Using two preferred retinal loci for different lighting conditions in patients with central scotomas. *Investigative Opthamalogy and Visual Science, 38*(9), 1812–1818.

Leigh, R. J., & Zee, D. S. (2006). *The neurology of eye movements* (4th ed.). Oxford, England: Oxford University Press.

Levi, D. M. (1992). Amblyopia: A development disorder of spatial vision. *Optometry and Visual Science, 69*, 123.

Marshall, R. S. (2009). Rehabilitation approaches to hemineglect. *Neurologist, 15*, 185–192.

Mash, C., & Dobson, V. (1998). Long-term reliability and predictive validity of the Teller acuity card procedure. *Vision Research, 38*(4), 619–626.

Massof, R. W., & Lidoff, L. (2000). *Issues in low vision rehabilitation*. New York, NY: American Foundation for the Blind Press.

Orr, A. L., & Huebner, K. (2001). Toward a collaborative working relationship among vision rehabilitation and allied health professionals. *Journal of Visual Impairment and Blindness, 95*(8), 468–482.

Ponchillia, P. E., Dewey, C., & Cymerant, J. (1988). Rehabilitation teachers and orientation and mobility instructors: Interprofessional perceptions. *Journal of Visual Impairment and Blindness, 82*(6), 411–414.

Rovner, B. W., & Ganguli, M. (1998). Depression and disability associated with impaired vision: The MoVies Project. *Journal of the American Geriatrics Society, 46*(5), 617–619.

Rovner, B. W., & Shmuely-Dulitzki, Y. (1997). Screening for depression in low-vision elderly. *International Journal of Geriatric Psychiatry, 12*(9), 955–959.

Scheiman, M. (2002). *Understanding and managing vision deficits: A guide for occupational therapists* (2nd ed.). Thorofare, NJ: Slack.

Scheiman, M., Scheiman, M., & Whittaker, S. G. (2007). *Low vision rehabilitation: A practical guide for occupational therapists.* Thorofare, NJ: Slack.

Schwartz, S. H. (2004). *Visual perception: A clinical orientation.* New York, NY: McGraw Hill.

Teller, D. Y., & Mavshon, J. A. (1986). Visual development. *Vision Research, 26,* 1483–1506.

Trobe, J. D. (2001). *The neurology of vision* (Vol. 60). Oxford, England: Oxford University Press.

Warren, M. (2001). *Occupational therapy practice guidelines for adults with low vision.* Bethesda, MD: AOTA.

Whittaker, S. G., & Lovie-Kitchin, J. E. (1993). Visual requirements for reading. *Optometry and Vision Science, 70*(1), 54–65.

Wiener, W. R., Welsh, R. L., & Blasch, B. B. (Eds.). (2010a). *Foundations of orientation and mobility: History and theory* (3rd ed., Vol. 1). New York, NY: American Foundation for the Blind Press.

Wiener, W. R., Welsh, R. L., & Blasch, B. B. (Eds.). (2010b). *Foundations of orientation and mobility: Instructional strategies and practical applications* (3rd ed., Vol. 2). New York, NY: American Foundation for the Blind Press.

Zoltan, B. (2007). *Vision, perception and cognition: A manual for the examination and treatment of the neurologically impaired adult* (4th ed.). Thorofare, NJ: Slack.

# Fall-Related Injuries

*Stephen M. Gagajewski*

## Synopsis of Clinical Condition

### Prevalence and Etiology

Among adults 65 years of age and older, falls are a major contributing factor for injuries and death. Fall-related-death rates have drastically increased over the past 10 years (Stevens, 2006). In 2005, about 15,800 people age 65 years and older died from injuries related to unintentional falls. In addition to increasing age, race and sex impact the fall fatality rate. Men are more likely to die from injuries sustained in a fall. In 2004, the fall fatality rate was 49% higher for men, after adjusting for age. The difference in fatal falls between African Americans and European Americans between the ages of 65 and 74 years is minimal. However, after the age of 75, European American men have the highest fatality rate, followed by European American women, African American men, and African American women (Stevens & Sogolow, 2005).

Fall rates and severity of injuries sustained in a fall increase with age. Fall injury rates for individuals age 85 years and older arc 4 to 5 times higher than those for adults between the ages of 65 and 74 years. One in three older adults falls each year; half of these will experience a second fall within 6 months. About 1.8 million adults over the age of 65 were treated in emergency departments for nonfatal injuries sustained in a fall.

Women are 67% more likely than men to experience a nonfatal fall injury. For older adults, 72% of those admitted to hospitals for hip fractures were women. Women who live alone experience more falls than do men who live alone. Women are more likely to report falls to their family or a health care provider. Women also demonstrate a greater fear of falling than do men (Painter & Elliott, 2009).

### Common Characteristics and Symptoms

The reasons for falls are multifactorial. Falls can occur at any place and any time. Some falls cannot be avoided; however, many falls are preventable. An unsafe environment, decreased safety awareness, and improper use of drugs and alcohol all contribute to the high number of preventable falls. Many medical issues can contribute to the risk of falls. However, with safety awareness training, patients and their family members/caregivers can reduce or eliminate the risk for falls.

Falls are the interaction (or lack of positive interaction) between intrinsic and extrinsic factors of the client. Intrinsic factors include the client's physical skills, sensory contributions, balance, mobility, medication routines, and psychological factors. Extrinsic factors relate to the environment: Throw rugs, poorly fitting shoes, clothing that could get caught up on other objects, the use of assistive devices, cluttered spaces, poor lighting, obstacles, and slippery surfaces are all part of the external physical environment that contributes to fall risks. The physical and psychological abilities of the client need to meet the demands of the environment in order to overcome the risk factors for safe mobility (Bergland & Wyller, 2004; Lord, Menz, & Sherrington, 2006; Peterson & Clemson, 2008).

The majority of falls occur during typical, everyday activities. Patients fall getting into and out of the shower or tub. Seniors report difficulty raising their legs to get over the side of the tub. They also report holding on to the shower curtain for support. Older adults admit to using towel racks and toilet paper racks as support during transfers. If they had a shower chair or safety bars in the tub/shower area and correct knowledge of safe transfer techniques, seniors could reduce the risk of falls.

Many older individuals report breaking an arm or a leg while reaching up for objects on a top shelf (mostly in the bathroom, kitchen, and bedroom). They take out a footstool, stand on their tiptoes, and shift their weight incorrectly, thus changing their center of gravity while reaching for an object. The result is a fall. If these patients had used a reacher and received training in item storage and retrieval, their falls could have been prevented. These are just some examples of fall-related injuries that could have been avoided with proper training and the use of adaptive equipment.

Multiple drug interactions are a significant contributor to increased fall risk among older adults. Patients take medications for pain, anxiety, sleep disturbances, high blood pressure, and personality disorders. While these patients are in the hospital, pharmacy and nursing staff members will closely monitor their use of these drugs. However, in the home, the drug routine is not as closely monitored. Patients may make mistakes and put themselves at increased risk for falls. Side effects of polypharmacy include feelings of giddiness, dizziness, somnolence, weakness, and fatigue; balance issues; equilibrium difficulties; and difficulty with postural adjustments.

Drugs also create difficulties with concentration and memory. This may not exemplify a true fall risk, but it does put the patient and his or her family members at a risk during meal preparation (e.g., the client forgets he put something on the stove, and the result is a fire). When medication routines are closely monitored to meet the needs of the client, falls may be reduced by 70% (Cooper & Burfield, 2009).

Improper footwear is a major preventable risk factor for falls. Somehow, fashion supersedes function when it comes to footwear. Worn-out shoes, shoes with no backs or sides, shoes without laces, and ill-fitting shoes are a significant contributor to falls. Shoes with a heel height greater than 2.5 centimeters can double the risk for falls (Tencer et al., 2004). Physical deformities of the feet increase the risk for falls. Bunions, toe deformities, ulcers, pain (especially from planter fasciitis), and deformed nails can predispose someone to falls. It is highly recommended that any fall assessment include a footwear inspection and regular visits to the podiatrist.

Postural hypotension also increases the risk for falls. Low blood pressure and cerebral hypoperfusion result in the loss of balance. Care must be taken during transfers (supine to sit, sit to stand). Patients should be instructed to take their time during transfers and give their body time to adjust to the change in position.

Nutritional intake also has an effect on fall rates in older adults. Higher fall rates have been noted in populations with vitamin D deficiency. Neuromuscular function as well as muscular strength can be impaired as a result of deficient vitamin D intake (Flicker et al., 2005).

Falls, fear of falling, and depression are interrelated. When a client decreases his or her participation in life, secondary to the fear of falling, feelings of depression will develop. Activity restrictions, especially for high-energy people, will result in decreased satisfaction with quality of life experiences. As the tendency toward fear of falling increases, the patient will experience a loss of autonomy. Malnutrition, sleep disturbance, gait dysfunctions, and decreased participation can manifest as depression (Thomas et al., 1998).

Sleep disturbances are associated with concerns for the individual's physical and psychological well-being. People with sleep disturbances will take medications to help them sleep. The combination of poor physical health, lack of sleep, and the taking of medications for sleep puts an individual at risk for falls (St. George, Delbaere, Williams, & Lord, 2009).

Poor hygiene and the need for catheterization may result in urinary tract infections (UTIs). About 30% of women and 10% of men over the age of 65 years will experience a UTI. These UTIs have a direct impact on fall rates in older adults. Fatigue develops because the body is fighting off the UTI. As a result, strength, balance, and reaction time may be affected. Patients may fall because they are in a rush to make it to the bathroom with a urinary emergency (Marquand, 2010). As therapists, we could instruct our clients in and review with them proper toileting and hygiene techniques. Safe and sanitary toileting techniques, the use of a commode at bedside, and the use of incontinence pads can reduce the need to rush to the toilet, thus reducing the possibility of a fall. Bladder retraining techniques could also be used to reduce hurried travel time to the toilet area.

Pain, chronic or acute, is another risk factor and predictor of falls. Two or more locations of musculoskeletal pain or polyarticular pain results in a greater occurrence of falls, and there are higher rates of falls when the pain is more intense and disabling. Pain that interferes with activities will result in increased falls

(Leveille et al., 2009). Pain results in problems with the physical, psychological, and social participation of the sufferer. Pain causes sleep disturbances, increased medication use, irritability, and poor appetite. All of these issues are predictors of future falls.

Cognitive impairments may also contribute to falls. Individuals with cognitive disabilities sometimes do not recognize that they are limited in their mobility skills. As a result, they may attempt to walk when they are physically limited by pain, balance, or motor planning difficulties. In addition, individuals with cognitive impairments may not be aware of safety concerns. For instance, they may get up in the middle of the night to use the bathroom and, not realizing that the sheets and blankets are around their ankles, trip over the blankets and injure themselves. Many older individuals are required to use assistive devices, such as walkers or canes, during mobility activities. Individuals with cognitive impairments may have greater difficulty recalling the proper use of these devices and will sometimes use them in an unsafe manner. Fall rates for individuals with cognitive impairments are twice those of persons without cognitive issues (Tinetti, Speechley, & Ginter, 1988; Van Dijk, Meulenberg, Van de Sande, & Habbema, 1993).

The ability to attend, sustain attention, and switch attention has a major impact on the rate of falls. It is more challenging for an older adult to engage in a cognitive task while simultaneously dealing with a balance issue. Performance of one task (recall of a phone number) may exclude the safe completion (balance adjustments) of another task. This trade-off is known as a *dual-task cost* (Lindenberger, Mariske, & Baltes, 2000; Maki, Zecevic, Bateni, Kirshenbaum, & McIlroy, 2001).

## Target Areas for Intervention

Areas of intervention should focus on the needs of the client. The causes of falls are multifactorial; therefore, interventions can take many approaches. From a physical view, intrinsic factors, such as strength, range of motion, balance, and endurance, should be addressed. A client presenting with cognitive concerns would benefit from a patient education–based program. One strategy is to provide the client with memory aids, such as a checklist for safe use of a walker or pictures posted in the client's room to show the proper sequence and positioning for correct dressing techniques. The risk of a fall may be increased by a cluttered environment. An environmental safety checklist could be used to address these extrinsic factors.

The client's roles can also have an impact on the interventions provided. If the patient is a caregiver for his or her spouse, patient education would benefit the client as well as his or her spouse. Reviews and instructions for safety and problem solving can be part of the cognitive/behavioral approach. This could include what to do after someone experiences a fall. For example, does the client know to dial 911 after a fall?

The goal of any type of intervention is to maximize function and participation. Research has demonstrated that combinations of interventions work the best in a fall-prevention program. This includes exercise, environmental adaptations, and cognitive/behavioral strategies. Intertwined within these approaches is the sensory processing component.

Does the client demonstrate over- or underreaction to sensory registration? It is important to understand the sensory processing abilities of the client to maximize safety during functional activities, such as activities of daily living (ADL) and mobility. To what types of cuing is the client most receptive? This could include tactile cues, verbal cues, and visual cues. It is important to address vestibular issues, auditory concerns, and proprioceptive difficulties, as all of these can contribute to falls.

## ⚙ Contextual Considerations

### Clinical

Assessments and information-gathering techniques will differ depending on the setting. Information can be obtained from a chart review, a computer review, or a report from the client. If the client is a poor historian, information could be obtained from a family member or caregiver.

A fall history should be obtained. This would include where, when, and why a fall occurred. The time of the day and surrounding circumstances should be recorded. What happened before the fall? What medications were being consumed? Did the client eat prior to the fall? Was the client rushing to complete an ADL task, such as toileting? Was the client upset before the fall? What was the physical environment like (e.g., lighting, clutter)? Did the client get injured during the fall? Is this this the first time there has been a fall, or have there been previous falls in the past? If there were previous falls, when were they, how many were there, and how far apart were they? Has the client experienced "almost" falls, where he was able to catch himself prior to hitting the ground? What did the client feel like before falling (e.g., short of breath, dizzy)? What type of clothing was the client wearing at the time of the fall? Was the client able to get up by himself after the fall? How long did the client stay on the floor after the fall? Does the client remember the fall?

A chart review will be initiated if the setting is in a hospital or nursing home. A complete medical history, including all diagnoses and comorbidities, the latest tests, and a current medication list, is important. A social history should also be obtained. This includes living arrangements. Does the client live with someone or by herself? Is the client employed and, if so, in what type of job? Does the client have a history of illegal drug use or excessive alcohol use? What type of transportation is available for the client? Is there family support? Does the client live in a house or an apartment? How many steps does the client take to get into the house and how many steps to get upstairs? Does the client use or have access to a commode, a walker, a wheelchair, crutches, a cane, a stair glide, a shower chair, or support bars around the tub/toilet area?

Physical skills of the client can be assessed with range of motion and manual muscle testing. *Timed Up and Go* (Podsiadlo & Richardson, 1991) and the *Tinetti Assessment Tool for Balance and Gait* (Tinetti, Williams, & Mayewski, 1986) can be used to assess safety during mobility. The risk for falls can be assessed with the *Modified Falls Efficacy Scale* (Cheal & Clemson, 2001) and the *Fall Risk Assessment for Older Adults: The Hendrich II Fall Risk Model* (Hendrich, Bender, & Nyhuis, 2003). Functional transfers and ADL skills can be assessed with the *Functional Independence Measurement* (FIM; Wright, 2000). The home environment should also be assessed. Apartment safety and design could be assessed with the *Gerontological Environmental Modifications* (Bakker, 2005).

Decreased cognition and feelings of depression are predictors for falls. The *Mini-Cog,* a quick and easy assessment for basic cognitive skills (Borson, Scanlan, Watanabe, Tu, & Lessing, 2005), the *Geriatric Depression Scale* (Sheikh et al., 1991), and the *Center for Epidemiologic Studies Depression Scale* (Hann, Winter, & Jacobsen, 1999) are good assessments for depression.

Falls and the fear of falling reduce participation in life. As a result, quality of life is diminished. The *Functional Status Questionnaire* (Jette et al., 1986), which examines physical, psychological, social, and role function, and the *Assessment of Occupational Functioning–Collaborative Version* (AOF-CV; Watts, 1996) can be used to assess quality of life after a fall. The AOF-CV is based on model of human occupation applications.

Changes in vision can put a client at risk for falls. Astigmatism can result in distorted or blurred images. Cataracts reduce light transportation in the retina. Macular degeneration may result in the loss of central field acuity. Glaucoma can cause anything from slightly decreased visual skills to complete blindness. Problems with depth perception, visual acuity, figure–ground, and visual memory can put one at risk for falls. Retinopathy, visual field cuts, and visual neglect increase the danger of falling while completing everyday tasks. As occupational therapists, we can use the *Motor-Free Visual Perception Test* (Colarusso & Hammill, 2002) and the *Beery–Buktenica Developmental Test of Visual–Motor Integration–Sixth Edition* (Beery, Buktenica, & Beery, 2010) to assess visual abilities. It is highly recommended that clients with visual disorders visit an ophthalmologist.

Changes in the auditory system can result in decreased reaction time when responding to safety warnings. Poor comprehension of verbal commands, including instructions for safe use of a walker and transfer techniques, caused by presbycusis, industrial noise exposure, or hearing loss secondary to disease, can put a patient at risk for falls. The *Brief Hearing Loss Screener* (Reuben, Walsh, Moore, Damesyn, & Greendale, 1998), the *Hearing Handicap Inventory for the Elderly* (Gates, Murphy, Rees, & Fraher, 2003), and the *Whispered Voice Test* (Swan & Browning, 1985) can be used to assess basic hearing issues. It is recommended that clients with hearing issues also be assessed by an audiologist.

## Family

The family has to be made aware that their loved one may require 24-hour supervision in order to return home. The patient may not need maximal help for transfers, mobility, and ADL, but the family should be aware that a major commitment is required to keep the patient safe. It is important that the family partake in the decision-making process because new responsibilities will be thrust upon the family members. Are they willing to be home when the therapists come to the house to provide therapy? Can they find the time to transport and stay with the family member if he or she goes to outpatient therapy? Culture and family dynamics have to be taken into consideration. What are the family members' roles related to the care of their loved one? Culture may dictate whether the male or female or younger or older family members are responsible for the help of the individual in need.

The family may experience financial strain because of the costs of the equipment needed for the patient's safety. Medicare may provide a walker and a commode, but that may be all. Bars in the tub area, a shower chair, a reacher, a sock donner, a handheld showerhead, a long-handled shoehorn, and a dressing stick may be required to prevent falls during ADL. The family needs to be made aware of the increased financial responsibilities that will come their way.

It is vital that the family be willing to participate in training to provide quality help for their loved one (especially if there are cognitive issues along with physical concerns). The family needs to encourage their loved one to participate in the home exercise program, to help prevent falls. Correct knowledge of the use of a walker, cane, and wheelchair is needed to ensure safe use of these items. Fall risks could actually increase if these items are not used correctly. Family members should be trained in how to go up and down stairs so they can correctly demonstrate this to the patient and provide help if needed. Can the caregivers help their family member get up safely from the ground if there is a fall?

Most important, the family must be willing to act as an advocate for their loved one. Professionals can make recommendations for equipment and treatments to help in fall prevention, but ultimately it is up to the family to obtain the equipment, use it correctly, and see that there is carryover of the home treatment plan.

A commitment is required on the part of the family. Family members need to be flexible, as habits, routines, and priorities may have to change to meet the demands of the new situation. It would help to provide the family with information about other families who are in similar situations. Respite care and support groups would be of great assistance for these families.

## Practice Setting

Fall prevention should be the concern of every health care provider, no matter what the setting. Any patient in the hospital, young or old, can experience a fall.

Of course, patients with some diagnoses are more predisposed to have a fall, for instance, older patients who have had a cerebral vascular accident, hip replacement, or knee replacement and patients with general overall weakness. The patient may not be in the hospital primarily because of a fall; the fall may be a secondary issue that the client has to deal with. Hospitals are much more concerned with falls than they used to be. Previously, if a client fell in the hospital and broke a leg, the patient's insurance would pay for it. Now, if a patient falls and breaks a leg in the hospital, the hospital is the party responsible for payment.

The setting dictates what can be done for fall prevention therapy. Patients in the intensive care unit (ICU) may have limitations secondary to medical issues. Some ICU patients who have had a coronary artery bypass graft can participate in exercises that strengthen the trunk and extremities. However, the therapist should maintain sternal precautions. Many patients in the ICU may not be responsive to fall prevention education because of an increased intake of drugs.

Subacute care, acute care, and acute rehabilitation patients can participate in all phases of fall prevention activities, including exercise, education, and environmental adaptations. The hospital room should be adapted to prevent falls (e.g., areas should be well lit; all tripping hazards, such as sheets, blankets on the floor, and IV poles, should be removed).

Outpatient therapy could address all three phases of fall prevention—exercise, education, and environmental adaptation. Clients could be taken outside to practice walking on uneven surfaces and maneuvering around obstacles. Assisted living centers and independent living centers could provide patient education, exercise programs, and environmental adaptations. The community centers and adult day care centers could provide all three phases of fall prevention. In these settings, activities are done in groups, which means patients can reinforce each other and encourage each other to participate.

The best setting for fall prevention is the home and the community. This is the natural environment of the participant. The client can adapt his or her own environment for safety, rearranging furniture without needing the permission of a director. Exercises could take place in the home, on the porch, or in the backyard. Other neighbors could be asked to join in. Clients could be taken to the stores they shop in, the churches they attend, and their places of business. They learn to move around obstacles, practice proper body mechanics, and correctly use assistive devices in a realistic setting.

## Sociopolitical

The 108th Congress recognized the increasing expenses for treating falls. Congress also realized that lives and money could be saved by fall prevention education. The Fall Prevention Act of 2003 increased research funding to help identify those at increased risk for falls. Funding was also provided for identifying protective factors as well as for providing interventions for treating falls. Funds were provided to evaluate the effectiveness of current community programs and programs in assisted living centers and nursing homes. A major component of the Act was to develop effective public educational strategies to reduce falls in older adults, and funding was obtained to expand current programs for preventing and treating these falls. The direct cost for falls is projected to reach $43.8 billion by the year 2020 (Centers for Disease Control and Prevention, 2010). The U.S. House of Representatives also approved the Safety of Seniors Act in 2007. This Act directed the Secretary of Health and Human Services to further develop research programs that addressed falls and the risk factors for falls in older adults in America.

## Lifestyle/Lifespan

People who experience falls may have to make some changes to their lifestyle, but this does not mean they have to stop enjoying life. Some people who fear falling give up the activities they enjoy. They stop going out for dinner, stop visiting family members, or stop going to church services. They develop a real fear of leaving the house and, in some cases, a fear of getting out of bed. This should not be the case. Some changes have to be made, and these might result in a slight loss of independence or feelings of grief and helplessness; however, those who experience falls can still participate in and enjoy life. If falls are the result of a neurological disorder, the individual may have to give up driving, but one can ask a friend for a ride, take a cab, or take a bus. Instead of going out alone, people can go out in groups to support each other. Individuals who experience falls may have to change their schedules to accommodate medicine routines, use walkers or canes for safety and balance, and take extra care when walking across uneven surfaces and steps, but they can still participate in many of the same activities. People can still walk, dance, and have fun. The pace just has to be somewhat slowed.

## Clinical Decision-Making Process

### Defining Focus for Intervention

The focus of treatment should depend on the underlying causes for falls and how falls are affecting the client's ability to participate in meaningful occupations. Intervention can focus on improving the client's strength, range of motion, and balance abilities. The cognitive/behavioral components for falls as well as the environmental contributions to increased fall risk might need to be addressed. In some cases, the intervention will need to address all these components, and in other cases, only one or two of the components will need to be addressed.

In order to maximize participation during the session, the therapist needs to discover the right challenge for the client by finding out what activities need to be addressed and whether they are important to the client. The client should be set up for success, meaning that activities chosen for therapy should be accomplishable but somewhat challenging. The client would make no gains and could become bored if activities are too easy. On the other hand, activities should not be too difficult, as this could put the client in danger. Activities that are beyond the client's abilities could result in failure and frustration, and the client's desire to participate could be diminished.

Prior to defining the focus of treatment, the needs of the client have to be determined. The focus of intervention should be based on information obtained from the occupational profile and the analysis of occupational performance. The collective influence (as related to falls) for the following areas should be considered for the focus of treatment: areas of occupation, client factors, activity demands, performance skills, performance patterns, and context/environment. In addition, intervention should focus on what is important to the client. For instance, if meal preparation is not important to the client, it should not be addressed. The client may have a family member or health care aide handle meal preparation. If bathing is important to the client, intervention could revolve around how falls make bathing difficult or dangerous and how to improve bathing skills, which are influenced by falls.

A variety of occupational interventions can be used in the treatment process. The therapeutic use of self (on the part of the practitioner) makes us unique in our approach. This involves the planned use of our personalities, perceptions, and insights in the therapeutic process. Types of possible interventions include occupation-based interventions, purposeful activity, preparatory methods, the consultation process, education process, and advocacy (American Occupational Therapy Association, 2008). There are also many possible approaches for intervention, including health promotion, remediation and restoration, maintaining current levels, compensation, adaptation, and disability prevention (American Occupational Therapy Association, 2008). The type of and approach to intervention should match the needs of the client and the setting.

## Establishing Goals for Intervention

Goals for intervention should be established via collaboration among the therapist (or the team, which might include professionals from other disciplines), the client, and possibly the client's family. Goals are based on the client's current skills, current medical stability, and previous skill levels prior to admission and the changes we want to see the client accomplish related to participation. The setting (e.g., hospital, acute care, acute rehabilitation, subacute care, assisted living center, home/community dwelling) can influence and determine the type of goals.

Strategies used to accomplish goals are based on the physical, psychological, social, and developmental stages of the client. If the client is going home, family input is vital for the success and safety of the client. The skills of the family members also need to be taken into consideration. For instance, can they provide the type of physical assistance required if the goal is moderate assistance for a tub transfer?

Insurance coverage can also determine the type of goals the team and client create. Insurance dictates where (i.e., in what type of setting) a client can be treated. The insurance provider also determines frequency and duration of treatment. If coverage is limited and finite, it might be best to provide family and staff training in fall prevention. Goals would be set accordingly.

The environment a client is discharged to can influence goals. For example, if the client has access to bars and railings around the tub area and a shower chair, a possible goal would be the following: "Mr. Z will be modified independent with a shower transfer." If there is no access to adaptive equipment, the goal would be downgraded: "Mr. Z will complete a shower with minimal assistance."

Goals for fall prevention can address many components, for example, the client's performance skills and areas of occupation. Whatever the needs are, the final goal for treatment should be functional and relate to participation (e.g., "Mr. Z will decrease falls by 50% when completing a tub transfer with minimal assistance"), rather than to biomechanics (e.g., "Mr. Z. will improve hip flexion by 10 degrees during a tub transfer").

## Designing Theory-Based Intervention

As occupational therapists, we have the potential to be leaders in addressing fall prevention. Using the frames of reference and occupational therapy models puts us in a unique position to address the physical, psychological, and social components of a fall-prevention program.

The person–environment–occupation (PEO) model addresses all the subcomponents needed for reducing and eliminating falls during participation in activities. The "person" component addresses active range of motion, strength, and endurance, as well as the sensory contributions required for safety during mobility, ADL, and transfers. This model also helps therapists understand the unseen factors that may contribute to falls. Psychological issues, including mood, depression, anger, and affect, and cognitive issues, which are important for recall of safe procedures for sequencing during transfers and the use of adaptive devices during mobility, are also explored. In addition, spiritual factors, if they are important to the client, are also part of the intervention process. For instance, some patients may feel that sickness is a punishment from the deity because of past sins. These issues need to be explored so they do not have a negative impact on the progress of the client. Most hospitals have a spiritual outreach group that could address these issues more fully.

The occupational and environmental factors contained within the PEO model have a direct impact on the progress a client makes toward fall elimination and reduction. Occupational demands could include activity expectations. Do the client's skills allow him or her to meet these expectations, or do modifications and adjustments have to be made? How does the danger of falls affect safe task completion? The environment also affects safety during the completion of any task. Is the environment safe for the client? What types of adjustments need to be made to make the environment appropriate for the client's skills? Does the client's skill level meet the demands of not only the physical environment but also the social, cultural, and institutional environments?

The biomechanical frame of reference can be used to address the physical concerns of a fall-prevention program. This frame of reference addresses the issues of range of motion, strength, and endurance and could specifically address the exercise portion of the program.

The sensory integration frame of reference could address the balance and proprioception concerns as well as the neuropathies that are associated with falls. Body awareness is important in fall prevention. The client needs to know how his or her body fits into and relates to the environment. The sensory integration frame of reference can address this issue and can help determine what types of cuing are most beneficial for the client.

The rehabilitation frame of reference could educate the participants in adapting the environment for safety. The patient and family are educated in the use of adaptive equipment, such as walkers, canes, reachers, dressing sticks, and sock aids. These devices help prevent falls during ADL and mobility. Many falls and injuries occur in the bathroom during ADL. Therapy can help in recommending commodes, grab bars, shower chairs, and bathtub safety rails. These devices reduce falls during functional transfers.

The model of human occupation addresses the will and desire to participate in occupation. The volition subsystem (personal causation, values, and interest) is the building block and foundation for occupational participation. Habituation (roles, habits, and routines) helps organize and maintain behaviors that are required to adapt to the demands of the environment. The performance subsystem builds on the physical, psychological, and communication/social skills needed for decreasing falls.

The cognitive disability frame of reference can be used for patient and family education. Issues addressed could be safe procedures during transfers and safe use of adaptive equipment. Clients can be educated in the use of nonthreatening clothing, especially safe footwear and well-fitting clothing. (This frame of reference could also be used to educate staff in hospitals, assisted living centers, and skilled nursing facilities and home-based aides.) The cognitive disability frame of reference is advantageous for addressing the different types of cuing required for those with advanced cognitive disabilities (based on Allen's cognitive levels [Allen et al., 2007]).

The cognitive disability frame of reference can be also be used for debriefing (e.g., talking about how an activity was accomplished, reviewing the strong points and areas that need improvement). Safe transfer techniques can be accomplished through rehearsals and repetitions. Many people fall because they are in a hurry. Time management skills could be addressed. Cognitive prosthetics (placing colored tape on the walker to show where the hands should be placed) may be beneficial for some clients. Environmental distractions and increased anxiety may result in falls. The cognitive disability frame of reference can be used to teach the client and family stress reductions techniques and provide them with instructions for creating a stress-free environment with minimal distractions.

The ecological model of occupation has four core constructs—person, tasks, context, and performance (Dunn, Brown, & Youngstrom, 2003). Each construct, individually or combined with another, may determine a person's risk factor for falls. The context takes into consideration where and when a task takes place. It examines the physical environment that may put one at risk for falls. The natural environment, such as hills, grassy surfaces, slippery surfaces, and wind, may contribute to the risk factors for falls. The built environment, which includes ramps, bathroom/kitchen designs, and parking availability, can contribute to fall reduction. The social and cultural environment may also contribute to an increase or decrease in falls. Risk factors that may contribute to falls in the cultural environment are views of adaptive devices (e.g., some cultures view adaptive devices, such as walkers, in a negative light) and gender roles. Some cultures, for example, see women as caretakers of the elderly and sick. Men are excluded from providing care to their older family members, which could increase the risk of falls.

## Evaluating Progress

Progress can be monitored in a variety of ways. Perhaps the most concrete manner is recording the number of falls and near-falls in the present and comparing them to pretreatment levels. The number of injuries, doctors' visits, and days spent in the hospital as a result of falls, along with formal assessment scores, can be recorded at present levels and compared to pretreatment days. Pretreatment and posttreatment quantitative levels of participation, quality of participation, and activity enjoyment could also be compared. Carryover of the home program (on the part of the client and his or her family members) can determine motivation for improvement and progress related to fall reduction.

Psychological issues, including the fear of falling, could also be reassessed. Fear of falling is a major contributor to decreased participation for social activities, such as going out for dinner, going to the movies, or attending religious services. Confidence levels related to functional mobility and transfers could be discussed.

Input from the entire team, including the client, family member, aides, and professionals, should be included for the evaluation of progress. Observations should be made in the natural environment while the client is completing functional tasks. A main component for progress in the treatment program comes from the client herself. How does the client view her own progress? Does she see room for improvement? Does she feel she is participating more in occupational activities? Perhaps the most important element in the reassessment process is the satisfaction of the client.

## Determining Change in or Termination of Treatment

Services are usually terminated when the long-term goals are accomplished and the client and team members are in agreement. Treatments or the intervention plan can be changed if there is progress toward the short-term goal but progress toward the long-term goal is slow in coming. New medical conditions (physical or psychological) may also require a change in treatment or cause a client to be put on hold. Changes on the part of the client, including a move to a new setting (e.g., acute care to acute rehabilitation setting) can also call for a change in treatment. New situations concerning the client's family can also result in a change of treatment, for example, if the family member is the primary person responsible for the carryover of the home program.

Treatment can be terminated when the patient plateaus and is no longer making progress. Prolonged and unexcused missed visits might be a reason for termination. However, all avenues should be explored because there might be an acceptable reason for numerous missed visits. Refusal on the part of the client to participate may cause termination of the program. Again, every opportunity should be provided to the client to participate in therapy. Some unknown issue may contribute to the patient's refusals.

Insurance companies can also determine the amount of therapy a client can receive. The number of visits is usually known in advance; therefore, there should be no surprises. In this case, the termination of services should result in an orderly discharge.

## Case Study

### Description

CM is an 86-year-old European American male admitted to the hospital with a transient ischemic attack (TIA). CM reported feeling dizzy while getting out of bed and then fell back onto the bed without any injuries. CM reported difficulty opening a toothpaste tube with his right hand (he is right-hand dominant) and, after brushing his teeth, CM was getting up from the commode and fell. Seven stitches were required to close the head wound. CM's spouse reported some slurred speech the morning of the incident.

Prior to admission, CM had an unremarkable medical history. He does have hypertension that is controlled by medications and diet. Ten years ago, he had a left total knee replacement secondary to degenerative joint disease. Prior to the TIA, he had never experienced any type of fall or near-fall. Presently, CM is taking medication for increased anxiety and depression. Two years ago, his son was killed in a drive-by shooting.

CM was independent with ADL, home management, and mobility. He will occasionally use a cane when he has pain in his left knee. CM lives in a two-story home with five steps to the entrance, and a handrail is on the right side of the steps. The bedroom and bathroom are on the second floor, and the family has a powder room on the first floor.

Initial assessments demonstrate a change in functional status. Grip strength in CM's right hand was significantly lower than in his left hand. The physical therapist reports decreased active range of motion and decreased strength in his right foot (decreased dorsiflexion and decreased planter flexion). CM requires minimal assistance with transfers (bed, commode, and tub transfers) and lower body dressing and bathing. Minimal help for the distal areas of the lower body is needed (per FIM scores). He did have a near-fall when putting on his pants. CM denies any falls, but his wife reports that he has had two falls (with no injuries) and two near-falls. Scores on the

*Tinetti Assessment Tool for Balance and Gait* demonstrate concerns for sit-to-stand activities, standing balance, and turning 360 degrees (staggers). The *Modified Falls Efficacy Scale* reveals concern for confidence in areas of dressing, functional transfers, and mobility within his house.

The *Mini-Cog* reveals no abnormal scores. The patient demonstrates orientation to person, place, time, and situation. Short-term memory is good. There are concerns for recalling the number of falls and near-falls. This may be a result of medications for hypertension, anxiety, and depression, or the client may be denying falls secondary to possible loss of independence and fears of being placed in a nursing home. A visual assessment was completed 2 weeks ago by an ophthalmologist. No visual concerns were noted.

CM does report decreased participation in activities he previously enjoyed, such as going to church services and dancing with his wife. He states that he is "afraid to do things because [he] might fall while in church and might trip over [his] own feet while dancing."

### Long- and Short-Term Goals

Long-term goals for CM are to participate in ADL, transfers and mobility, and leisure activities without falling. CM will maintain current levels of participation in his social life without decreasing his involvement secondary to the fear of falling.

Short-term goals for CM are the following:

1. Within 2 weeks, CM will complete a commode transfer with modified independence, without falling, 100% of the time.
2. CM will complete a tub transfer, with supervision and without falling, 100% of the time, within 3 weeks.
3. During lower body dressing, CM will use a dressing stick and a sock aid, with modified independence, without falling, 100% of the time, within 2 weeks.
4. CM and his family will demonstrate good carryover of his home program for exercise, cognitive/behavioral strategies to prevent falls, and environmental adaptations, 100% of the time.
5. CM and his family will complete the fall prevention medication review checklist provided by the therapist and review it with the pharmacist within 1 week.
6. Within 3 weeks, CM will walk the two blocks to his church, with supervision and a rolling walker, without falling, 100% of the time.
7. CM will dance with his wife, with modified independence, without falling, within 2 weeks.

### Therapist Goals and Strategies

1. Upgrade/downgrade activities to instill confidence in client and subsequently decrease fear of falling and anxiety.
2. Increase active range of motion and strength of trunk to increase balance and postural adjustments and prevent falls.
3. Increase strength and active range of motion of proximal and distal joints to prevent falls.
4. Address protective reactions to cut back on injuries if there is a fall.

5. Educate patient on correct techniques for functional transfers and correct use of adaptive devices, such as walkers, canes, and shower/tub chairs to prevent falls.

6. Educate patient on carryover of home program for cognitive/behavioral strategies and address drug interactions to prevent balance dangers during mobility and transfer activities. Provide the family with a checklist for home adaptations for safety. This list will include ideas to cut back on clutter in the environment. In addition, provide CM and his family with a fall-prevention medication review checklist to cut back on possible balance issues related to drug intake.

## Activity: Dancing

CM enjoys dancing with his wife. This activity includes all components of the *Occupational Therapy Practice Framework* (American Occupational Therapy Association, 2008), which addresses concerns for balance, falling, the fear of falling, and activity participation. Areas of occupation, which can be influenced by falls, include ADL, instrumental ADL, play, and leisure activities.

Specific client factors, required to decrease falls, improve balance, and increase activity participation, can be addressed by a dance program. This includes specific and global mental function for remembering dance steps. These mental functions could be generalized into remembering safe techniques for transfers and correct use of adaptive devices. Dancing requires input from the sensory system. Hearing functions, vestibular functions, and proprioceptive functions are addressed by dancing and can be applied to functional mobility in the home (for transfers and balance during ADL) and within the community. Dancing requires neuromusculoskeletal and movement-related functions. Joint mobility, joint stability, muscle power, tone, and endurance are required for a client to maintain balance and function safely within the environment. Dancing provides all of these components.

Performance skills needed for balance, fall reduction, and activity participation can be found in a dance program. These include motor and praxis skills, sensory perceptual skills, cognitive skills, and emotional regulation skills. The emotional regulation skills experienced during a dance routine can be generalized to identify and manage feelings concerning the fear of falling during activity participation.

Dancing can provide activities to address performance patterns—habits, routines, and roles. For instance, if a couple has been going dancing on Friday nights for years, this routine provides structure as well as the anticipation of an enjoyable event. The couple now has something to look forward to.

Those who have experienced falls or near-falls report a fear of participation. They fear possible injury from another fall, but they also speak of embarrassment as a result of a fall. Social isolation may be the result. Dancing can reduce or eliminate social isolation by increasing activity participation gained by positive interactions in social, physical, personal, and cultural environments.

## Treatment Objectives

CM and his wife will understand how dancing (an activity they both enjoy) can help with balance, strength, and endurance. By the end of the session, they will see how skills found in the dance routine will decrease or eliminate falls. They will also discover that the dance routine can be upgraded or downgraded to meet CM's current level of functioning and to challenge him to move to the next level.

# Resources

American Geriatric Society. (2010). *Prevention of falls in older persons.* Retrieved from http://www.americangeriatrics.org/health_care_professionals/clinical_practice/clinical_guidelines_recommendations/2010

American Occupational Therapy Association. (2006). *Occupational therapy and prevention of falls.* Retrieved from http://www.aota.org/Practitioners/PracticeAreas/Aging/Tools/38513.aspx?FT=.pdf

Center for Healthy Aging: www.healthyagingprograms.org

Center for Universal Design: www.ncsu.edu/ncsu/design/cud

Centers for Disease Control and Prevention. (n.d.). *What you can do to prevent falls.* Retrieved from http://www.cdc.gov/ncipc/pub-res/toolkit/Falls_ToolKit/Desktop-PDF/English/brochure_Eng_desktop.pdf

Centers for Disease Control and Prevention. (2006). *Check for safety: A home fall prevention checklist for older adults.* Retrieved from http://www.cdc.gov/ncipc/pub-res/toolkit/CheckListForSafety.htm

Fall Prevention Center of Excellence: www.stopfalls.org

National Institute on Aging. (2009). *Age page: Falls and fractures.* Retrieved from http://www.nia.nih.gov/healthinformation/publications/falls.htm

# References

Allen, C., Austin, S., David, S., Earhart, C., McCraith, D., & Riska-Williams, L. (2007). *Manual for the Allen Cognitive Level Screen–5 (ACLS-5) and Large Allen Cognitive Level Screen–5 (LACLS-5).* Camarillo, CA: ACLS and LACLS Committee.

American Occupational Therapy Association. (2008). Occupational therapy practice framework: Domain & process. *The American Journal of Occupational Therapy, 62,* 625–683.

Bakker, R. (2005). *Gerontological environmental modifications.* Retrieved from http://www.cornellaging.com/gem/enviro_assessment.pdf

Beery, K. E., Buktenica, N. A., & Beery, N. A. (2010). *Beery–Buktenica developmental test of visual–motor integration* (6th ed.). San Antonio, TX: Pearson Assessments.

Bergland, A., & Wyller, T. (2004). Risk factors for serious fall-related injuries in elderly women living at home. *Injury Prevention, 10,* 308–313.

Borson, S., Scanlan, J., Watanabe, J., Tu, S., & Lessing, M. (2005). Simplifying detection of cognitive impairment: Comparison of the Mini-Cog and Mini-Mental State Examination in a multiethnic sample. *Journal of the American Geriatrics Society, 5,* 871–874.

Centers for Disease Control and Prevention. (2010). *Costs of falls among older adults.* Retrieved from http://www.cdc.gov/HomeandRecreationalSafety/Falls/fallcost.html

Cheal, B., & Clemson, L. (2001). Older people enhancing self-efficacy in fall-risk situations. *Australian Occupational Therapy Journal, 48,* 80–91.

Colarusso, R., & Hammill, D. (2002). *Motor-free visual perception test* (3rd ed.). Novato, CA: Academic Therapy Publications.

Cooper, J., & Burfield, A. (2009). Medication interventions for fall prevention in the elder adult. *Journal of the American Pharmacists Association, 49*(3), e70–e84.

Dunn, W., Brown, C., & Youngstrom, M. (2003). Ecological model of occupation. In P. Kramer, J. Hinojosa, & C. Brasic Royeen (Eds.), *Perspectives in human occupation: Participation in life* (pp. 222–263). Baltimore, MD: Lippincott, Williams & Wilkins.

Fall Prevention Act of 2003, 42 U.S.C. § 241 (2003).

Flicker, L., MacInnis, R. J., Stein, M. S., Scherer, S. C., Mead, K. E., Nowson, C. A., . . . Wark, J. D. (2005). Should older people in residential care receive vitamin D to prevent falls? Results of a randomized trial. *Journal of the American Geriatric Society, 53,* 1881–1888.

Gates, G. A., Murphy, M., Rees, T. S., & Fraher, A. (2003). Screening for hearing loss in the elderly. *Journal of Family Practice, 52,* 56–62.

Hann, D., Winter, K., & Jacobsen, P. (1999). Measurement of depressive symptoms in cancer patients: Evaluation of the Center for Epidemiologic Studies Depression Scale (CES-D). *Journal of Psychosomatic Research, 46,* 437–443.

Hendrich, A. L., Bender, P. S., & Nyhuis, A. (2003). Validation of the Hendrich II Fall Risk Model: A large concurrent CASE/control study of hospitalized patients. *Applied Nursing Research, 16,* 9–21.

Jette, A. M., Davies, A. R., Cleary, P. D., Calkins, D., Rubenstein, L. V., Fink, A., . . . Delbanco, T. L. (1986). The Functional Status Questionnaire: Reliability and validity when used in primary care. *Journal of General Internal Medicine, 1,* 143–149.

Leveille, S., Jones, R., Kiely, D., Hausdorff, I., Shmerling, R., Guralnik, J., . . . Bean, J. (2009). Chronic musculoskeletal pain and the occurrence of falls in an older population. *The Journal of the American Medical Association, 302*(20), 2214–2221.

Lindenberger, V., Marsiske, M., & Baltes, M. (2000). Memorizing while walking: Increase in dual-task costs from young adulthood to old age. *Psychology and Aging, 15,* 417–436.

Lord, S. R., Menz, H. B., & Sherrington, C. (2006). Home environment risk factors for falls in older adults and the efficacy of home modification. *Age and Ageing, 35*(2), 55–59.

Maki, B., Zecevic, A., Bateni, H., Kirshenbaum, N., & McIlroy, W. (2001). Cognitive demands of executing postural reactions: Does aging impede attention switching? *Neuroreport, 12,* 3583–3587.

Marquand, B. (2010, January 18). The infection-fall connection: UTI goeth before a fall. *Today in Physical Therapy,* pp. 20–21.

Painter, J., & Elliott, S. (2009). Influence of gender on falls. *Physical and Occupational Therapy in Geriatrics, 27*(6), 387–404.

Peterson, E., & Clemson, L. (2008). Understanding the role of occupational therapy in fall prevention for community-dwelling older adults. *OT Practice, 13*(3), CE1–CE7.

Podsiadlo, D., & Richardson, S. (1991). The timed "Up & Go": A test of basic functional mobility for frail elderly persons. *Journal of the American Geriatrics Society, 39,* 142–148.

Reuben, D., Walsh, K., Moore, A., Damesyn, M., & Greendale, G. (1998). Hearing loss for community-dwelling older persons: National prevalence data and identification using simple questions. *Journal of the American Geriatrics Society, 56*(8), 1008–1011.

Safety of Seniors Act of 2007, Pub. L. No 110-202 122 §1, Stat. 697 (2008).

Sheikh, J. I., Yesavage, J. A., Brooks, J. O. III, Friedman, L. F., Gratzinger, P., Hill, R. D., . . . Crook, T. (1991). Proposed factor structure of the Geriatric Depression Scale. *International Psychogeriatrics, 3,* 23–28.

Stevens, J. A. (2006). Fatalities and injuries from falls among older adults–United States, 1993–2003 and 2001–2005. *Morbidity and Mortality Weekly Report, 55*(45), 1221–1224.

Stevens, J. A., & Sogolow, E. D. (2005). Gender differences for non-fatal unintentional fall related injuries among older adults. *Injury Prevention, 11,* 115–119.

St. George, R., Delbaere, K., Williams, P., & Lord, S. (2009). Sleep quality and falls in older people living in self- and assisted-care villages. *Gerontology, 55*(2), 162–168.

Swan, I. R., & Browning, G. G. (1985). The Whispered Voice as a screening test for hearing impairment. *Journal of the Royal College of General Practice, 35,* 197.

Tencer, A., Koepsell, T., Wolf, M., Frankenfeld, C., Buchner, D., Kukull, W., . . . Tautvydas, M. (2004). Biomechanical properties of shoes and the risk of falls in older adults. *Journal of the American Geriatric Society, 52,* 1840–1846.

Thomas, P., Hazif, T., Billon, R., Peix, R., Fauglron, P., & Clement, J. (1998). Depression and frontal lobe dysfunction: Risk for the elderly? *L'encephale, 35*(4), 361–369.

Tinetti, M. E., Speechley, M., & Ginter, S. F. (1988). Risk factors for falls among the elderly persons living in the community. *New England Journal of Medicine, 319,* 1701–1707.

Tinetti M. E., Williams, T. F., & Mayewski, R. (1986). Fall Risk Index for elderly patients based on number of chronic disabilities. *American Journal of Medicine, 80,* 429–434.

Van Dijk, P. T., Meulenberg, O. G., Van de Sande, H. J., & Habbema, J. D. (1993). Falls in dementia patients. *Gerontologist, 33*(2), 200–204.

Watts, J. (1996). *Assessment of occupational functioning–Collaborative version.* Retrieved from Virginia Commonwealth University, Department of Occupational Therapy website: http://www.sahp.vcu.edu/occu/ot/aofinstrument2.pdf

Wright, J. (2000). *The FIM(TM).* Retrieved from The Center for Outcome Measurement in Brain Injury website: http://www.tbims.org/combi/FIM

# Cerebral Vascular Accident (CVA)

*Marlene J. Morgan*

## 🕮 Synopsis of Clinical Condition

### Prevalence and Etiology

The World Health Organization (n.d.) defined a cerebral vascular accident (CVA), or stroke, as an interruption of the blood supply to the brain, usually because a blood vessel bursts or is blocked by a clot. This cuts off the supply of oxygen and nutrients, causing damage to the brain tissue. Brain cells are susceptible to death when deprived of adequate blood and oxygen.

There are two broad categories of stroke: ischemic and hemorrhagic. Ischemic strokes are the result of emboli to the brain. An emboli, or clot, which causes blockages to the circulation in the brain, may originate in the heart or anywhere in the arterial circulation (Bartels, 2004). Risk factors for ischemic stroke include age, race, gender, heredity, hypertension, diabetes, cardiac disease, smoking, obesity, stress, and a sedentary lifestyle (American Heart Association, 2009). In a hemorrhagic stroke, a vessel ruptures, causing leakage of blood into the surrounding structures. Hemorrhagic strokes account for approximately 20% of strokes. While less common than ischemic strokes, hemorrhagic strokes have a higher mortality rate (American Heart Association, 2009).

The effects of a stroke depend on the location and the mechanism of vascular damage. Cerebral vascular accident may result in a complex cluster of symptoms, including motor paralysis, sensory disturbances, speech and language disorders, and intellectual and personality changes (World Health Organization, n.d.). The most common symptom of a stroke is sudden weakness or numbness of the face, arm, or leg, most often on one side of the body. Other symptoms include confusion, difficulty speaking or understanding speech, difficulty seeing with one or both eyes, difficulty walking, dizziness, loss of balance or coordination, severe headache with no known cause, and fainting or unconsciousness (American Heart Association, 2009).

Each year in the United States, approximately 795,000 individuals experience either a first or a recurrent stroke. This positions stroke as the third leading cause of death after heart disease and cancer. Stroke is a leading cause of serious long-term disability in the United States. Specifically, in stroke survivors, 48% experience hemiparesis, 22% are nonambulatory, between 24% and 53% experience difficulty with activities of daily living (ADL), 12% to 18% experience aphasia, and 32% exhibit signs of depression (American Heart Association, 2009).

## Common Characteristics and Symptoms

In a stroke, the neurological deficits persist longer than 24 hours. Some individuals may experience intermittent signs and symptoms associated with stroke that last for a few minutes to 24 hours. These episodes are classified as *transient ischemic attacks* (Bartels, 2004).

The specific presentation of the patient who has sustained a stroke depends on the artery involved. The anterior cerebral artery, the middle cerebral artery, and the posterior cerebral artery supply blood to the brain. Using diagnostic techniques such as a computerized tomography (CT) scan and a positron emission tomography (PET) scan allows the physician to determine which anatomic structures are involved (Bartels, 2004).

Interruption of the blood flow in the middle cerebral artery is the most common cause of CVA (Bartels, 2004). Characteristics of middle cerebral artery involvement include hemiplegia on the contralateral side, aphasia if the lesion is on the dominant side, and sensory and perceptual deficits if the lesion is in the nondominant hemisphere. Interruption of blood flow in the anterior cerebral artery produces weakness in both the upper and the lower extremity contralaterally. Typically, weakness in the lower extremity is more severe than weakness in the upper extremity. Related changes may include apraxia; incontinence of bowel and bladder; sensory loss; changes in intellectual function, such as disorientation; and the reemergence of primitive reflexes. Symptoms of interruption of blood flow in the posterior cerebral artery are more difficult to anticipate. This artery supplies blood to a number of important regions, such as the upper brain stem, the temporal lobe, and the occipital lobe. Some patients with posterior cerebral artery lesions exhibit involuntary movement, such as tremor. Memory loss, homonymous hemianopsia, and topographical disorientation may also be present (Aminoff, Greenberg, & Simon, 2005; Bartels, 2004).

The complicated nature of stroke requires that the therapist be aware of complications and precautions that may accompany the primary diagnosis. Complications and precautions to be aware of include deep venous thrombosis (DVT), shoulder subluxation, impaired sensation, visual field deficits, and impaired communication (Bartels, 2004; Brandstater, 2005; Roth, 1991). DVT is the formation of blood clots in the deep leg veins. They frequently form secondary to immobility. Physicians fear that the thrombosis may produce a pulmonary embolus. Pulmonary embolism is the most common cause of death in patients with CVA and is apt to occur 30 days after the incident. Management of DVT includes drug therapy, the use of compressive stockings, and movement (Roth, 1991). Changes in tone and strength in the muscles of the shoulder girdle after a stroke may result in a subluxation at the glenohumeral joint. Subluxation is a malalignment and instability of the glenohumeral joint. It typically results from a malalignment between the scapula and the trunk. Because the subluxed shoulder is unstable, it is important that it is handled and positioned carefully. Positioning with pillows, a lap tray, and taping are all suggested approaches to carefully handling a subluxed shoulder (Andrews & Bohannon, 2000; Bartels, 2004; Bohannon & Andrews, 1990; Carr & Kenny, 1992).

Sensory impairment that occurs after a stroke may result in the patient demonstrating decreased protective sensation. Limited awareness of and decreased protective sensation in an affected extremity may subject the patient to the risk of injury. Patients and family members must be made aware of sensory impairments and be taught compensation techniques. Such compensation techniques may include using vision to monitor the affected arm and hand and/or using the sound side to test the temperature of the water before bathing or showering (Brandstater, 2005).

CVA may create visual field deficits. A patient with a visual field deficit receives limited or no information from a specific area of the visual field. Limited visual information creates an unsafe situation as the patient moves in and interacts with the environment. The patient and his or her family must be made aware of the presence and implications of any visual field deficit. The patient may be taught to use head turning in combination with visual scanning to compensate for a visual field deficit. The patient and his or her family may also be taught to modify the environment or activity by moving objects into the functioning visual field (Warren, 1999).

A stroke may impact a patient's ability to communicate. The most common poststroke communication impairment is aphasia. Aphasia is a language disorder that results in a loss of language skills, slowed or slurred speech, impaired auditory comprehension, or difficulty retrieving words (Halper & Mogil, 1986). The occupational therapist may model for the family a system for communicating with an aphasic patient, which includes using a patient tone of voice and using short, simple sentences. Use of demonstrations and gestures may also aid understanding.

## Target Areas for Intervention

Each patient who presents with a stroke will demonstrate an individual complement of signs and symptoms. Additionally, a stroke will affect each patient's life roles and activities in a unique way. Despite individual presentations, occupational therapy intervention for a stroke survivor can be summarized into the following areas of intervention focus:

- Improve motor control to support functional independence in ADL and instrumental ADL (IADL).

- Improve perceptual abilities to support functional independence in ADL and IADL.
- Improve cognitive abilities to support functional independence in ADL and IADL.
- Support psychosocial processes and adjustment to disability in support of independent ADL and IADL.

## Contextual Considerations

### Clinical

The occupational therapist collects information related to the patient's premorbid life roles and activities. This may be accomplished through an interview with the patient and/or family. The impact that the stroke has had on a patient's level of functioning in ADL and IADL can be measured using an assessment such as the *Canadian Occupational Performance Measure* (COPM; Law et al., 2005), the *Functional Independence Measure* (FIM; Wright, 2000), or the *Assessment of Motor and Process Skills* (AMPS; Fisher, 2006). The COPM, using an interview format, yields information about the patient's perspective of the impact of the stroke on his or her life by eliciting goals, information about his or her current level of performance, and his or her level of satisfaction with current performance. The FIM provides information on the patient's level of independence in basic ADL on 18 items, including self-care and mobility. The FIM provides scoring on a 7-point scale, which characterizes the amount of physical assistance, adaptive equipment and techniques, or cuing that is required to support performance. The AMPS provides information on the impact of motor and process skills on function.

Assessment of the patient's motor control is based on observation. The therapist assesses the presence of any abnormal reflexes during movement. Abnormal patterns of muscle tone are identified and compared to the typical pattern of deformity that is found in patients after a stroke. Specifically, the therapist looks for evidence of neck flexion to the weak side, neck rotation to the sound side, scapular retraction, trunk flexion to the affected side, wrist flexion with ulnar deviation, finger flexion and adduction, elbow flexion, pelvis rotation up and back, hip extension and adduction and internal rotation, ankle plantar flexion, foot inversion, and toe flexion and adduction (Bobath, 1990).

Assessment of upper extremity status may include tests for range of motion, subluxation, sensation, coordination, and upper extremity function. Range of motion is assessed in both the affected and the unaffected extremities through observation and/or goniometry. The presence of subluxation is tested for by first locating the head of the humerus in the glenoid fossa. The therapist attempts to insert one or two fingers in the space between the humeral head and the scapula. The number of fingers that the therapist is able to insert into the space describes the presence of a subluxation (Anderson, 1985).

A sensory test is completed to identify the pattern and degree of sensory awareness in the affected extremity. The therapist makes careful note of the areas in which protective sensations, such as sharp/dull and hot/cold, are absent or impaired (Dellon, 1981). Coordination may be formally assessed through the *Jebsen Hand Function Test* (Jebsen, Taylor, Trieschmann, Trotter, & Howard, 1969) or through clinical observation. Upper extremity function, specifically the role that the affected extremity is able to play in bimanual tasks, can be assessed using the *Functional Test for the Hemiparetic Extremity,* which allows the therapist to evaluate the effectiveness of the affected extremity as a stabilizer, holder, or fine motor assist (Wilson, Baker, & Craddock, 1984).

The patient's perceptual status is assessed through a combination of functional observations and tests. During functional tasks, such as dressing and cooking, the therapist observes for perceptual deficits, which may include body scheme disorders, disorders in spatial relations, apraxias, and agnosias. A patient demonstrating a body scheme disorder may have difficulty recognizing the relationship between his or her body parts. The patient may be unable to put his or her arm into the sleeve of a shirt without demonstration. Spatial relation disorders may limit the patient's ability to recognize the characteristics of an object, such as its position, form, or depth. A patient with distorted spatial relations may have difficulty finding a fork in a utensil drawer. Patients with apraxia demonstrate an inability to complete certain skilled movements, even though the components of muscle strength, sensation, and coordination are present. Finally, agnosia is an inability to recognize objects, even though sensation is intact. The patient with agnosia may be unable to recognize his own clothes, even though sight is intact. Formal tests such as the *Motor-Free Visual Perception Test* (Colarusso & Hammill, 2002) may be used to assess specific perceptual skills.

Cognitive skills may be assessed using tests such as the *Mini-Mental State Examination* (Folstein, Folstein, & McHugh, 1975) and the *Lowenstein Occupational Therapy Cognitive Assessment* (Katz, Itzkovich, Averbauch, & Elazer, 1989). Such tests provide insight into higher level cognitive function. Results of formal tests provide valuable insights and a foundation for interpreting difficulty that the patient may be experiencing in ADL and IADL.

Psychological adjustment to disability is a critical area to assess. Psychological adjustment may affect the patient's willingness to participate in treatment, as well as his or her interaction with family and friends (Eriksson et al., 2004). Occupational therapists may look to psychology or neuropsychology for guidance on how to address these issues. They may also administer tests such as the *Beck Depression Inventory* (Beck, Steer, & Brown, 1996), which requires the patient to provide a self-rating of attitudes and behaviors related to depression.

Assessments of home safety and accessibility are completed as discharge planning progresses. Clinical observation in combination with assessments such as the *Kohlman Evaluation of Living Skills* (Kohlman-Thompson, 1992) will alert the therapist to potential safety hazards at discharge. Clinical information, test results, and interview data from the patient and family may point to the need for a home visit or a referral to a home care agency.

## Family

Assessment of the family's reaction to the stroke is key. Since a stroke may have a major impact on the roles that the patient resumes, preparing for its effect on the family system is important. Family members may be called on to provide psychological support or direct physical care for the patient. It is critical that they understand the ramifications of the diagnosis to prepare them for ongoing interactions with the patient after discharge. Since the majority of stroke survivors exhibit some degree of long-term effects from the insult, family members must be prepared for a potentially long period of adjustment (Evans, Hendricks, Haselkorn, Bishop, & Baldwin, 1992).

## Practice Setting

Occupational therapists may provide services to stroke survivors in a variety of treatment settings, including acute care hospitals, rehabilitation centers, outpatient facilities, home care, skilled nursing facilities, nursing homes, and specialized programs, such as those in work hardening or driving. Because recovery from stroke may be slow and progressive, a single patient may receive care in more than one practice setting.

In acute care, the occupational therapy program focuses on early assessment, beginning treatment, and determining the subsequent level of care required to benefit the patient. The alternatives may include a rehabilitation unit, skilled nursing facility, nursing home, or home care setting. A rehabilitation admission provides the patient with the opportunity to participate in a program designed to determine the motor, sensory, perceptual, cognitive, and psychological effects of the stroke and the impact that each has had on ADL an IADL function. It is during the rehabilitation stay that decisions are made as to whether deficits can be remedied or if the patient will benefit from adaptive equipment and techniques. Inpatient rehabilitation requires that the patient be able to participate actively in 3 hours of combined therapy per day (Braveman, 2006).

Stroke survivors who are making slow but steady progress may benefit from admission to a skilled nursing facility. In skilled nursing facilities, the intensity of therapy is reduced, allowing the patient to progress at a slower pace. Outpatient and home care programs provide opportunities for the stroke survivor to apply the skills and techniques acquired in the rehabilitation strategy designed to manage independence in IADL (Braveman, 2006).

## Sociopolitical

Because the majority of stroke survivors are 65 years old or older, Medicare coverage and rules serve as a critical backdrop to much of the care in both inpatient and outpatient settings (American Heart Association, 2009). Terms and limitations on services and equipment provided through Medicare and commercial insurers pose a challenge for health care providers, the patient, and the family. The age of many stroke survivors makes them eligible for senior services, such as senior centers, adult day care, and Meals on Wheels. These services may be factored into a comprehensive plan. In addition, many community-based support groups exist for stroke survivors and their families. These groups provide social, educational, recreational, and advocacy opportunities.

The Americans With Disabilities Act of 1990 (ADA) ensures community accessibility for stroke survivors. For those patients returning to work, ADA ensures reasonable accommodations to the workplace and job to facilitate the important worker role.

## Lifestyle/Lifespan

Most individuals who have a stroke will experience residual effects that impact their lives on an ongoing basis. The stroke may limit or change the roles that a person is able to play within the family. For example, a grandmother who provided care for grandchildren when her daughter was at work may be unable to continue in that role. Adapting to the limitations in activity imposed by the stroke may be a long process. The patient may experience challenges, and activities that were simple and comforting in the past may become difficult. For example, a stroke survivor who looked forward to making cookies twice a year with her church group may find that she is only able to participate in a limited way.

The cost of living with a long-term disability may be high, and this may impact the family's financial status and plans. In addition to the cost of medications, patients may be faced with the cost of additional therapy, adaptive equipment, and the cost of making home modifications for accessibility and safety.

A severe stroke may limit opportunities for a patient to return to work or seek employment in a related field. The extraction of such an important role from a person's life will create a void of time and activity that must be filled. After a stroke, a patient may experience residual motor, perceptual, or cognitive disability that makes driving unsafe. Many individuals rely on driving, even short distances, for shopping, keeping appointments, and meeting friends. Inability to drive may result in increased dependence on others, increased fear of dependence, and social isolation (Fisk, Owsley, & Pulley, 1997).

## ⚕ Clinical Decision-Making Process

### Defining Focus for Intervention

The focus for occupational therapy intervention is guided primarily by a combination of the results of the functional assessments, such as the COPM and the FIM. These assessments target the areas of intervention that are most important to the patient. In the next stage of the process, the therapist carefully examines the results of specific assessments of motor control, perception, cognition, and psychosocial reaction. The relationship and impact of each of these areas to overall function is analyzed. Initial treatment will focus on the deficit areas that impact overall performance.

Practice area affects the focus of occupational therapy intervention. During an acute hospitalization, the primary role of occupational therapy intervention may be positioning the patient to prevent deformity and facilitate function. The therapist also completes an initial assessment. The assessment in acute care may be used to determine the best course of treatment after discharge: home, rehabilitation, outpatient, or skilled nursing facility. The length of stay in acute care for patients who have had a stroke is very limited. This triage function is critical.

A poststroke inpatient rehabilitation stay is typically limited to several weeks. During this time, the focus is to work concurrently with the family and patient both to upgrade the patient's level of independence and to train the family to provide required care at home. For more specialized settings, such as those for work hardening or driver rehabilitation, the focus of the occupational therapy program is on the individual IADL.

## Establishing Goals for Intervention

Establishing goals for a patient after a stroke involves an ongoing process of assessment and reassessment. In establishing goals for intervention, the therapist examines the options for improvement that are available. Initially, the therapist sets goals that will require the patient to demonstrate improvement in motor, sensory, perceptual, or cognitive areas. Such is the case when the therapist indicates that a patient's goal is to be "independent in upper extremity dressing." This indicates that the patient will develop the motor control and skills to complete the activity without equipment or assistance.

If the patient does not develop the required skills, the therapist then adjusts his or her thinking and amends the goals to focus on compensatory training. Such is the case when the therapist states that the patient will "complete upper extremity dressing using one-handed techniques, sitting at the edge of the bed." The therapist may also amend the goal to focus on the use of adaptive equipment. In this case, the goal becomes to "complete upper extremity dressing using a buttonhook." In cases where the patient will require assistance, goals are written to reflect the type and degree of cuing or physical assistance required. The process of goal setting for this population is one that changes as the prognosis for neurological recovery from the stroke becomes more apparent.

## Designing Theory-Based Intervention

The complex nature of the signs and symptoms of a stroke in combination with the long recovery period requires that the occupational therapist give careful consideration to designing a treatment plan that meets the needs of the patient throughout. Because a stroke has the potential to impact so many areas of function, an integrated frame of reference, such as the model of human occupation, can serve as an overarching frame. The model of human occupation requires the therapist to examine all aspects of the patient's life (e.g., values, habits, routines, roles); thus, it ensures that a comprehensive treatment plan is developed (Kielhofner, 2008). For issues related to psychosocial adjustment to disability, the model of human occupation can be used to guide the selection of activities to reinforce motivation and engagement in activity.

The focus for occupational therapy intervention, as noted earlier, includes attention to deficits in motor control, perceptual processing, cognitive processes, and issues of adjustment. Deficits in one of more of these areas may impact ADL and IADL. Each of these areas is best addressed by a different frame of reference.

Motor control deficits in patients who have had a stroke may be addressed by the neurodevelopmental, motor learning and motor control, biomechanical, or rehabilitation frames of reference (Carr & Shepherd, 1987; Kielhofner, 2009). During the initial period of recovery, the patient may demonstrate abnormal reflexes or abnormal muscle tone. It is at this time when a neurodevelopmental frame of reference and techniques may be used. In the neurodevelopmental frame of reference, the focus is on inhibiting abnormal tone and movement and facilitating normal movement. As motor control improves and the patient's underlying motor control is normalized, the frame of reference may shift to biomechanical. Using the biomechanical frame of reference, the therapist can address problems of residual muscle weakness and limitations in range of motion and coordination. Should the patient fail to regain the motor control necessary for completing ADL and IADL, the rehabilitation frame of reference can guide the therapist in the choice of adaptive devices and techniques. Such an approach would include the use of an adapted cutting board to compensate for the limited use of the affected upper extremity as a stabilizer.

Perceptual and cognitive deficits may be addressed using the cognitive and/or rehabilitation frames of reference. During the period of recovery immediately after the stroke, a cognitive approach may be used to remediate specific perceptual or cognitive deficits. Such an approach may include graded training activities to improve memory or sequencing. Should the patient fail to regain the perceptual or cognitive skills necessary to participate in ADL and IADL safely and successfully, the rehabilitation frame of reference again can be used to guide the choice of adaptive equipment and strategies. One example may be the use of a memory book or planner to facilitate keeping appointments.

Several new approaches have been developed and are being integrated into current occupational therapy practice for stroke survivors in an effort to improve motor function. One approach is the use of technology, including the NESS H200 and NESS L300, the Saebo Arm Training Program, and the Myomo and InMotion2 and InMotion3 robotic systems. Robotic therapy devices are designed to promote the return of movement and function in a paralyzed limb.

These devices are sophisticated exercise machines that guide the user through repeated movements. Botulinum toxin injections are often used by physicians to treat spasticity or muscle stiffness in stroke survivors. Constraint-induced movement therapy (CIMT) consists of an intensive upper limb exercise program, coupled with placing the unaffected arm in a restrictive mitt to encourage use of the weak upper limb. Classic CIMT includes 6 hours of supervised therapy 5 days per week for a 2-week period. Modified versions of CIMT may involve less intensive therapy programs over a longer period of time. Dynamic splinting has been developed for the wrist and hand to mechanically assist stroke survivors in extending their wrist and fingers. The Saebo Arm Training Program is an example of this type of device. Electrical stimulation of the nerves or muscles in the arm or leg can cause movement of the weak limb. Functional electrical stimulation devices used for the upper limb include the NESS H200 and the NeuroMove. Therapists are encouraged to keep abreast of the latest research and emerging approaches being developed to treat stroke survivors.

## Evaluating Progress

Evaluation of progress occurs throughout the recovery from stroke. The most comprehensive evaluation of progress is seen as the patient improves in functional measures, such as the FIM and COPM. An increase in the FIM score implies more independent performance on the part of the patient and a decreased need for adaptive equipment, physical assistance, or cuing. On the COPM, a higher score indicates improved performance and satisfaction on the part of the patient.

For the components of the program addressing motor control, improvement in the neurodevelopmental frame of reference is noted as abnormal reflexes and patterns of movement are extinguished and the patient's movement becomes more normal. As motor control moves into the biomechanical frame of reference, improvement is noted in strength, range of motion, sensation, and coordination.

In the components of the program addressing perception and cognition, improvement is noted as the patient requires fewer verbal, tactile, or environmental cues to be successful. In the rehabilitation frame of reference, progress is noted as the patient demonstrates the ability to integrate adaptive equipment and devices into daily routines and generalize the use of equipment and techniques to new situations.

## Determining Change in or Termination of Treatment

The thinking and decision-making process regarding changes in or termination of treatment for this group of patients closely parallels that of goal setting. Initially, the focus is on remediation of components and the integration of new skills to support ADL and IADL. An example of this approach is teaching the stroke patient to incorporate scapular protraction and elbow extension by positioning the affected upper extremity between his knees and leaning forward during dressing.

The expectation in this approach is that the control of upper extremity spasticity will be developed and improved, thereby supporting increased function at discharge.

If, during the course of the treatment, it becomes apparent that the remedial approach to developing skills is not working, the therapist should change the approach to include adaptive strategies, adaptive equipment, and family teaching. The initial emphasis is to facilitate optimal neurological and functional recovery prior to teaching compensation or planning for ongoing family caregiving.

## Case Study

### Description

RP is a 70-year-old female who sustained a left CVA 1 week ago, affecting the middle cerebral artery. This resulted in a right hemiplegia. During her time in the acute care hospital, RP was seen by an occupational therapist. At that time, she presented with low muscle tone in her right upper extremity (dominant), exhibited poor trunk control, and appeared alert and oriented. Observations noted during ADL indicated that she may be having difficulty with visual–spatial skills. This was evidenced by difficulty locating and positioning items on her tray when eating. RP needed physical assistance to complete all aspects of ADL. Physical therapy issued RP a standard wheelchair, and she required assistance to push it. These symptoms and observations were consistent with the location of her lesion. The occupational therapist established a positioning program to prevent deformity and facilitate function in the upper extremity. The acute care occupational therapist further determined that RP could benefit from admission to the rehabilitation unit.

Upon admission to the rehabilitation unit, RP presented with a synergy pattern in her right upper extremity. She positioned her right upper extremity in a posture of scapular retraction, adduction and internal rotation, elbow flexion, forearm pronation, and wrist and finger flexion. She was able to feed herself but had difficulty opening containers and cutting meat. RP continued to require physical assistance for all other ADL, and the suspected visual–spatial problems continued to persist. She had difficulty with positioning her clothing correctly while dressing, among other things.

RP is single and lives in a two-story house with her sister. Her bedroom and bathroom are on the second floor. She is very motivated to be independent. Prior to admission, RP was responsible for most of the cooking and housekeeping. She enjoys gardening and going to the local senior center to play bingo. She has been referred for an initial 2-week rehabilitation stay to increase independence in ADL, mobility, home management, and adjustment to disability.

### Long- and Short-Term Goals

RP's long-term goal is to demonstrate competence in the ADL and IADL that are necessary for her to perform at her highest functional level. RP's short-term goal, which supports her long-term goal, is to be independent in upper extremity dressing. This goal will be reached in part through RP demonstrating the ability to complete upper extremity dressing sitting at the edge of the bed, incorporating tone reduction strategies.

### Therapist Goals and Strategies

The therapist's goals include the following:

1. Reduce spasticity in the affected right upper extremity.
2. Facilitate the use of the right upper extremity as a functional assist.
3. Facilitate safe sitting balance.
4. Facilitate functional mobility.
5. Teach the patient tone reduction strategies.
6. Improve ADL independence.

The therapist's strategies include the following:

1. Apply selected neurodevelopmental techniques to reduce spasticity and improve function.
2. Train RP to incorporate mobility aids (e.g., cane, walker) into ADL.
3. Train RP in use of selected adaptive devices to promote independence and participation in meaningful activities.

### Activity: Planting Spring Bulbs in a Window Box

Prior to starting the activity, the therapist collects the following equipment and supplies: a small window box filled with soft soil, a bulb planter, an assortment of spring bulbs (such as miniature tulips and hyacinths), and a small stool. The planter box is positioned in front of RP on the low stool. RP sits at the edge of a mat or chair and straddles the planter box and stool. RP places the bulb planter in her right upper extremity. The bulbs are placed in a small container on a tray table to her left. To plant each bulb, RP will grasp the bulb with her left hand, lean forward, and use the bulb planter to dig a hole. She will place the bulb in the hole with her left hand and cover the bulb with dirt. She will continue until each bulb has been planted.

This activity meets the requirements described above. Sitting and leaning will challenge RP's dynamic sitting balance. Grasping and reaching for each bulb with her left upper extremity will require trunk rotation. By leaning forward, she is encouraging scapular protraction and elbow extension. Digging the hole requires elbow extension and supination. Each of these aspects of the activity supports a neurodevelopmental approach. The visual demands of the task are low. Finally, the motor control required in this task mimics that which is required to integrate neurodevelopmental principles into upper extremity dressing.

In designing an activity for RP, it is important to consider that she has two broad areas of deficit that appear to be impacting ADL—limited motor control and visual–spatial problems. As the therapist designs a treatment session for RP, he or she will complete an analysis of each activity that is being considered, keeping a careful eye on the motor challenges of the activity as well as its visual–spatial challenges. In structuring the treatment session, the therapist will design tasks that have high motor demands and limited visual–spatial demands. The therapist will also design tasks that have high visual–spatial demands and limited motor demands. The thinking behind this approach to activity analysis and creation becomes clear when RP is reexamined. Because RP is having difficulty with both motor control and visual–spatial skills, she will be unable to successfully complete a task if that task is designed to provide a maximum challenge to her motor skills and visual–spatial skills concurrently. Therefore, the therapist designs a series of activities that are incorporated into the treatment session, which alternately challenges motor control and visual–spatial skills. The goal for this sample activity is to provide RP with an opportunity to improve her motor control.

*Treatment Objective*

The treatment objective for this session is to have RP demonstrate the ability to complete self-inhibition techniques for her right upper extremity.

## Resources

American Heart Association: www.americanheart.org

American Occupational Therapy Association: www.aota.org

Stroke Association: www.strokeassociation.org

## References

American Heart Association. (2009). *Heart disease and stroke statistics—2009 update.* Dallas, TX: Author.

Americans With Disabilities Act of 1990, 42 U.S.C. § 12101 *et seq.* (1990) (amended 2008).

Aminoff, M., Greenberg, D., & Simon, R. (2005). *Clinical neurology* (6th ed.). New York, NY: Lange Medical Books/McGraw-Hill.

Anderson, L. (1985). Shoulder pain in hemiplegia. *American Journal of Occupational Therapy, 9,* 11–19.

Andrews A., & Bohannon, R. (2000). Distribution of muscle strength impairments following stroke. *Clinical Rehabilitation, 14,* 79–87.

Bartels, M. (2004). Pathophysiology and medical management of stroke. In G. Guillen & A. Burkhardt (Eds.), *Stroke rehabilitation: A function based approach* (2nd ed., pp. 1–30). St. Louis, MO: Mosby.

Beck, A., Steer, R., & Brown, K. (1996). *Beck Depression Inventory manual II.* New York, NY: The Psychological Corporation.

Bobath, B. (1990). *Adult hemiplegia: Evaluation and treatment* (3rd ed.). London, England: Heinemann Medical.

Bohannon, R., & Andrews, A. (1990). Shoulder subluxation and pain in stroke patients. *American Journal of Occupational Therapy, 44,* 506–509.

Brandstater, M. (2005). Stroke rehabilitation. In J. A. DeLisa et al. (Eds.), *Physical medicine and rehabilitation principles and practice* (4th ed., pp. 1655–1676). Philadelphia, PA: Lippincott, Williams & Wilkins.

Braveman, P. (2006). Health disparities and health equity: Concepts and measurement. *Annual Review of Public Health, 27,* 167–194.

Carr, J., & Kenney, F. (1992). Positioning of the stroke patient: A review of the literature. *International Journal of Nursing Studies, 29,* 355–369.

Carr, J., & Shepherd, R. (1987). *A motor re-learning programme for stroke* (2nd ed.). Rockville, MD: Aspen.

Colarusso, R., & Hammill, D. (2002). *Motor-free visual perception test* (3rd ed.). Novato, CA: Academic Therapy Publications.

Dellon, A. (1981). *Evaluation of sensibility and re-education of sensation in the hand.* Baltimore, MD: Lippincott, Williams & Wilkins.

Eriksson, M., Asplund, M., Glader, E., Norrving, B., Stegmayr, B., Terent, A., Asberg, K., & Wester, P. (2004). Self-report depression and use of antidepressants after stroke: A national survey. *Stroke, 35,* 936–941.

Evans, R., Hendricks, R., Haselkorn, J., Bishop, D., & Baldwin, D. (1992). The family's role in stroke rehabilitation. *American Journal of Physical Medicine and Rehabilitation, 71,* 135–139.

Fisher, A. (2006). *Assessment of motor and process skills. Vol. 1: Development, standardization, and administration manual* (6th ed.). Fort Collins, CO: Three Star Press.

Fisk, F., Owsley, C., & Pulley, L. (1997). Driving after stroke: Driving exposure, advice and evaluations. *Archives of Physical Medicine and Rehabilitation, 78,* 1338–1345.

Folstein, M. F., Folstein, S. E., & McHugh, P. R. (1975). Mini-mental state: A practical method for grading the cognitive state of patients for the clinician. *Journal of Psychiatric Research, 12*(3), 189–198. doi:10.1016/0022-3956(75)90026-6.

Halper, A., & Mogil, S. (1986). Communication disorders: Diagnosis and treatment. In P. Kaplan & B. Cerullo (Eds.), *Stroke rehabilitation* (pp. 12–13). Boston, MA: Butterworth.

Jebsen, R., Taylor, N., Trieschmann, R., Trotter, M., & Howard, L. (1969). An objective and standardized test of hand function. *Archives of Physical Medicine and Rehabilitation, 50*(6), 311–319.

Katz, N., Itzkovich, M., Averbuch, S., & Elazer, B. (1989). Lowenstein occupational therapy cognitive assessment battery for brain-injured patients: Reliability and validity. *American Journal of Occupational Therapy, 43,* 184–192.

Kielhofner, G. (2008). *Model of human occupation.* Philadelphia, PA: Lippincott, Williams & Wilkins.

Kielhofner, G. (2009). *Conceptual foundations in occupational therapy* (3rd ed.). Philadelphia, PA: FA Davis.

Kohlman-Thompson, L. (1992). *The Kohlman evaluation of living skills* (3rd ed.). Bethesda, MD: American Occupational Therapy Association.

Law, M., Baptiste, S., Carswell, A., McColl, M. A., Polatajko, H., & Pollock, N. (2005). *Canadian occupational performance measure* (4th ed.). Bethesda, MD: AOTA.

Roth, E. (1991). Medical complications encountered in stroke rehabilitation. *Physical Medicine and Rehabilitation Clinics of North America, 2*(3), 563–577.

Warren, M. (1999). *Evaluation and treatment of visual perceptual dysfunction in adult brain injury, part 1* (continuing education handbook). Birmingham, AL: visAbilities Rehabilitation.

Wilson, D., Baker, L., & Craddock, J. (1984). Functional test for the hemiparetic upper extremity. *American Journal of Occupational Therapy, 38*(3), 159–164.

World Health Organization. (n.d.). *Stroke, cerebrovascular accident.* Retrieved from http://www.who.int/topics/cerebrovascular_accident/en/

Wright, J. (2000). *The FIM(TM).* Retrieved from the Center for Outcome Measurement in Brain Injury website: http://www.tbims.org/combi/FIM

# Dementia

*Christine L. Hischmann*

*James Siberski*

## 🌿 Synopsis of Clinical Condition

### Prevalence and Etiology

There are numerous definitions for *dementia*. According to the *Diagnostic and Statistical Manual of Mental Disorders–Fourth Edition* (DSM–IV; American Psychiatric Association, 2000), dementia is a syndrome that may be caused or characterized by multiple neurocognitivie deficits, including memory impairment. Dementia is a progressive, often irreversible disease that impairs cognitive and functional abilities and results in a decrease in the ability to perform daily activities. The diagnosis of dementia usually includes aphasia, apraxia, agnosia, and disturbances in behavior regulation as well as in social and occupational function. A more inclusive definition, proposed by Mendez and Cummings (2003), is "an acquired, persistent impairment in multiple areas of intellectual function not due to delirium" (p. 4). A minimum of three of the following areas of mental activity must be compromised: memory, language, perception, praxis (the ability to execute learned purposeful movements on verbal command), calculations, executive function, personality, and emotional awareness. These compromises would be noted by clinical examination through objective tests, assessments, or clinical scales (Mendez & Cummings, 2003). Therefore, when an individual's assessment shows three or more persistent deficiencies in the aforementioned activities, which had been previously accomplishable, the individual is said to have a dementia.

The most common causes of irreversible dementia are pure Alzheimer's disease, vascular dementia with Alzheimer's disease, dementia with Lewy bodies, frontotemporal dementia, and Parkinson's disease with dementia. These dementias account for 90% of all dementias that occupational therapists will likely encounter in older clientele (Malhotra & Desai, 2010). Medication-induced dementia and dementias due to hypothyroidism, B12 deficiency, thyroid disorders, and systemic infections are considered reversible dementias.

The prevalence of dementia is about 5% to 7% at the age of 65 years, 15% to 20% at age 75 years, and 25% to 50% at age 85 years. Perhaps 9 million plus individuals in the United States have some form of dementia (Agronin, 2008). The prevalence is sure to increase as 78 million baby boomers come of age. In fact, the medical community will experience a shocking increase in the demands, and strain will soon be placed on care resources. Individual, family, and governmental budgets will be stressed beyond anticipation. Unless cures for these dementias are discovered, there may be a dementia crisis in the United States.

## Common Characteristics and Symptoms

### Pure Alzheimer's Disease

The Alzheimer's Association currently estimates that someone is diagnosed with Alzheimer's disease every 72 seconds. Today, the average cost of caring for someone with Alzheimer's disease is $174,000 over a lifetime (National Institutes of Health, 2003). Alzheimer's disease affects activities of daily living, behavior, and cognition, and the course of the disease varies with each individual. Typically, the disease is divided into three stages. The preclinical stage is the initial 1 to 3 years. In this stage, new learning is impaired. During Stage II, which can last 2 to 10 years, the symptoms from the preclinical stage continue to worsen. In Stage III, the symptoms from Stage II continue to progress and deteriorate and physical problems become dominant. In the preclinical stage, the losses are mild, with the loss of the ability to learn new information most noticeable. For example, an individual may be able to use his or her old clock radio but incapable of mastering the use of a new clock radio. The most apparent losses late in the preclinical stage are the inability to complete complex tasks, such as balancing a checkbook, planning an event or a meeting, or working at a demanding job. As the dementia progresses and neuropathological damage becomes more pervasive, a person may not recognize a spouse; understand how to use everyday objects, such as utensils; or be able to identify any type of hazard or emergency situation. It is not uncommon for individuals encountering Stage II, the middle stage of Alzheimer's disease, to become lost in familiar surroundings, experience hallucinations, or need moderate to maximal assistance with personal hygiene. In addition, these individuals experience cognitive degeneration, exacerbated balance and ambulation problems, eating difficulties, and bowel and bladder issues. Stage III is marked by total dependence and inactivity (Mendez & Cummings, 2003).

Current treatment revolves around reducing the risk of developing Alzheimer's disease and the drugs that can modify the expression of the disease. Lifestyles that encompass intellectual, social, and physical stimulation are believed to create excess brain capacity, or a protective cognitive reserve to postpone the development of symptoms of Alzheimer's disease (Agronin, 2008). Research has shown that individuals who adhere to a Mediterranean diet, as well as those who exercised for 30 minutes at least 3 times a week, have a reduced risk of Alzheimer's disease. In addition, those who either attain college degrees or practice lifelong learning exhibit fewer symptoms of Alzheimer's disease than do those with lower educational achievement (Malhotra & Desai, 2010).

The future of dementia will be in its prevention. Identifying the modifiable risk and protective factors to potentially reduce, minimize, or delay the risk of developing dementia is vital. For this population, the occupational therapist's goal is to get brain span to equal lifespan. The current drug interventions for Alzheimer's disease include Aricept, Exelon, and Razadyne. These drugs are believed to increase the levels of acetylcholine in the brain, a deficiency of which is hypothesized to be responsible for the cognitive impairment in Alzheimer's disease. Although medications do not cure Alzheimer's disease, some of their many benefits include improving or stabilizing cognition for 10 to 12 months, delaying nursing home placement, and decreasing caregiver stress. They are not effective in all individuals and can create gastrointestinal side effects. Namenda, a drug approved for moderate to severe Alzheimer's disease, works with the neurotransmitter glutamate. Its side effects include sedation, confusion, and constipation. It can be used as a monotherapy or in combination with the previously discussed drugs.

## Vascular Dementia With Alzheimer's Disease
Pure vascular dementia accounts for about 10% of all cases of dementia. Vascular disease occurs when blood vessels are damaged and oxygen fails to get to the brain. Without the necessary oxygen, the brain cells are likely to die, which results in a series of ministrokes (infarcts) and possible vascular dementia. Approximately 15% of the time, vascular dementia and Alzheimer's disease occur together. As a comorbid condition, vascular dementia may worsen the dementia of Alzheimer's disease.

With vascular dementia, the cognitive changes are likely to have a clear starting date. The symptoms usually progress slowly after each attack, suggesting that small strokes have been occurring. Since any area of the brain can be affected by the ministrokes, the symptoms vary and include severe depression, mood swings, epilepsy, and cognitive or physical deficits. Some cognitive abilities may be relatively unaffected.

## Dementia With Lewy Bodies
Dementia with Lewy bodies, the third most common cause of dementia, accounts for 15% of all dementias (Mendez & Cummings, 2003). Dementia with Lewy bodies is similar to Alzheimer's disease in that it is caused by the degeneration and death of nerve cells in the brain. However, it is due to the abnormal collection of protein, known as Lewy bodies, within the brain cells. Although memory impairment does not necessarily occur in the early stages, it becomes more prominent as the disease progresses. The core features of dementia with Lewy bodies are fluctuating cognition with significant variation in attention and alertness, recurrent visual hallucinations, and the spontaneous motor features of Parkinson's disease.

Falls, sensitivity to antipsychotic medication, and delusions may also occur at the onset. Recent literature suggests that dementia with Lewy bodies may respond to Aricept, Exelon, or Razadyne (Green, 2005).

## Frontotemporal Dementia

Frontotemporal dementia, one of the least common causes of dementia, accounts for 5% of dementia. It typically develops at 40 to 50 years of age and is generally underdiagnosed. The frontal lobe of the brain is particularly affected, and a progressive decline in mental abilities usually occurs over 8 to 11 years. Damage to brain cells is more localized than in Alzheimer's disease and usually begins in the frontal lobe, which is the area that controls executive functioning, social skills, reasoning, judgment, and the ability to take initiative. Individuals with frontal lobe dementia often lack flexibility in thinking and are unable to carry a project through to completion. However, there are no lapses of memory, as in Alzheimer's disease.

Failure of executive functions may increase safety risks, as individuals may be unable to plan appropriate actions or inhibit inappropriate actions. Changes in personality, the ability to concentrate, social skills, motivation, and reasoning are common with this form of dementia. These symptoms are often confused with psychiatric disorders. Although memory, language, and visual perception are usually not impaired for the first 2 years, as the disease progresses and spreads to other areas of the brain, they, too, may become affected. Mood and behavior may become fixed and difficult to change, making patients seem selfish and unfeeling. The person afflicted with frontal lobe dementia may appear to have difficulty in many areas of cognitive function. The ability to maintain attention and concentration and the ability to organize information are also affected with frontal lobe dementia. Since the psychological, social, family, and financial issues that affect individuals with frontal lobe dementia occur earlier in life, issues such as job security or caring for a family become paramount. Driving is usually unsafe for individuals with this diagnosis. A particularly troubling symptom of frontotemporal dementia is Klüver–Bucy syndrome, which features compulsive behaviors, such as counting aloud, humming, hand rubbing, trichotillomania, hyperorality, and hypersexuality. There is no specific treatment for frontotemporal dementia. Individuals are disinhibited, and some of their actions (such as requesting sex) will disturb staff members, who need to remember that it is not deviant, but diseased, behavior (Agronin, 2008).

## Parkinson's Disease With Dementia

About 50% of the time, individuals with Parkinson's disease will experience dementia in the late stages of the disease. Initially, the cognitive changes are not dramatic. Depression and sleep issues are also present in a significant number of individuals. Aricept, Exelon, and Razadyne can be useful for individuals experiencing dementia related to Parkinson's disease (Mendez & Cummings, 2003).

## Target Areas for Intervention

When developing interventions for individuals with dementia, it is important to keep in mind that they are "first of all, persons: Persons worthy of respect with a treasured life story who *also happen* to have a dementing condition" (Hellen, 1998, p. 2). Occupational therapy has routinely focused on using occupations to maintain functional skills, which can slow deterioration. However, the strengths of the person with dementia must be the focus as the occupational therapist works with the person and the caregiver to maintain competence through adapting familiar and valued tasks, modifying the environment to support function, and providing support for the caregiver.

# Contextual Considerations

## Clinical

The *Occupational Therapy Practice Framework–Second Edition* summarizes the approach that needs to be the focus of occupational therapy with persons with dementia: "supporting health and participation in life through engagement in occupation" (American Occupational Therapy Association, 2008, p. 214). Thus, the occupational therapist views the person with dementia as someone with abilities, not just disabilities.

Choosing how to assess the abilities and need areas of a person with dementia frequently depends on the context of the intervention. Is the person living at home? Is she or he a participant in a day program? If in a residential care setting, what kinds of assistance are offered? How does the environment influence function or lack thereof? In many instances, the choice of assessment will be guided by the referral.

A variety of assessments are available to the occupational therapist. The *Montreal Cognitive Assessment* (www.mocatest.org) focuses on all four lobes of the brain, providing information on the areas of concern for both mild cognitive impairment and mild dementia; it has a sensitivity and specificity in the 90% area and only takes about 10 minutes to administer. The *Montreal Cognitive Assessment*, including the instrument and instructions in several different languages, can be found online and may be reproduced without permission by universities, foundations, health professionals, clinics, and public health institutes. The *Allen Cognitive Levels Test* is a screening tool for assessing new learning (Allen & Earhart, 1992). Specific assessments for daily living skills, both basic and instrumental, include the *Performance Assessment of Self-Care Skills* (Holm & Rogers, 2006) and the *Kitchen Task Assessment* (Baum & Edwards, 1993). The *Mini-Mental State Examination* (MMSE; Folstein, Folstein, & McHugh, 1975) is an assessment that provides information regarding the level of orientation, memory, attention span, registration, ability to follow commands, constructional ability, and communication. It takes about 10 minutes to administer. The MMSE does not have a very good ability to pickup mild cognitive impairment and lacks the sensitivity and specificity of the *Montreal Cognitive Assessment*. It is frequently used by various health care professionals. The *Geriatric Depression Scale* (Yesavage et al., 1983) is a good instrument to use to evaluate for the presence of depression. It has a true–false format and is very easy and quick to administer.

The occupational therapist should not overlook a method of assessment that can offer multiple areas of information: observation during routine tasks. Individuals with dementia frequently become confused, frightened, or hostile when asked to perform tasks that are outside their area of experience. Additionally, when cognitive awareness remains, these individuals may be anxious about what such a test may reveal. Perhaps the biggest fear of the majority of older people is that an evaluation, a hospitalization, a fall, or any event that results in injury or decline will lead to placement in a nursing home. Therefore, merely observing the person in a familiar setting completing routine tasks, such as dressing, grooming, mobility, eating, and/or meal preparation, can provide a wealth of information as to the person's strengths and needs. In addition, the physical changes that frequently accompany aging, such as decreased strength and coordination, decreased ability to be mobile, and decreased vision and hearing, can be evaluated during the observation of routine occupations.

Assessment must also include the person's concerns. What does she or he identify as problematic or upsetting? What are the concerns of the caregiver? As stated succinctly in the *Occupational Therapy Practice Framework*, "Collaboration must occur with client and/or family/caregiver for occupational therapy intervention to be successful" (American Occupational Therapy Association, 2008, p. 236).

## Family

No discussion of intervention for individuals with dementia can begin without taking into consideration the role of the family and/or caregiver. Indeed, for the person with dementia, the family is the unit of care, regardless of whether the person resides at home or in a care facility and whether the disease is mild or severe. Families may experience many strong emotions regarding the losses and decline of their family member. When the person lives at home, the care is typically provided by family members, most often daughters, daughters-in-law, sisters, and granddaughters. This is true regardless of whether the person with dementia is a woman or a man. In evaluating the person with dementia, the abilities and concerns of the caregiver must be included in any plan of intervention.

Support for the caregiver should include listening empathically, as many caregivers feel isolated and overwhelmed. In addition to addressing what may be helpful to the caregiver, the occupational therapist can offer other options for support, such as local support groups. Many groups are sponsored by the Alzheimer's Association (www.alz.org). Caregivers can also seek support through a professional geriatric care manager, a health and human services specialist who helps families who are caring for older relatives. Professional geriatric care managers are trained and experienced in any of several fields related to long-term care, including nursing, gerontology, social work, occupational therapy, and psychology, with a specialized focus on issues related to aging and elder care. Programs such as the Alzheimer's Family Relief Program provide financial assistance when no other means are available. In addition, the American Health Assistance Foundation is a nonprofit, charitable organization that has dedicated over 30 years to funding research on age-related and degenerative diseases, educating the public about these diseases, and providing emergency financial assistance to Alzheimer's disease patients and their caregivers.

Some concrete strategies that may assist the caregiver include modifying occupations of importance to the person with dementia and/or the caregiver. Such adaptations or modifications may include arranging bathing and grooming areas to reduce distractions, creating a system for dressing that involves reducing the number of choices to increase focus and decision making, and planning meals around finger foods with snack items to increase intake and decrease distractibility. Environmental adaptations may include decreasing the number of items in living areas to reduce confusion; improving lighting in hallways and bathrooms; providing nightlights to assist in nighttime navigation; and providing solutions for safety, such as installing alarms for doors, using identification bracelets, and coordinating with local law enforcement if wandering is a problem. Many such solutions may be found on the websites listed at the end of this chapter. The Safe Return program has a national information and photo database. Designed for individuals with dementia who wander, Safe Return operates 24 hours a day, 7 days a week, with a toll-free crisis line. The program works through the Alzheimer's Association, law enforcement, and emergency responders. For a modest, one-time fee, the family will receive educational materials, entry of their loved one's data into the national database, jewelry, wallet cards, and clothing labels to be used with the wandering individual. All items come with a toll-free number to facilitate the safe return of the individual. Many such solutions may be found at the Alzheimer's Store (http://www.alzstore.com).

## Practice Setting

Occupational therapists treat individuals with dementia in a variety of settings, ranging from the person's home environment, adult day care facilities, assisted living facilities, and long-term care centers. As stated in the first part of this chapter, intervention needs to be initiated as early as possible to slow the progression of the disease. The person's home is the ideal place to begin intervention, as it is a setting filled with familiar items and people. As the disease progresses, caregivers may choose to use day care programs or respite services to provide an option for a break from caregiving. Caregivers may use their local Area Agency on Aging to locate services. The focus of recent funding for such agencies has been to help older persons remain in their homes for as long as possible. Such funding can supply home health aides, homemaker or handyman services, or social services to assist in negotiating the complexities of our health care system. When caregivers are no longer able to meet the needs of the person with dementia, placement in an assisted living setting or long-term care facility may be considered. This can be a difficult decision for families who vowed never to place the family member in a nursing facility. Enlisting the support of family members and health care providers may ease the burden of guilt and smooth the transition. The role of the occupational therapist in all of these stages is to be a good listener, providing information about resources and assisting the family in identifying the strengths of the person, as well as areas of need (Hellen, 1998).

## Sociopolitical

As previously mentioned, caring for a person with dementia is very expensive, in terms of both the financial cost and the human cost of caring for a person with a severe disability. A year in a long-term care facility can cost $80,000, and assisted living centers usually charge $40,000 per year. A personal care assistant can cost $20,000 per year. At the time of this writing, Medicaid can be used for payment for long-term care but not for assisted living, and this is only after personal resources have been exhausted. The long-term care lobby has worked very diligently to ensure that Medicare dollars are directed for long-term care and not for care at home, but this may be changing with the health care reform legislation. There are 78 million reasons why occupational therapists should be concerned, as this is the number of baby boomers who may experience dementia and who will, in many instances, require the assistance of a professional in geriatric medicine, rehabilitation, or psychosocial care. The occupational therapist will need to gain the knowledge, values, and skills needed to treat and care for these individuals, ensuring the delivery of quality care and an optimal quality of life to the aging baby boomer generation, as well as the current population of older individuals.

## Lifestyle/Lifespan

The nature of dementia affects both the client and the family support system. As the patient's level of function deteriorates, intervention shifts to the caregivers. It is important that caregivers continue to participate in social and leisure activities consistent with a satisfying life. At the later stages of the disease, long-term care may be required in an assisted living or nursing home setting.

# Clinical Decision-Making Process
## Defining Focus for Intervention

The *Occupational Therapy Practice Framework* clearly outlines what guides the direction for intervention: "Who is the client? Why is the client seeking services?

What occupations and activities are successful or causing problems? What contexts and environments support or inhibit desired outcomes? What is the client's occupational history? What are the client's priorities and targeted outcomes?" (American Occupational Therapy Association, 2008, p. 236). As mentioned earlier, with dementia, the family is the unit of care; therefore, another set of concerns, strengths, need areas, and histories need to be taken into consideration. While the occupational therapy practitioner may believe that the person with dementia should be dressing himself every morning, assisting her spouse in getting dressed may be an important role for his wife. She may be more interested in her husband improving his food intake and managing eating utensils, and the client may not express an opinion about the importance of either activity. Therefore, learning about the person with dementia, the family, their roles prior to the onset of illness, and routines that had been established will guide the occupational therapy practitioner to plan an intervention that meets the needs of the person and the family.

## Establishing Goals for Intervention

In addition to the priorities established by the person with dementia and his or her family, goal setting is frequently dependent on the setting in which the person lives, the stage of the disease, and the best available evidence. Considering that dementia results in ongoing gradual cognitive and physical deterioration over time, the focus of occupational therapy is to maintain existing skills and/or modify the context or activity (American Occupational Therapy Association, 2008). Typically, the occupational therapist is asked to provide intervention in activities of daily living, instrumental activities of daily living, leisure, and social participation. Interventions may include identifying hazards and making recommendations to increase safety, setting up a routine for morning dressing and grooming, and providing adaptations to permit accomplishment of valued tasks, such as gardening. This would apply to a person in Stage I or II, regardless of the setting. In Stage III, the occupational therapist may provide consultation on positioning to increase functional participation in meals and other activities and sensory stimulation to engage all senses to increase awareness of others and the environment.

## Designing Theory-Based Intervention

Many models of practice can be used to guide intervention with persons with dementia. However, the person–environment–occupation model, otherwise known as the Canadian model of occupational performance, addresses issues that specifically affect individuals with dementia. This model has as its central theme the belief that practice must be client centered. Drawing on the theories of Rogers (1951), who first described client-centered practice, this model envisions occupational performance as a dynamic relationship between the person, the environment, and the occupation. The person is at the center of this model, with spiritual, social, and cultural experiences shaping meanings and connections to others. The environment is defined as contexts and situations (Law et al., 1997). This theory also includes a developmental aspect, describing how a person's occupations change in relation to the environment and others.

This model comports well with the needs of the person with dementia. Using the concept of client-centered practice, the person, family, and/or caregivers are the unit of care. The person's values, beliefs, culture and social choices, and valued occupations can help the occupational therapist make choices in selecting occupations that have meaning for the client. Context is vital to interventions with persons with dementia, as the environment can have a significant effect on function, be it life enhancing or deleterious. As expressed by Polatajko (1992), practice is conceptualized as a cooperative process between the client and the occupational therapy practitioner—intervention is completed *with* a client, not *to* a client. The focus is in listening to the client, believing that the client knows her/his needs better than anyone, and supporting the client in those choices. As the illness progresses, the challenge for the occupational therapist is to continue to provide choices based on interests and values while limiting choices enough so that success can occur. Additionally, the context of intervention increases in importance, as abilities diminish and need for adaptation increases.

## Evaluating Progress

Objective evaluations and guided observation establish baseline functional levels. Repeating such assessments in 3-month intervals can provide a picture of where strengths remain intact or have improved through skillful adaptation of contexts and tasks. They can also indicate where skills have deteriorated, providing opportunities for adaptation. The occupational therapist needs to be alert for the potential for excessive disability—where disability occurs through disuse.

## Determining Change in or Termination of Treatment

In addressing the issues of the person with dementia, the occupational therapist must be cognizant that the progression of the disease is one of deteriorating abilities, meaning that *progress* is defined differently with dementia than with other conditions. Progress with a person with dementia may mean stabilizing wandering behavior through a guided exercise program, serving several small meals throughout the day to increase nutritional intake, or reducing excessive stimuli when bathing to decrease distractibility. As the disease progresses and abilities are lost, the goal for the person changes based on needs. A person who is able to eat independently now may need assistance with cutting food and may eventually need assistance with positioning while being fed. This makes the role of the occupational therapist that of a consultant—one who assists the person and/or caregivers to adapt to the changing abilities throughout the course of the disease. Therefore, discontinuing and then restarting intervention may happen several times during the person's life. In many cases, the role of the occupational therapist is to assess, provide adaptation, teach caregivers, and then return when the next level of disease interferes with function.

## Case Study

*Description*

VF is a 78-year-old woman who is married and lives with her husband in a one-bedroom apartment in an assisted living center. VF and her husband, GF, moved here 6 months ago, when caring for VF and their two-story house and yard became overwhelming for GF. At the assisted living center, meals are provided in a dining room, and an aide assists VF with bathing, dressing, and grooming. At this point, VF is able to dress and groom with verbal cues, if choices are limited.

The issue that triggered the move to the assisted living center was VF's wandering behavior. VF had frequently left the house "just to take a little walk" and would become lost. While their suburban neighborhood was fairly safe and did not have much traffic, VF would immediately become disoriented. It became increasingly difficult for GF to keep track of her. As they live in the Midwest, VF's wanderings in the winter were cause of concern for her safety.

At the assisted living center, VF spends much of her day walking the hallways, going into other residents' apartments, and attempting to leave the facility. This has caused an uproar with other residents, who are annoyed at this intrusive behavior. All of the doors at the facility are equipped with alarms, other than the front door, which is monitored 24 hours a day.

*Long- and Short-Term Goals*

VF will decrease aimless wandering and limit attempts to elope from the facility. VF's short-term goal is to participate in one structured walking activity per day, with others offered during the day at intervals.

*Therapist Goals and Strategies*

The therapist's goal is to increase awareness of VF and caregivers regarding options for reducing aimless wandering through structured walking activities.

The therapist's strategies are as follows:

1. Meet with VF and GF to determine VF's interests so as create a better fit between VF's walking activities and her prior interests.
2. Provide a laundry list of walking and moving activities for VF and GF and other caregivers to consider for the daily activity. Such activities could include the following:
   - participating in daily walking group with other residents
   - assisting staff to deliver mail, laundry, or newspapers
   - dancing
   - participating in exercise groups with simple demonstration
   - assisting in the yard and garden—raking, sweeping
   - assisting with care of the apartment—vacuuming, sweeping
   - walking the facility dog accompanied by a staff member, GF, or a responsible resident

*Activity*

During a discussion with VF and GF, the occupational therapist learned that VF had sold Avon cosmetics during her middle years. Thus, delivering items was a familiar and valued task for her. With the approval of the staff, VF was given the position of assistant to the person who delivered mail and newspapers each morning. VF was provided with a cart to push and was also offered the opportunity to deliver the newspapers to the residents at their apartments. As this is a large facility with three buildings and 100 apartments in each building, this task consumed the better part of each morning. This activity was followed by lunch, after which VF was usually tired and needed to take a nap.

This activity was chosen for the following reasons:

1. The task redirects aimless and potentially unsafe wandering into a purposeful task.
2. The task relates to resident's prior role of delivering cosmetics.
3. The task addresses safety concerns for VF and also decreases aimless wandering into the apartments of others.
4. The task reduces GF's need to constantly monitor VF and provides respite for him.
5. The task uses large muscle groups and ambulation to maintain muscle tone and walking abilities.

*Treatment Objectives*

1. VF will participate in a task that will redirect her wandering into a purposeful activity.
2. GF will be given a period of respite from hypervigilance for VF's safety.

# Resources

Alzheimer's Association: www.alz.org

Alzheimer's Disease Education and Referral Center: www.nia.nih.gov/alzheimers

Alzheimer's Disease Health Center on WebMD: www.webmd.com/alzheimers

Alzheimer's Disease International: www.alz.co.uk

Alzheimer's Disease Research, American Health Assistance Foundation: www.ahaf.org/alzheimers

National Family Caregivers Association: www.thefamilycaregiver.org

National Hospice and Palliative Care Organization: www.nhpco.org

# References

Agronin, M. E. (2008). *Alzheimer's disease and other dementias.* Philadelphia, PA: Lippincott, Williams & Wilkins.

Allen, C., & Earhart, C. (1992). *Occupational therapy treatment goals for the physically and cognitively disabled.* Rockville, MD: AOTA.

American Occupational Therapy Association. (2008). Occupational therapy practice framework: Domain and process (2nd ed.). *American Journal of Occupational Therapy, 62*(6), 213–256.

American Psychiatric Association. (2000). *Diagnostic and statistical manual of mental disorders* (4th ed., text rev.). Washington, DC: Author.

Baum, C., & Edwards, D. F. (1993). Cognitive performance in senile dementia of the Alzheimer's type: The Kitchen Task Assessment. *American Journal of Occupational Therapy, 47*(5), 431–436.

Folstein, M., Folstein, S., & McHugh, P. (1975). Mini-mental state: A practical method for grading the cognitive state of patients for the clinician. *Journal of Psychiatric Research, 12,* 189–198.

Green, R. C. (2005). *Diagnosis and management of Alzheimer's disease and other dementias* (2nd ed.). West Islip, NY: Professional Communications, Inc.

Hellen, C. R. (1998). *Alzheimer's disease—Activity focused care.* Boston, MA: Butterworth-Heinemann.

Holm, M. B., & Rogers, J. C. (2006). Assessing and documenting function: Performance Assessment of Self-Care Skills. *Gerontology Special Interest Section Quarterly, 29*(1), 1–3.

Law, M., Polatajko, H., Baptiste, S., & Townsend, E. (1997). Core concepts of occupational therapy. In E. Townsend (Ed.), *Enabling occupations: An occupational therapy perspective* (pp. 29–56). Ottawa, Ontario, Canada: CAOT Publications.

Malhotra, R. K., & Desai, A. K. (2010). Healthy brain aging: What has sleep got to do with it? *Clinics in Geriatric Medicine, 26*(1), 45–56.

Mendez, M. F., & Cummings, J. L. (2003). *Dementia: A clinical approach* (3rd ed.). Philadelphia, PA: Butterworth-Heinemann.

Polatajko, A. J. (1992). Naming and framing occupational therapy: A lecture dedicated to the life of Nancy B. *Canadian Journal of Occupational Therapy, 59*(4), 189–200.

Rogers, C. R. (1951). *Client-centered therapy: Its current practice, implications and theory.* Boston, MA: Houghton-Mifflin.

Yesavage, J. A., Brink, T. L., Rose, T. L., Lum, O., Huang, V., Adey, M., & Leirer, V. O. (1983). Development and validation of a geriatric depression screening scale: A preliminary report. *Journal of Psychiatric Research, 17,* 37–49.

# About the Editors

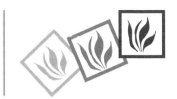

**Donna Weiss, PhD, OTR/L, FAOTA,** is an associate professor emeritus in the Occupational Therapy Program of the Department of Rehabilitation Sciences in the College of Health Professions and Social Work at Temple University in Philadelphia, Pennsylvania. Dr. Weiss has taught courses in pediatrics, group dynamics, clinical education and fieldwork supervision, outcomes measurement, and leadership, and is a consultant in the areas of group dynamics, interpersonal communication, and leadership.

**Marlene J. Morgan, EdD, OTR/L,** is the program director of the Department of Occupational Therapy in the Panuska College of Professional Studies at The University of Scranton in Scranton, Pennsylvania. Dr. Morgan teaches in the areas of physical rehabilitation, gerontology, and research. Her research is concentrated in the areas of maintaining independence in community-dwelling seniors and interdisciplinary education.

**Moya Kinnealey, PhD, OTR/L, FAOTA,** is an associate professor emeritus in the Occupational Therapy Program of the Department of Rehabilitation Sciences in the College of Health Professions and Social Work at Temple University in Philadelphia, Pennsylvania. Dr. Kinnealey's clinical, teaching, and research activities are focused on infants, children, and youth. Her research interests include the effects of sensory processing disorders on adults and developing intervention models for enhancing quality of life for adults with sensory processing issues.